CT Angiography

Editors

PETER S. LIU
JOEL F. PLATT

RADIOLOGIC CLINICS
OF NORTH AMERICA

www.radiologic.theclinics.com

Consulting Editor
FRANK H. MILLER

January 2016 • Volume 54 • Number 1

ELSEVIER

1600 John F. Kennedy Boulevard • Suite 1800 • Philadelphia, Pennsylvania, 19103-2899

http://www.theclinics.com

RADIOLOGIC CLINICS OF NORTH AMERICA Volume 54, Number 1
January 2016 ISSN 0033-8389, ISBN 13: 978-0-323-41468-5

Editor: John Vassallo (j.vassallo@elsevier.com)
Developmental Editor: Donald Mumford

Radiologic Clinics of North America (ISSN 0033-8389) is published bimonthly by Elsevier Inc., 360 Park Avenue South, New York, NY 10010-1710. Months of issue are January, March, May, July, September, and November. Periodicals postage paid at New York, NY and additional mailing offices. Subscription prices are USD 460 per year for US individuals, USD 784 per year for US institutions, USD 100 per year for US students and residents, USD 535 per year for Canadian individuals, USD 1002 per year for Canadian institutions, USD 660 per year for international individuals, USD 1002 per year for international institutions, and USD 315 per year for Canadian and foreign students/residents. To receive student and resident rate, orders must be accompanied by name of affiliated institution, date of term and the signature of program/residency coordinatior on institution letterhead. Orders will be billed at individual rate until proof of status is received. Foreign air speed delivery is included in all *Clinics* subscription prices. All prices are subject to change without notice. **POSTMASTER:** Send address changes to *Radiologic Clinics of North America*, Elsevier Health Sciences Division, Subscription Customer Service, 3251 Riverport Lane, Maryland Heights, MO63043. **Customer Service: Telephone: 1-800-654-2452** (U.S. and Canada); **1-314-447-8871** (outside U.S. and Canada). **Fax: 1-314-447-8029. E-mail:** journalscustomerservice-usa@elsevier.com **(for print support);** journalsonlinesupport-usa@elsevier.com **(for online support).**

Reprints. For copies of 100 or more of articles in this publication, please contact the Commercial Reprints Department, Elsevier Inc., 360 Park Avenue South, New York, New York 10010-1710. Tel.: +1-212-633-3874; Fax: +1-212-633-3820; E-mail: reprints@elsevier.com.

Radiologic Clinics of North America also published in Greek Paschalidis Medical Publications, Athens, Greece.

Radiologic Clinics of North America is covered in *MEDLINE/PubMed (Index Medicus), EMBASE/Excerpta Medica, Current Contents/Life Sciences, Current Contents/Clinical Medicine, RSNA Index to Imaging Literature, BIOSIS, Science Citation Index,* and *ISI/BIOMED.*

Printed in the United States of America.

Contributors

CONSULTING EDITOR

FRANK H. MILLER, MD
Chief, Body Imaging Section and Fellowship
Program; Medical Director of MRI; Professor,
Department of Radiology, Northwestern
University Feinberg School of Medicine,
Chicago, Illinois

EDITORS

PETER S. LIU, MD
Staff Radiologist, Abdominal Imaging, Imaging
Institute, Cleveland Clinic, Cleveland, Ohio

JOEL F. PLATT, MD
Professor of Radiology, Director, Abdominal
Imaging Division, Department of Radiology,
University of Michigan Medical Center, 1500
East Medical Center Drive, Ann Arbor, Michigan

AUTHORS

SUHNY ABBARA, MD
Chief, Cardiothoracic Imaging Division;
Professor of Radiology, Southwestern
Medical Center, University of Texas, Dallas,
Texas

MOHIT AGARWAL, MD
Division of Neuroradiology, Department of
Radiology, Medical College of Wisconsin,
Milwaukee, Wisconsin

DAVID M. BIKO, MD
Assistant Professor of Clinical Radiology,
Perelman School of Medicine, University of
Pennsylvania; Department of Radiology,
The Children's Hospital of Philadelphia,
Philadelphia, Pennsylvania

ANNE S. CHIN, MD
Assistant Professor of Radiology,
University of Montreal, Montreal, Quebec,
Canada

JONATHAN H. CHUNG, MD
Assistant Professor of Radiology, National
Jewish Health, Denver, Colorado

TESSA SUNDARAM COOK, MD, PhD
Assistant Professor of Radiology, Perelman
School of Medicine, University of
Pennsylvania, Philadelphia, Pennsylvania

RADHIKA B. DAVE, MD
Department of Radiology, Stanford
University Medical Center, Stanford,
California

LUKE A. FALESCH, MD
Instructor, Department of Radiology, Medical
College of Wisconsin, Milwaukee, Wisconsin

ELLIOT K. FISHMAN, MD
Professor of Radiology, Johns Hopkins
University, Baltimore, Maryland

DOMINIK FLEISCHMANN, MD
Professor of Radiology, Stanford University
School of Medicine; Chief of Cardiovascular
Imaging, Department of Radiology; Director
Computed Tomography, Stanford Health Care;
Medical Director Stanford University 3D
Imaging Laboratory, Stanford, California

WILLIAM DENNIS FOLEY, MD
Professor, Department of Radiology, Medical
College of Wisconsin, Milwaukee, Wisconsin

BRIAN B. GHOSHHAJRA, MD, MBA
Service Chief, Cardiovascular Imaging;
Assistant Professor of Radiology,
Massachusetts General Hospital, Harvard
Medical School, Boston, Massachusetts

RICHARD HALLETT, MD
Department of Radiology, Stanford University
School of Medicine, Stanford, California

NEIL J. HANSEN, MD
Assistant Professor of Radiology, University of
Nebraska Medical Center, Omaha, Nebraska

JEFFREY H. KOZLOW, MD, MS
Clinical Assistant Professor, Section of
Plastic Surgery, Department of Surgery,
University of Michigan Health System, Ann
Arbor, Michigan

PETER S. LIU, MD
Cleveland Clinic, Cleveland, Ohio; Assistant
Professor, Departments of Radiology and
Vascular Surgery, University of Michigan
Health System, Ann Arbor, Michigan

SUYASH MOHAN, MD, PDCC
Division of Neuroradiology, Department of
Radiology, Perelman School of Medicine,
University of Pennsylvania, Philadelphia,
Pennsylvania

LIOR MOLVIN, RT, MBA
Department of Radiology, Stanford Health
Care, Stanford Medicine Imaging Center, Palo
Alto, Stanford, California

ANDREW MONG, MD
Assistant Professor of Clinical Radiology,
Perelman School of Medicine, University of
Pennsylvania; Department of Radiology, The
Children's Hospital of Philadelphia,
Philadelphia, Pennsylvania

RYAN B. O'MALLEY, MD
Assistant Professor, Department of
Radiology, University of Washington Medical
Center, Seattle, Washington

MANUEL PATINO, MD
Division of Abdominal Imaging,
Massachusetts General Hospital, Boston,
Massachusetts

MELISSA PRICE, MD
Division of Abdominal Imaging,
Massachusetts General Hospital, Boston,
Massachusetts

BRYAN PUKENAS, MD
Division of Neuroradiology, Department of
Radiology, Perelman School of Medicine,
University of Pennsylvania, Philadelphia,
Pennsylvania

SIVA P. RAMAN, MD
Assistant Professor of Radiology, Johns
Hopkins University, Baltimore, Maryland

TRACY J. ROBINSON, MD, MS
Seattle Radiologists, Seattle, Washington

DUSHYANT SAHANI, MD
Division of Abdominal Imaging,
Massachusetts General Hospital, Associate
Professor of Radiology, Harvard Medical
School, Boston, Massachusetts

DAVID SAUL, MD
Department of Radiology, The Children's
Hospital of Philadelphia, Philadelphia,
Pennsylvania

JONATHAN A. SCHESKE, MD
Clinical Instructor of Radiology, Massachusetts
General Hospital, Harvard Medical School,
Boston, Massachusetts

JIA WANG, PhD
Environmental Health and Safety, Stanford
University, Stanford, California

Contents

The principles of computed tomography angiography (CTA) remain the following with modern-day computed tomography (CT): high-resolution volumetric CT data acquisition, imaging at maximum contrast medium enhancement, and subsequent angiographic two- and three-dimensional visualization. One prerequisite for adapting CTA to ever evolving CT technology is understanding the principle rules of contrast medium enhancement. Four key rules of early arterial contrast dynamics can help one understand the relationship between intravenously injected contrast medium and the resulting time-dependent arterial enhancement. The technical evolution of CT has continued with many benefits for CT angiography. Well-informed adaptations of CTA principles allow for leveraging of these innovations for the benefit of patients with cardiovascular diseases.

Video of prosthetic aortic valve endocarditis with sinus of valsalva pseudoaneurysm; normal aortic motion throughout the cardiac cycle; aortic isthmic traumatic pseudoaneurysm; and aortic root anatomy and orientation for preprocedural evaluation of transcatheter aortic valve replacement accompanies this article

This article reviews the multidetector-row computed tomography (MDCT) imaging appearance of common entities that are part of the wide spectrum of diseases involving the thoracic aorta. Electrocardiogram-gated MDCT is poised to become the reference standard method in assessing the thoracic aorta. Reproducible images of the aorta can be acquired independent of operator skill.

Computed tomographic (CT) angiography (CTA) has become the preferred imaging test of choice for various aortic conditions because of its excellent spatial resolution, rapid image acquisition, and its wide availability. CTA provides a robust tool for planning aortic interventions and diagnosing acute and chronic vascular diseases in the abdomen. CTA is the standard for imaging aneurysms before intervention and evaluating the aorta in the acute setting to assess traumatic injury, dissection, and aneurysm rupture. Knowledge of the imaging features of these disease processes, inflammatory vasculitides, and occlusive atherosclerotic disease is essential for guiding surgical and medical management of patients.

Although lower extremity CTA is most commonly performed in patients with peripheral artery disease or trauma affecting the lower extremities, it also plays a role in the workup of nonischemic etiologies such as vasculitis, aneurysms, and congenital vascular malformations. CT scan protocols should adjust bolus timing and multiphasic imaging to account for the clinical question of interest, and 3-dimensional postprocessing plays an important role in the visualization and interpretation of these high-resolution imaging examinations.

Computed Tomography Angiography for Preoperative Thoracoabdominal Flap Planning   131

Ryan B. O'Malley, Tracy J. Robinson, Jeffrey H. Kozlow, and Peter S. Liu

Mastectomy rates have increased, coinciding with more advanced reconstruction options. Deep inferior epigastric perforator (DIEP) flaps decrease abdominal donor site morbidity, but require considerable technical expertise. Preoperative computed tomography angiography (CTA) can accurately demonstrate DIEA anatomy and perforator courses, facilitating preoperative planning and flap design, allowing for more targeted intraoperative microdissection. Patients who undergo CTA before DIEP flap have better clinical outcomes with shorter operative times and hospital length of stay, which can decrease overall associated health care costs. Future directions include selected imaging of the thoracic anatomy and recipient vasculature, allowing for additional preoperative planning and customization.

Computed Tomography Angiography of the Neurovascular Circulation   147

Suyash Mohan, Mohit Agarwal, and Bryan Pukenas

Computed tomography angiography of the head and neck is a powerful tool for imaging and diagnosis of a plethora of disorders of the cervicocerebral vasculature. This article reviews the technique, indications, and interpretation of many of these disorders. A standard report checklist is also presented.

Pediatric Considerations in Computed Tomographic Angiography   163

David Saul, Andrew Mong, and David M. Biko

Cardiovascular disease in children comprises a diverse collection of diseases involving multiple organ systems. Abnormality in children is predominately congenital but also may be acquired. Although noninvasive vascular imaging modalities such as magnetic resonance angiography and ultrasound lack ionizing radiation, with improving technology and an increased focus on radiation dose reduction, computed tomographic angiography (CTA) continues to have a role in evaluating cardiovascular disease in pediatric patients. This review focuses on specific considerations of CTA that the radiologist or ordering provider should consider when imaging the pediatric cardiovascular system.

PROGRAM OBJECTIVE

The objective of the *Radiologic Clinics of North America* is to keep practicing radiologists and radiology residents up to date with current clinical practice in radiology by providing timely articles reviewing the state of the art in patient care.

TARGET AUDIENCE

Practicing radiologists, radiology residents, and other health care professionals who provide patient care utilizing radiologic findings.

LEARNING OBJECTIVES

Upon completion of this activity, participants will be able to:
1. Review the main principles and technical updates in the use of CT angiography.
2. Discuss methods of CT angiography of circulation to the abdominal organ systems and the extremities.
3. Recognize special considerations for CT angiography in the pediatric population.

ACCREDITATION

The Elsevier Office of Continuing Medical Education (EOCME) is accredited by the Accreditation Council for Continuing Medical Education (ACCME) to provide continuing medical education for physicians.

The EOCME designates this enduring material for a maximum of 15 *AMA PRA Category 1 Credit*(s)™. Physicians should claim only the credit commensurate with the extent of their participation in the activity.

All other health care professionals requesting continuing education credit for this enduring material will be issued a certificate of participation.

DISCLOSURE OF CONFLICTS OF INTEREST

The EOCME assesses conflict of interest with its instructors, faculty, planners, and other individuals who are in a position to control the content of CME activities. All relevant conflicts of interest that are identified are thoroughly vetted by EOCME for fair balance, scientific objectivity, and patient care recommendations. EOCME is committed to providing its learners with CME activities that promote improvements or quality in healthcare and not a specific proprietary business or a commercial interest.

The planning committee, staff, authors and editors listed below have identified no financial relationships or relationships to products or devices they or their spouse/life partner have with commercial interest related to the content of this CME activity:

Suhny Abbara, MD; Mohit Agarwal, MD; David M. Biko, MD; Anne S. Chin, MD; Jonathan H. Chung, MD; Radhika B. Dave, MD; William Dennis Foley, MD; Luke A. Falesch, MD; Elliot K. Fishman, MD; Anjali Fortna; Brian B. Ghoshhajra, MD; Richard Hallett, MD; Neil J. Hansen, MD; Jeffrey H. Kozlow, MD, MS; Peter S. Liu, MD; Frank H. Miller, MD; Suyash Mohan, MD, PDCC; Andrew Mong, MD; Ryan B. O'Malley, MD; Manuel Patino, MD; Joel F. Platt, MD; Melissa Price, MD; Bryan Pukenas, MD; Siva P. Raman, MD; Tracy J. Robinson, MD, MS; Dushyant Sahani, MD; David Saul, MD; Erin Scheckenbach; Jonathan A. Scheske, MD; Karthik Subramaniam; Tessa Sundaram Cook, MD, PhD; John Vassallo; Jia Wang, PhD.

The planning committee, staff, authors and editors listed below have identified financial relationships or relationships to products or devices they or their spouse/life partner have with commercial interest related to the content of this CME activity:

Dominik Fleischmann, MD is a consultant/advisor for Bracco Diagnostic Inc., with research support from Siemens AG and General Electric Company.
Lior Molvin, RT, MBA is a consultant/advisor for General Electric Company.

UNAPPROVED/OFF-LABEL USE DISCLOSURE

The EOCME requires CME faculty to disclose to the participants:
1. When products or procedures being discussed are off-label, unlabelled, experimental, and/or investigational (not US Food and Drug Administration [FDA] approved); and
2. Any limitations on the information presented, such as data that are preliminary or that represent ongoing research, interim analyses, and/or unsupported opinions. Faculty may discuss information about pharmaceutical agents that is outside of FDA-approved labelling. This information is intended solely for CME and is not intended to promote off-label use of these medications. If you have any questions, contact the medical affairs department of the manufacturer for the most recent prescribing information.

TO ENROLL

To enroll in the *Radiologic Clinics of North America* Continuing Medical Education program, call customer service at 1-800-654-2452 or sign up online at http://www.theclinics.com/home/cme. The CME program is available to subscribers for an additional annual fee of USD 315.

METHOD OF PARTICIPATION

In order to claim credit, participants must complete the following:

1. Complete enrolment as indicated above.
2. Read the activity.
3. Complete the CME Test and Evaluation. Participants must achieve a score of 70% on the test. All CME Tests and Evaluations must be completed online.

CME INQUIRIES/SPECIAL NEEDS

For all CME inquiries or special needs, please contact elsevierCME@elsevier.com.

RADIOLOGIC CLINICS OF NORTH AMERICA

THE CLINICS ARE AVAILABLE ONLINE!
Access your subscription at:
www.theclinics.com

Preface
CT Angiography

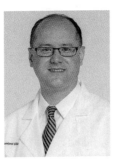   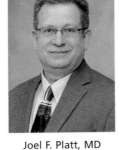

Peter S. Liu, MD   Joel F. Platt, MD
Editors

In modern clinical practice, computed tomographic angiography (CTA) has become a robust tool for evaluation of the vascular system in all territories. CTA offers an unmatched combination of outstanding spatial resolution, ultrashort acquisition times, and high repeatability in numerous systems/practice setups. In many clinical algorithms, CTA has replaced catheter angiography as the test of choice for evaluating the vessels in a particular organ system. In fact, this utility is two-fold, as CTA not only provides excellent diagnostic information about the vascular system itself but also yields important information about supplied and adjacent parenchymal tissues as well—previously, this had to be evaluated via secondary features on catheter angiography or through an additional cross-sectional examination. Therefore, CTA has assumed a primary role for a broad spectrum of clinical questions, including intrinsic vascular disease such as abdominal aortic aneurysm and thoracic aortic dissection, and clinical situations that may have a vascular component or cause, such as dyspnea due to pulmonary embolism or abdominal pain from mesenteric ischemia.

Because of the frequency with which CTA is utilized in current clinical practice, it is hard to believe that this technology was considered a nascent technique just over 10 years ago. Several critical technical developments in CT technology have made this astronomical growth possible, including slip-ring CT technology, evolution of multidetector CT arrays, and marked advancement in computer processing power. This growth has pushed the limits of high temporal and spatial resolution imaging in a test that is much easier and safer to perform than conventional diagnostic angiography, allowing catheter angiography to be better allocated for indeterminate cases or interventional/therapeutic goals.

The rapid growth of CTA has not been without some growing pains, including indication creep due to ease of access, an increased radiation dose to patients, and educational deficits in both clinical use and technique. It is this latter problem that this issue of *Radiologic Clinics of North America* seeks to address: by providing a singular resource that discusses up-to-date technical issues and diagnostic considerations in CTA across all parts of the body, this issue will help prepare the reader for CTA utilization in modern clinical practice. The first article, from Drs Fleischmann, Chinn, Molvin, and Hallett, reviews the basic technical principles of CTA, which are globally applicable to all circulations and provide the reader with a baseline understanding of the various parameters relevant to CTA studies. Each subsequent article then covers the primary diagnostic considerations and technical questions relevant to various CTA studies, which may provide a platform for further investigation or reading about niche topics. Aortic disease is described in two parts: first, thoracic aortic pathology by Drs Scheske, Chung, Abbara, and Ghoshhajra; and second, abdominal aortic pathology by Dr Hansen. The visceral circulation of the abdomen is divided among three different articles, given the importance of vascular contributions to the various organ systems of the abdomen. Drs Price, Patino, and Sahani discuss

Radiol Clin N Am 54 (2016) xi–xii
http://dx.doi.org/10.1016/j.rcl.2015.10.001
0033-8389/16/$ – see front matter © 2016 Published by Elsevier Inc.

CTA applications in hepatic, pancreatic, and splenic circulations, followed by a review of CTA uses in the renal circulation by Drs Falesch and Foley, and concluding with CTA utilization in the small bowel and mesentery authored by Drs Raman and Fishmann. The emergence of CTA for evaluation of the extremities is then discussed, including the upper extremity circulation by Drs Dave and Fleischmann, and the lower extremity circulation by Dr Cook. The novel use of CTA for planning microvascular surgical flaps is described by Drs O'Malley, Robinson, Kozlow, and Liu. An overview of the use of CTA for investigation of the neurovascular circulation is provided by Drs Mohan, Agarwal, and Pukenas. Finally, Drs Saul, Mong, and Biko provide an excellent review of the clinical uses and modifications for CTA use in the pediatric population.

We believe that this issue will be an important educational piece for many practitioners eager to implement or optimize CTA for modern practice, including key technical and interpretative clinical points. We appreciate the hard work of all of the contributing authors as well as that of the editorial staff at Elsevier, particularly Don Mumford. We hope you enjoy reading this issue of *Radiologic Clinics of North America* as much as we have.

Peter S. Liu, MD
Staff Radiologist, Abdominal Imaging
Imaging Institute, Cleveland Clinic
9500 Euclid Avenue, L10
Cleveland, OH 44195, USA

Joel F. Platt, MD
University of Michigan Medical Center
1500 East Medical Center Drive
Ann Arbor, MI 48109, USA

E-mail addresses:
liup3@ccf.org (P.S. Liu)
jplatt@med.umich.edu (J.F. Platt)

Computed Tomography Angiography
A Review and Technical Update

Dominik Fleischmann, MD[a],*, Anne S. Chin, MD[b],
Lior Molvin, RT, MBA[c], Jia Wang, PhD[d], Richard Hallett, MD[e]

KEYWORDS

- Computed tomography angiography • CT technology • Technology assessment
- Iodinated contrast • Contrast enhancement • Iterative reconstruction

KEY POINTS

- The principles of (CTA) are the acquisition of a high-resolution volumetric dataset at maximum contrast medium enhancement, and image post-processing including 2D and 3D visualization.
- This article explains the technical aspects of CTA, including early contrast medium dynamics to understand the physiology of early arterial enhancement.
- The effects of technical advances in x-ray tube design, detector design, dual source technology, dual-energy technology, and iterative reconstruction on CTA are elucidated.

INTRODUCTION

Computed tomography angiography (CTA) was introduced shortly after spiral computed tomography (CT) was launched in the early 1990s. The initial technical challenges of acquiring high-resolution volumetric CT datasets within a single breath-hold during the first-pass of arterial contrast enhancement were completely overcome in little more than a decade. By the early 2000s, CTA had toppled conventional angiography, the undisputed diagnostic reference standard for vascular disease for the prior 70 years, as the preferred modality for the diagnosis and characterization of most cardiovascular abnormalities.[1]

The principles of CTA, however, have remained the same since its inception, and are explained in this article. Understanding the principles of contrast dynamics is particularly important for any cardiovascular CT application. The last 10 to 15 years have again seen dramatic changes in CT technology, with many opportunities and practical consequences for CTA. The key technical developments are also discussed in this article. It is important to understand the principles of modern CT technology to adapt and further advance the use of CTA for noninvasive cardiovascular imaging.

BASIC PRINCIPLES

The technologic development that enabled CT to become a noninvasive vascular imaging technique was the introduction of spiral- or helical CT in the early 1990s.[2,3] Spiral CT transformed CT from a

Disclosure statement: PI, research grant, Siemens Medical Solutions; Co-PI, research grant, General Electric Healthcare; Advisory Board: Bracco Diagnostics (D. Fleischmann).
[a] Stanford University 3D Imaging Laboratory, Department of Radiology, Computed Tomography, Stanford Hospital and Clinics, Stanford University School of Medicine, 300 Pasteur Drive, Room S-072, Stanford, CA 94305-5105, USA; [b] University of Montreal, 3840 Saint Urbain, Montreal, Quebec H2W 1T6, Canada; [c] Department of Radiology, Stanford Health Care, Stanford Medicine Imaging Center, 451 Sherman Avenue, Palo Alto, CA 94306, USA; [d] Environmental Health and Safety, 480 Oak Road, Stanford, CA 94305, USA; [e] Department of Radiology, Stanford University School of Medicine, 300 Pasteur Drive, Room S-072, Stanford, CA 94305-5105, USA
* Corresponding author.
E-mail address: d.fleischmann@stanford.edu

Radiol Clin N Am 54 (2016) 1–12
http://dx.doi.org/10.1016/j.rcl.2015.09.002

two-dimensional (2D) to a true three-dimensional (3D) imaging modality: the continuous rotation of the CT gantry using slip-ring technology combined with the continuous transport of the patient table through the gantry allowed much faster acquisition speeds than 2D step-and-shoot CT. Acquisition times decreased from several minutes to well less than 1 minute, which allow for capturing of the arterial phase of contrast medium (CM) enhancement. Subsequent generation of angiography-like images from the CT datasets requires the use of image postprocessing techniques. Modern CTA technique is still based on these three enduring principles: (1) fast, high-resolution volumetric CT data acquisition; (2) strong CM enhancement; and (3) 2D, 3D, or four-dimensional (4D) image postprocessing.

These principles still apply even as ongoing technical developments in all aspects of CT technology have expanded the possibilities of CTA. These developments range from advancements in x-ray tubes, detector materials, and design, and CT acquisition modes. This section first reviews basic CT principles that lay the foundation for discussing novel technologies later in the article.

Principles of Computed Tomography Angiography Data Acquisition

The acquisition of a high-resolution dataset in a short period of time posed a significant challenge to early single detector-row CTA. Anatomic coverage of vascular territories larger than a few centimeters often required trading off spatial resolution versus scan time[4] (**Box 1**).

The introduction of multiple detector-row CT scanners soon overcame these initial challenges. Modern CT equipment (eg, any 64-detector-row CT system, introduced in 2002) can easily acquire

---

Box 1
Principles of CTA data acquisition

- High-resolution volumetric dataset
  - Isotropic volume elements (voxels), submillimeter
  - Typically requires submillimeter section spacing
  - Ideally acquired with submillimeter detector
- Fast acquisition speed
  - Within a single breath-hold (<10–20 second)
  - Synchronized with arterial contrast enhancement (first-pass)

---

submillimeter isotropic 3D datasets within a single breath-hold, during the first pass of CM enhancement, of virtually any vascular territory. For large aneurysms or patients with peripheral artery disease, it is necessary to deliberately slow down the acquisition speed to allow adequate opacification of the diseased arteries.[5]

Although isotropic submillimeter datasets can routinely be acquired with thin CT sections, further improvements of spatial resolution would also require improvement of in-plane (X-Y) resolution. The inherent physical limitation of spatial resolution of any CT system is the size of the focal spot and the size of each detector element; hence, further improvements in spatial resolution are linked to x-ray tube technology and detector design.

Principles of Contrast Medium Enhancement for Computed Tomography Angiography

Synchronizing the CT data acquisition with strong arterial CM enhancement requires a fundamental understanding of early arterial CM dynamics.[6,7] Building and optimizing CM injection protocols for any CTA application and for any new CT technology still needs to account for the physiologic boundaries of the circulatory system. The basic principles of early arterial CM enhancement following the intravenous injection of iodinated CM for CTA are summarized in four key rules (**Box 2**).[8]

The most important concept in understanding arterial CM enhancement is to think of any CM injection in terms of CM injection rate (milliliter per second) multiplied by the injection duration (second), rather than in terms of CM volume and CM injection rate. For example:

- Injection A: instead of 100 mL CM injected at 5 mL/s, think of 5 mL/s CM injected over 20 seconds
- Injection B: instead of 60 mL CM injected at 6 mL/s, think of 6 mL/s CM injected over 10 seconds

This concept is meaningful because the two dimensions of the injection (injection rate in milliliter per second, injection duration in seconds) translates roughly into strength of enhancement, and the expected duration of adequate enhancement. In the example, Injection A results in strong enhancement over 20 seconds. Note, the enhancement is brighter toward the end of the 20 seconds. Even a slow scanner could acquire a CTA of the thoracic and abdominal aorta in 20 seconds. Injection B results in a strong enhancement, but for only 10 seconds or less. Such a protocol is used for scanning a small anatomic territory or a larger territory with a fast scanner.

The first two key rules (see **Box 2**) actually reflect the principle of considering an injection as the combination of injection rate and injection duration. The theoretic and experimental underpinnings are described in detail elsewhere.[9,10] For the mathematically inclined reader, the relationship between time-dependent CM injection and time-dependent arterial enhancement of key rules 1 and 2 is given by

$$enh(t) = \int_{0}^{t} pat(s - t) \cdot inj(s) \cdot ds$$

where the time-dependent arterial enhancement *enh(t)* is the time integral of a patient's specific enhancement response *(pat)* multiplied by the intravenously injected CM *(inj)* over time.

Basic Contrast Injection Protocol

There is no single best CM injection protocol for CTA. A good protocol integrates the physiology of arterial enhancement with the scanner capabilities, and the expected pathologic findings, with ease of use and practicality. A basic robust protocol for body CTA is as follows **Table 1**:

- Scan time: 10 seconds
- Injection duration: 18 seconds
- Injection rate: weight based (5 mL/s for an average 75-kg patient: 90 mL)
- Scan timing: automated bolus triggering; scan initiated 8 seconds after contrast arrival is detected

Table 1
Basic 64-channel CT acquisition and injection protocol for CTA of the thoracic, abdominal, or thoracoabdominal aorta

Acquisition	64 × 0.6 mm (channels × channel width); automated tube current modulation (250 mAs reference mAs)		
Pitch	Variable (depends on volume coverage, usually <1.0)		
Scan time	Fixed to 10 s (all patients)		
Injection duration	Fixed to 18 s (all patients)		
Scanning delay	t_{CMT} + 8 s (scan starts 8 s after CM arrival, as established by automated bolus triggering)		
Contrast medium	High concentration (350–370 mg I/mL)		
Injection flow rates and volumes	*Individualized to body weight*		
	Body weight (kg)	*CM Flow Rate (mL/s)*	*CM Volume (mL)*
	≤55	4.0	72
	56–65	4.5	81
	66–85	5.0	90
	86–95	5.5	99
	>95	6.0	108

A scan time of 10 seconds is relatively slow for modern scanners. However, a single basic protocol with a fixed scan time of 10 seconds simplifies protocols and can even be used for CTAs with variable anatomic ranges (chest, abdomen, or chest-abdomen-pelvis) by varying the pitch. A slow scan time also has the benefit of not exceeding milliampere limitations of the x-ray tube, and thus providing power-reserves that can be used in obese individuals or for using lower kilovolt (peak) (kV[p]) settings in slim individuals. The rationale for using an injection duration that is longer than the scan time, combined with an extra 8 seconds scan delay after contrast arrival, is that this allows the arterial territory of interest to fill adequately, even if significant pathology is present (eg, an aneurysm or substantial obstructive disease; see key rule #4). The injection flow rate should be adjusted for body size (see key rule #3); this is done according to body weight (eg, milliliter per kilogram body weight) or by weight groups.

Principles of Image Postprocessing

Viewing of axial source CTA images is neither efficient nor intuitive. Visualization of vascular anatomy and pathology requires angiography-like visualization, often in the form of maximum intensity projections or as a 3D display using volume rendering techniques. In addition, numerous 2D and 3D postprocessing tools are used to interrogate vascular pathology in CTA datasets, such a multiplanar reformats, single path or multipath curved planar reformations,[11] and 4D visualization of cardiac-gated or time-resolved CTA acquisitions.

Powerful 3D workstations allowing real-time, interactive interrogation of CTA datasets are a prerequisite for interpretation, communication, and documentation of normal and abnormal vascular anatomy and pathology.

Image postprocessing is an integral part of CTA, even billing and reimbursement. It is the last link in the chain of events resulting in images for viewing and interpretation. Optimization of CTA technique must therefore account not only for the individual effects of acquisition, reconstruction, and contrast parameters on axial source images, but also on their downstream effects on the postprocessing technique being used for interpretation.

COMPUTED TOMOGRAPHY ANGIOGRAPHY: TECHNICAL UPDATE

With the introduction and subsequent wide availability of 64-detector-row CT systems more than 10 years ago, CTA has become a well-established, robust, noninvasive cardiovascular imaging technique. CTA (and MR angiography) has replaced diagnostic catheter angiography in all vascular territories, with the exception of the coronary arteries.[1] Continued major advancements in CT technology over the last decade have important implications for CTA, and for cardiovascular imaging in general. At the same time, cardiovascular imaging is a driving force for technical developments. Some of the recent technical developments are not intuitive, and confounded by the marketing driven claims by vendors. An overview of technical parameters for the latest models of the four major CT vendors is given in **Table 2**.

X-ray Tube Technology

The power requirements of modern CT x-ray tubes mounted on fast rotating gantries have increased

---

Table 2
Technical parameters of latest CT equipment by four major vendors

	X-Ray Tube Power Rating and Max. mA	Detector Design (Rows × mm)	Detector Bank Width	Channels (n)	Gantry Rotation (ms)	Temporal Resolution (ms)
GE revolution (Waukesha, WI)	103 kW 740 mA	256 × 0.625	16 cm	512	270 ms (200 ms)[a]	135 ms (100 ms)[a]
Phillips iCT (Best, The Netherlands)	120 kW 1000 mA	128 × 0.625	8 cm	256	270 ms	135 ms
Siemens FORCE (Erlangen, Germany)	2[b] × 120 kW 2[b] × 1300 mA	2[b] × 96	5.8 cm	2[b] × 192	250 ms	66 ms
Toshiba ONE (Otawara, Japan)	100 kW 900 mA	320 × 0.5	16 cm	640	275 ms	138 ms

[a] Faster gantry rotation announced.
[b] Indicates dual-source technology.

substantially (**Box 3**). To generate enough photons, modern CT x-ray tubes have power ratings up to 120 kW, and can deliver up to 1300 mA. Ten years ago, typical power ratings were 75 kW and maximum milliampere was approximately 800 mA. This allows not only faster acquisitions and higher temporal resolution, but also provides ample power reserves required for imaging at tube voltages lower than the traditional 120 kV(p). Another requirement of modern CT x-ray tubes, exposed to large g-forces, is the need for electronic control of the focal spot position and size. Rapid (within milliseconds) electronic flipping of the focal spot in the x-y plane results in a higher sampling rate and in-plane resolution. Similarly, rapid flipping of the focal spot between two alternate positions in the z-direction improves through-plane resolution.[12] Because two separate projection datasets are generated for each detector row, the number of data channels of slices acquired is sometimes reported to be double the number of physical detector rows, a somewhat confusing practice that is now adopted by all vendors:

- Detector configuration (n × d) 32 × 0.6 mm, with z-focal spot flipping: 64-slice CT (Siemens Definition)
- Detector configuration 128 × 0.625, with z-focal spot flipping: 256-slice CT (Phillips iCT)
- Detector configuration 256 × 0.625, with focal spot flipping: 512-slice CT (GE Revolution)

Dual-Source Technology

One of the CT manufacturers (Siemens) offers CT scanners equipped with two x-ray tubes and two detector arrays mounted on the CT gantry.[13,14] The latest iteration of this technology, its third generation, was launched recently.[15] The main advantage of dual-source technology over standard single-source CT is the substantially improved temporal resolution.

The geometry of dual-source CT technology also allows for the use of a pitch substantially larger than two, resulting in the fastest acquisition times for volumes greater than the largest detector banks. Finally, dual-source technology can be used for dual-energy acquisitions by operating the two x-ray-tubes at different tube potentials (eg, 140 kV[p], and 100 kV[p]). Adding a specific filter (tin) to reduce low-energy photons from the spectrum of the high-energy tube results in excellent spectral separation of the two x-ray beams.

Detector Technology

All modern CT scanners are equipped with sophisticated detector systems (**Box 4**). Highly sensitive detector materials are combined with miniaturized electronics to minimize electronic noise, and tiled together into larger detector arrays. The in-plane number of detector elements is typically between

---

Box 3
Properties of modern CT x-ray tubes

- High power rating (up to 120 kW) and maximum tube current (up to 1300 mA)
  - Enables adequate photon output at fast gantry rotations
  - Enables CT acquisitions at low kilovolt (peak) (as low as 70 kVp)
- Electronic focal spot control
  - Enables rapid focal spot shifting in x-y plane: improved in-plane sampling rate and spatial resolution
  - Enables rapid focal spot shifting in z (through-plane): improved sampling and spatial resolution in the z-axis; doubles the number of slices for a given number of detector rows
- Rapid kilovolt (peak) switching
  - Enables near simultaneous acquisitions of high (eg, 140 kVp) and low (eg, 80 kVp) energy x-ray photons for dual-energy CT

Box 4
Properties of CT detector banks and detector configurations

- CT detector bank
  - Describes the physical number of detectors in-plane (x-y), the number of detector rows (in z), and their respective widths for a given CT system. Most modern detectors have detector rows of equal width, but older CT systems may have smaller-width detector rows in the center (z) of the detector, and wider detector rows at the periphery of the detector.
- Detector configuration
  - Refers to the specific combination of detector rows and their width used for a specific acquisition. A CT acquisition may use the entire detector bank or illuminate only a subset of detector rows: for example, when used in spiral mode, only the central 64 detector rows of a larger detector bank (eg, 64 of 128 × 0.625 mm physical detector rows) may be used. The detector configuration would be 64 × 0.625.

700 and 900, spaced approximately 1 mm (at iso-center). The number of detector rows and their respective widths in z varies between scanner models and manufacturers and ranges from 96 × 0.6 mm (Siemens FORCE) to 320 × 0.5 mm (Toshiba One).

The total width of the detector (ie, the product of the number of detector rows and detector row width) has important implications for the scan mode and the acquisition speed. The largest CT detectors currently available are 16 cm in z coverage (Toshiba One, 320 × 0.5 mm; GE Revolution, 256 × 0.625). The Phillips system has an 8-cm detector (iCT, 128 × 0.625 mm), the smallest detector width in z is less than 6 cm (Siemens Force, 96 × 0.6 mm = 57.6 mm), albeit on a third-generation dual-source system.

The specific detector configuration used for a CTA acquisition does not necessarily illuminate the entire detector bank available, particularly if a helical acquisition is used for large-volume coverage rather than a step-and-shoot approach with a wide detector array (see **Box 4**).

Computed Tomography Acquisition Speed Versus Temporal Resolution

The speed of the CT acquisition with modern equipment is typically not a major limitation in CTA. Fast acquisitions in general reduce motion artifacts, particularly from breathing and involuntary patient motion. To some extent, faster acquisitions also allow reduced duration of contrast injection and thus the total contrast volume needed. This relationship, however, is not linear (ie, half the scan time does not translate into half the CM needed).

For building CTA protocols it is important to be able to calculate the acquisition speed of a protocol, because it affects the strategy of how the CTA data acquisition is synchronized with maximum arterial enhancement. In helical CT, the scan time simply equals the number of gantry rotations needed to cover the volume of interest, multiplied by the gantry rotation time. The number of rotations equals the scan range divided by the product of the total width of the illuminated detector bank multiplied by the pitch.

- T (scan) = number of rotations × gantry rotation time
- Number of rotations = anatomic coverage [mm]/(detector bank width [mm] × pitch)

The scan time for a CTA of the chest-abdomen-pelvis (ie, 700 mm in length) with a detector configuration of 64 × 0.625 mm (total width, 40 mm) at a pitch of 1.375 and a gantry rotation of 0.5 seconds

is 6.35 seconds: 12.7 rotations of 55 mm (40 mm × 1.375) are needed to cover 700 mm in length. A total of 12.7 rotations at 0.5 seconds rotation time take 6.35 seconds. Accordingly, if one aims for a total scan time of 10 seconds, the gantry rotation time is set to 0.8 seconds.

For step and shoot acquisitions of volumes that are smaller than the detector bank, the scan time equals the gantry rotation time. For electrocardiogram (ECG) triggered scans of the heart, the scan time is just slightly more than half the gantry rotation time. If step-and-shoot scanning is used for larger volumes, the scan times for each scan must also be added to the sum of the interscan time intervals needed for table repositioning.

It is important to understand the difference between scan time and temporal resolution. The scan time (discussed previously) is the time it takes to acquire all the projection data for the entire anatomic volume scanned. Temporal resolution is understood as the time window needed to acquire the projection data needed to reconstruct one (of many) CT image of a dataset. This temporal window can be much shorter than the scan time: in CT, the temporal resolution equals approximately half the gantry rotation time in single-source CT systems, but it is as short as a quarter of the gantry rotation time in dual-source CT systems.

Electrocardiogram Synchronization Techniques for Computed Tomography Angiography

The principles of prospectively or retrospectively synchronizing the CT acquisition with the patient's ECG signal have been conceived in the 1970s.[16,17] The combination with low-pitch multidetector spiral CT technology and, more recently, with wide-detector step and shoot CT technology is the basis for modern coronary CTA.[18]

ECG synchronization also has important advantages for noncoronary CTA: suppression of the notorious motion artifacts in CTA of the thoracic aorta allows for differentiation between pulsation artifacts and subtle thoracic aortic lesions in patients with acute aortic syndromes.[19] ECG gating is also critical for preoperative and postoperative imaging of aortic root aneurysms.[20] ECG gated CTA has also become the imaging technology of choice for device sizing in patients with severe aortic stenosis before transcatheter aortic valve replacement (TAVR).[21] Of note, the aortic applications of ECG gating do not require premedication with β-blockers or nitroglycerine, nor do they necessarily require submillimeter resolution.

The selection of ECG gating techniques (prospective gating, retrospective gating, or high-pitch gated mode[14]) mainly depends on the CT scanner model. Large detectors (8 cm or more) can use prospective triggering and still cover the entire thorax in a few seconds. If smaller detectors are used (4 cm width or less), helical acquisitions are faster than prospective triggering, even at low pitch. There is minimal to no dose penalty for retrospective gating if rigorous ECG-based tube current modulation is used. The most important consideration for any ECG synchronized acquisition of the thoracic aorta is the selection of the width of the exposure window relative to the cardiac cycle. For surveillance of patients with ascending aortic and aortic root aneurysms, this window is minimized (eg, only at diastole or systole). Prospective triggering, retrospective gating, or a high-pitch mode (dual-source) is used. If both systolic and diastolic phases of the cardiac cycle need to be visualized, such as for patients immediately pre and post aortic root repair, or patients scanned for TAVR planning, prospective or retrospective gating with wider exposure windows are needed. With modern scanners, the radiation exposure is less determined by the mode of ECG synchronization used (prospective/retrospective), but more so by the proportion of cardiac phases that need to be evaluated to answer the clinical question.

Low Tube Potential (Kilovolt [Peak]) for Computed Tomography Angiography

The powerful x-ray tubes of modern CT equipment allow for the use of lower peak tube voltages (kilovolt [peak]) than the traditional 120 kV(p). The apparent benefit for cardiovascular CT comes from the relatively increased x-ray absorption of iodine at lower kilovolt (peak), which translates into higher attenuation values (HU) of CM-enhanced vessels or organs.[22] Because a greater fraction of lower energy x-ray photons is absorbed in tissue, low kilovolt (peak) scanning requires substantially higher tube currents (milliampere) to maintain the same image noise.

It is useful to remember the order of magnitude of change in attenuation of iodine with different kilovolt (peak) settings, to allow an educated guess of what to expect when kilovolt (peak) is changed. The simple experimental data in **Table 3** show that iodine enhancement increases roughly 25% per kilovolt (peak) step. The most common scenario is trying to decrease the tube voltage from 120 kV(p) to 100 kV(p), 80 kV(p), or 70 kV(p), which increases the iodine attenuation by approximately 25%, 50%, or more than 75%, respectively.

These same relationships can also be used to adapt protocols: if a routine 120 kV(p) CTA protocol results in adequate enhancement, one can expect similar contrast enhancement with approximately 40% less CM volume when the scan is acquired at 80 kV(p). The injection duration, the scan time, and the scan-delay must remain the same, however, and the injection flow rate should be reduced by 40% as well (eg, 3 mL/s instead of 5.0 mL/s). Furthermore, to maintain overall image quality, the x-ray tube must be powerful enough to generate a tube current (milliampere) approximately four times higher (depending on body size), typically approximately double for each kilovolt (peak) step. If, however, the contrast volume remains reduced by 40% but tube current limitations only allow for kilovolt (peak) to be reduced to 100 kV(p), the vascular enhancement is not as strong as in the original routine 120 kV(p) protocol. In this case, one can expect approximately 63% of the original enhancement (50% because of half of contrast volume/flow rate, but add 25% of the reduced signal because of the lowering of kilovolt [peak] from 120 to 100).

Table 3
Attenuation change (% HU) per kilovolt (peak) step

Change from - to	70 kV(p)	80 kV(p)	100 kV(p)	120 kV(p)	140 kV(p)
70 kV(p)	—	−15%	−35%	−45%	−55%
80 kV(p)	+15%	—	−25%	−40%	−50%
100 kV(p)	+55%	+30%	—	−20%	−30%
120 kV(p)	+88%	+62%	+25%	—	−20%
140 kV(p)	+125%	+90%	+45%	+20%	—

Attenuation change (in percent) because of changing kilovolt (peak) settings, calculated from a phantom of diluted contrast medium (1:50 of iopamidole 370 mg/mL), scanned at different tube potential settings on a second-generation dual-source scanner. Starting at 120 kV(p), attenuation increases by 88% (70 kV[p]), 62% (80 kV[p]), 25% (100 kV[p]), and decreases by 20% (140 kV[p]).

Automated Kilovolt (Peak) Selection for Cardiovascular Computed Tomography

Although the previously discussed guidelines are helpful, selecting the best kilovolt (peak) for a given patient and application is not intuitive or straightforward, mainly because of the nonlinear effect of patient size on x-ray absorption. Automated kilovolt (peak) selection software installed on modern CT equipment can accomplish this task.[23] The patient size information needed to calculate optimal kilovolt (peak) for a given imaging task (eg, CTA) is obtained from the digital radiograph (topogram). It is important to understand that for optimization of CTA the algorithm assumes good contrast enhancement of the vasculature.[23] Because iodine attenuation strongly increases with lower kilovolt (peak), a favorable signal-to-noise ratio is achieved even though image noise increases as well. Under the assumption of good vessel enhancement, the algorithm allows for noisier images to be generated. In a situation where very low volumes and flow rates of CM are used, such as in an attempt to reduce the risk of contrast medium induced nephrotoxicity (CIN), these conditions do not apply. If the intravascular iodine concentration is not as high as for a typical CTA, then the increase in image noise will exceed the intravascular signal gain, resulting in potentially inadequate image quality.

Disadvantages and Limitations of Low Kilovolt (Peak) Computed Tomography Angiography

There are several potential limitations and caveats related to using lower tube voltage for cardiovascular CT. The most problematic of these occurs when attempting to reduce CM volume in patients with chronic kidney disease: although the signal gain from lower kilovolt (peak) acquisitions can compensate for the lower arterial iodine concentration, a slight increase of image noise is often accepted mainly because of tube power limitations. The argument is typically that iterative reconstructions reduce the noise. Of note, this is done at the cost of decreased spatial resolution or artifacts. The required increase of milliampere at low kilovolt (peak) imaging results in a larger focal spot size, resulting in decreased spatial resolution.[24] This is further aggravated by the more prominent blooming of vascular calcifications with lower kilovolt (peak), and potentially worse beam hardening and motion artifacts. This may be problematic in situations where accurate measurements have to be obtained, such as for TAVR treatment planning.

Another commonly overlooked limitation of low kilovolt (peak) imaging is that cardiovascular CT studies are not exclusively reviewed as transverse images, but also using 2D, 3D, or 4D image postprocessing. Many postprocessing algorithms, such as maximum intensity projections (MIPs) and thin-slab MIPs inherently amplify image noise. This is particularly problematic when small vessels are not strongly enhanced, and can thus be completely obscured by image noise.

Dual-Energy Computed Tomography

The potential of dual-energy CT to differentiate between materials with high atomic number (eg, iodine) versus those with lower atomic number (eg, calcium) has been proposed by Hounsfield.[25] Commercial CT scanners capable of acquiring data at two different kilovolt (peak) settings have only recently become available, with several technical solutions on the market, all with their specific advantages and limitations.[13,14,26,27] Dual-source technology acquires two datasets using two separate x-ray tubes operated simultaneously at different kilovolt (peak) settings. The rapid kilovolt (peak) switching technique changes the tube potential, alternating between high and low kilovolt (peak) within milliseconds, resulting in two sets of projection data. The most recent dual-energy acquisition technique uses a single x-ray tube with a dual-layer detector.[27] The upper layer of the detector absorbs low-energy photons, whereas higher energy photons are detected in the deeper layer of the detector.

The theoretic benefits of dual-energy CT include the possibility of reconstructing virtual images at very low photon energy (kiloelectron volt),[28] with benefits similar to and possibly better than low kilovolt (peak) CT acquisitions. The increased sensitivity to iodine might be exploited for low-contrast dose acquisitions, or might translate into improved detectability of sources of bleeds. Dual-energy CT also allows the reconstruction of virtual noncontrast images by subtracting the iodine signal from the data.[29] This can obviate acquisition of nonenhanced images. The ability to separate iodine from calcium has been used to help subtract bone or calcified plaque in CTA datasets.[30,31]

Although overall promising, dual-energy CT has several limitations, the most critical being the cumbersome workflow, which has so far prevented this technology from becoming widely adopted outside of academic centers.

Iterative Image Reconstruction for Computed Tomography Angiography

CT image reconstruction refers to solving the fundamental problem of reconstructing an unknown cross-sectional image from its measured projections. The two major classes of image reconstruction algorithms are algebraic (iterative) techniques and analytical algorithms.[32]

Algebraic reconstructions, in their simplest form, are mathematical trial and error procedures, gradually converging to the correct answer (the image) over multiple iterations. The first CT images were reconstructed using such an algebraic reconstruction technique.[25,33] A major disadvantage of this class of algorithms is that they are computationally demanding and thus much slower than analytical solutions. Iterative reconstruction techniques can account for the stochastic nature of the projection data. This is a great advantage at low photon counts, hence iterative reconstructions are typically used in emission tomography reconstructions.[34]

Analytical image reconstructions are fundamentally different: if the relationship between the projection data and the corresponding image can be exactly described analytically, then for a given set of projections there is one exact solution (image).[35,36] Analytical methods, such as filtered back-projection (FBP),[37] are thus inherently faster, allowing near real-time reconstruction speeds of CT images (which is needed every day, for example, in any bolus tracking technique).

Iterative image reconstructions have recently regained interest,[38] and all major vendors have implemented iterative reconstruction algorithms on their commercial CT systems.[39–42] With computational power no longer an insurmountable limitation, iterative reconstructions have two advantages over or when combined with analytical techniques. First the stochastic nature of the projection data is accounted for in the image reconstruction process, which is used to decrease image noise, particularly at low dose. All modern iterative image reconstructions include a statistical noise model. Algorithms that address only the image noise are sometimes referred to as statistical iterative reconstructions. Second, in addition to accounting for photon statistics, advanced iterative algorithms can include other models.[43] The image reconstruction is more accurate if more details of the scanner geometry (focal spot size and shape, detector element size) are built into the model, which can translate into improved spatial resolution.[44] Algorithms that include models beyond simple photon statistics are often referred to as model-based iterative reconstructions.

A comprehensive review of current iterative reconstruction techniques is provided elsewhere.[42]

ADVANTAGES, LIMITATIONS, AND COMMON MISCONCEPTIONS

The main advantage of iterative reconstruction is the ability to decrease image noise. Advanced model-based iterative reconstructions may also improve spatial resolution (**Table 4**).[44] Both of these advantages can synergistically benefit CTA, which relies on high spatial resolution, and is vulnerable to image noise (notably in postprocessed images, such as MIP). Iterative reconstructions also have their limitations, and it is fundamentally important to understand these because inexperienced use of these techniques may jeopardize image quality.

The most important difference between analytical (FBP) and iterative image reconstruction is related to image noise: in FBP, image noise is predictably related to dose and an important image quality parameter. Lowering radiation dose results in higher noise and vice versa. Spatial resolution is not affected at lower dose with FBP. In iterative reconstructions, image noise is predetermined and thus cannot be a measure of image quality, or a measure of dose-reduction potential. Although lowering radiation dose does not increase image noise, the price to pay is a decrease of spatial resolution and image quality.

The dose-reduction potential of iterative reconstructions has been dramatically exaggerated in the literature and in marketing material, mainly by ignoring that low image noise in iterative reconstruction does not equal good image quality. It is safe to say, however, that advanced iterative image reconstructions result in similar image quality at 40% to 60% of the dose when compared with FBB.[45] Even 40% dose reduction at maintained image quality is a substantial benefit. When advanced iterative reconstructions are used at the same doses as filtered back-projection, this translates into improved image quality because it results not only in lower noise but also in improved spatial resolution. This advantage works synergistically with optimal CM enhancement and low kilovolt (peak) imaging, because the potential to improve spatial resolution in iterative reconstructions depends on the inherent signal in the raw data: the brighter the CM enhancement of small vessels, intensified by lowering kilovolt (peak), the better that small vessels can be resolved in the image reconstruction.

The flip side of this relationship is, however, that one cannot expect equal image quality when the radiation dose is reduced more than approximately 50%. Image quality is lower despite the apparently low image noise. Also, if the arterial

Table 4
Properties of analytical and iterative image reconstructions for CT

	Analytical Reconstruction (Filtered Back Projection)	Iterative Reconstructions
Principle	One-on-one (exact) relationship between projection data and the corresponding CT image	Trial and error procedure gradually approaching the best solution in several iterations
Characteristics	Linear Exact	Nonlinear Probabilistic
Image noise	• Predictable relationship to dose (Noise variance ≈ 1/dose) • Noise characterizes image quality • Noise reduction can be converted into dose reduction	• Noise variance is not related to dose • Noise does not characterize image quality • Noise reduction cannot be converted into dose reduction
Spatial resolution	Spatial resolution is independent of dose and contrast	Spatial resolution depends on the signal-to-noise ratio of raw data (ie, dose and inherent contrast of objects)
Effect of lowering radiation dose	• Increase of image noise • Unchanged spatial resolution • Overall predictable decrease of image quality	• Image noise remains constant • Spatial resolution deteriorates and artifacts occur at low dose • Overall image quality better than filtered back-projection but deteriorates with low dose as well
Effect at same dose	N/A (baseline)	Overall improved image quality because of lower noise and better spatial resolution

contrast enhancement is low, iterative reconstructions may not improve spatial resolution.

SUMMARY

CTA has evolved from its early steps in the late 1990s to a robust and widely available noninvasive cardiovascular imaging tool by the early 2000s. Ongoing technical developments in CT technology are continuing to expand the wealth of information obtained from a modern cardiovascular CTA, as much as cardiovascular CTA is driving CT technology. A robust understanding of basic principles and technical advancements will best leverage this technology for the benefit of many patients with cardiovascular disease.

REFERENCES

1. Rubin GD, Leipsic J, Joseph Schoepf U, et al. CT angiography after 20 years: a transformation in cardiovascular disease characterization continues to advance. Radiology 2014;271:633–52.
2. Crawford CR, King KF. Computed tomography scanning with simultaneous patient translation. Med Phys 1990;17:967–82.
3. Kalender WA, Seissler W, Klotz E, et al. Spiral volumetric CT with single-breath-hold technique, continuous transport, and continuous scanner rotation. Radiology 1990;176:181–3.
4. Rubin GD, Dake MD, Napel SA, et al. Three-dimensional spiral CT angiography of the abdomen: initial clinical experience. Radiology 1993;186:147–52.
5. Fleischmann D, Rubin GD. Quantification of intravenously administered contrast medium transit through the peripheral arteries: implications for CT angiography. Radiology 2005;236:1076–82.
6. Fleischmann D. Contrast medium administration in computed tomographic angiography. In: Rubin GD, Rofsky NM, editors. CT and MR angiography. Philadelphia: Lippincott Williams & Wilkins; 2009. p. 129–54.
7. Fleischmann D, Rubin GD, Bankier AA, et al. Improved uniformity of aortic enhancement with customized contrast medium injection protocols at CT angiography. Radiology 2000;214:363–71.
8. Fleischmann D. Present and future trends in multiple detector-row CT applications: CT angiography. Eur Radiol 2002;12(Suppl 2):S11–5.
9. Fleischmann D, Paik D, Napel S, et al. Quantitative CT angiography of the abdominal aorta in healthy adults. Eur Radiol 1999;9:S548.
10. Hittmair K, Fleischmann D. Accuracy of predicting and controlling time-dependent aortic enhancement from a test bolus injection. J Comput Assist Tomogr 2001;25:287–94.

11. Roos JE, Fleischmann D, Koechl A, et al. Multipath curved planar reformation of the peripheral arterial tree in CT angiography. Radiology 2007;244:281–90.

12. Kyriakou Y, Kachelriess M, Knaup M, et al. Impact of the z-flying focal spot on resolution and artifact behavior for a 64-slice spiral CT scanner. Eur Radiol 2006;16(6):1206–15.

13. Flohr TG, McCollough CH, Bruder H, et al. First performance evaluation of a dual-source CT (DSCT) system. Eur Radiol 2006;16:256–68.

14. Petersilka M, Bruder H, Krauss B, et al. Technical principles of dual source CT. Eur J Radiol 2008;68:362–8.

15. Meyer M, Haubenreisser H, Raupach R, et al. Initial results of a new generation dual source CT system using only an in-plane comb filter for ultra-high resolution temporal bone imaging. Eur Radiol 2015;25:178–85.

16. Harell GS, Guthaner DF, Breiman RS, et al. Stop-action cardiac computed tomography. Radiology 1977;123:515–7.

17. Sagel SS, Weiss ES, Gillard RG, et al. Gated computed tomography of the human heart. Invest Radiol 1977;12:563–6.

18. Earls JP, Berman EL, Urban BA, et al. Prospectively gated transverse coronary CT angiography versus retrospectively gated helical technique: improved image quality and reduced radiation dose. Radiology 2008;246:742–53.

19. Fleischmann D, Mitchell RS, Miller DC. Acute aortic syndromes: new insights from electrocardiographically gated computed tomography. Semin Thorac Cardiovasc Surg 2008;20:340–7.

20. Fleischmann D, Liang DH, Mitchell RS, et al. Pre- and postoperative imaging of the aortic root for valve-sparing aortic root repair (v-sarr). Semin Thorac Cardiovasc Surg 2008;20:365–73.

21. Leipsic J, Hague CJ, Gurvitch R, et al. MDCT to guide transcatheter aortic valve replacement and mitral valve repair. Cardiol Clin 2012;30:147–60.

22. Newton TH, Potts DG. One of the titles. In: Newton TH, Potts DG, editors. Radiology of the skull and brain: technical aspects of computed tomography. St Louis (MO): Mosby; 1981.

23. Yu L, Fletcher JG, Grant KL, et al. Automatic selection of tube potential for radiation dose reduction in vascular and contrast-enhanced abdominopelvic ct. AJR Am J Roentgenol 2013;201:W297–306.

24. Oh LC, Lau KK, Devapalasundaram A, et al. Efficacy of 'fine' focal spot imaging in CT abdominal angiography. Eur Radiol 2014;24:3010–6.

25. Hounsfield GN. Computerized transverse axial scanning (tomography). Part 1. Description of system. Br J Radiol 1973;46:1016–22.

26. Marin D, Nelson RC, Schindera ST, et al. Low-tube-voltage, high-tube-current multidetector abdominal CT: improved image quality and decreased radiation dose with adaptive statistical iterative reconstruction algorithm–initial clinical experience. Radiology 2010;254:145–53.

27. Gabbai M, Leichter I, Mahgerefteh S, et al. Spectral material characterization with dual-energy CT: comparison of commercial and investigative technologies in phantoms. Acta Radiol 2014;56(8):960–9.

28. Silva AC, Morse BG, Hara AK, et al. Dual-energy (spectral) CT: applications in abdominal imaging. Radiographics 2011;31:1031–46 [discussion: 1047–50].

29. De Cecco CN, Buffa V, Fedeli S, et al. Dual energy CT (DECT) of the liver: conventional versus virtual unenhanced images. Eur Radiol 2010;20:2870–5.

30. Johnson TR, Krauss B, Sedlmair M, et al. Material differentiation by dual energy CT: initial experience. Eur Radiol 2007;17:1510–7.

31. Tran DN, Straka M, Roos JE, et al. Dual-energy CT discrimination of iodine and calcium: experimental results and implications for lower extremity CT angiography. Acad Radiol 2009;16:160–71.

32. Macovski A, Herman GT. Principles of reconstruction algorithms. St Louis (MO): Mosby; 1981.

33. Ambrose J, Hounsfield G. Computerized transverse axial tomography. Br J Radiol 1973;46:148–9.

34. Rockmore AJ, Macovski A. A maximum likelihood approach to emission image reconstruction from projections. IEEE Trans Nucl Sci 1976;23:1428–32.

35. Cormack AM. Reconstruction of densities from their projections, with applications in radiological physics. Phys Med Biol 1973;18:195–207.

36. Radon J. Über die bestimmung von funktionen durch ihre integralwerte längs gewisser mannigfaltigkeiten. Berichte Sächsische Acadamie der Wissenschaften 1917;69:262.

37. Shepp LA, Logan BF. The Fourier reconstruction of a head section. IEEE Trans Nucl Sci 1974;NS21:21–34.

38. Fleischmann D, Boas FE. Computed tomography: old ideas and new technology. Eur Radiol 2011;21:510–7.

39. Marin D, Nelson RC, Samei E, et al. Hypervascular liver tumors: low tube voltage, high tube current multidetector CT during late hepatic arterial phase for detection. Initial clinical experience. Radiology 2009;251:771–9.

40. Pontana F, Duhamel A, Pagniez J, et al. Chest computed tomography using iterative reconstruction vs filtered back projection (part 2): image quality of low-dose CT examinations in 80 patients. Eur Radiol 2011;21:636–43.

41. Yadava G, Kulkarni S, Rodriguez Colon Z, et al. Tu-a-201b-03: dose reduction and image quality benefits using model based iterative reconstruction (MBIR) technique for computed tomography. AAPM Annual Meeting 2010;37:3372.

42. Beister M, Kolditz D, Kalender WA. Iterative reconstruction methods in x-ray ct. Phys Med 2012;28: 94–108.

43. Boas FE, Fleischmann D. Evaluation of two iterative techniques for reducing metal artifacts in computed tomography. Radiology 2011;259:894–902.

44. Thibault JB, Sauer KD, Bouman CA, et al. A three-dimensional statistical approach to improved image quality for multislice helical ct. Med Phys 2007;34: 4526–44.

45. Olcott EW, Shin LK, Sommer G, et al. Model-based iterative reconstruction compared to adaptive statistical iterative reconstruction and filtered back-projection in CT of the kidneys and the adjacent retroperitoneum. Acad Radiol 2014;21: 774–84.

Computed Tomography Angiography of the Thoracic Aorta

Jonathan A. Scheske, MD[a], Jonathan H. Chung, MD[b],
Suhny Abbara, MD[c], Brian B. Ghoshhajra, MD, MBA[a,*]

KEYWORDS

- Thoracic aorta • Computed tomography • Angiography • Aneurysm • Dissection
- Acute aortic syndrome

KEY POINTS

- Electrocardiogram gating should be considered for evaluation of the aortic root and ascending aorta and is required for accurate evaluation of the aortic valve and annulus.
- Acute aortic syndrome should be evaluated for important additional findings, such as extension to the coronary arteries or aortic valve, occlusion of major branches, or evidence of aortic rupture, because these factors can influence patient management.
- Familiarity with the normal postoperative appearance of the aorta will prevent misdiagnoses such as mistaking elephant trunk for dissection or surgical pledget for pseudoaneurysm.

▶ Video of prosthetic aortic valve endocarditis with sinus of valsalva pseudoaneurysm; normal aortic motion throughout the cardiac cycle; aortic isthmic traumatic pseudoaneurysm; and aortic root anatomy and orientation for preprocedural evaluation of transcatheter aortic valve replacement accompanies this article http://www.radiologic. theclinics.com/

INTRODUCTION

The aorta is the largest artery in the human body, pumping up to 200 million liters of blood through the body in an average lifetime. Thoracic aortic disease presentation ranges from asymptomatic (as in an aneurysm incidentally detected on imaging) to severe acute chest pain (as in acute aortic dissection). The recent increased prevalence of aortic disease in Western countries is a result of increased clinical awareness and longer life spans. Multidetector-row computed tomography (MDCT)

of the aorta can be used to diagnose various acute and chronic conditions of the aorta, including aortic aneurysms, aortic dissections, intramural hematomas, penetrating atherosclerotic ulcers, traumatic injuries, inflammatory disorders, and congenital abnormalities.

In the early 1990s, single-detector spiral computed tomography (CT) was introduced into routine clinical imaging, allowing excellent visual assessment of vessels from any angle as opposed to catheter-based projectional angiography.[1–3] However, single-detector spiral CT had limitations,

Funding Support: None.
[a] Department of Radiology, Massachusetts General Hospital, Harvard Medical School, 55 Fruit Street, GRB-295, Boston, MA 02114, USA; [b] Department of Radiology, National Jewish Health, 1400 Jackson Street, Denver, CO 80206, USA; [c] Department of Radiology, Southwestern Medical Center, University of Texas, 5323 Harry Hines Boulevard, Dallas, TX 75390, USA
* Corresponding author.
E-mail address: bghoshhajra@mgh.harvard.edu

Radiol Clin N Am 54 (2016) 13–33
http://dx.doi.org/10.1016/j.rcl.2015.08.004

such as long breath holds, motion artifacts from slow gantry rotation time, and limited coverage in z-dimension.[1–3] In the late 1990s, MDCT was introduced. MDCT significantly improved image quality with improved through-plane resolution, faster gantry rotation, increased coverage along the z-axis, and increased table speed.[4]

Modern 64 detector-row and newer-generation CT scanners can evaluate the entire aorta, including its smaller branches, with one short breath hold. Compared with catheter angiography, extravascular structures are also well assessed with MDCT.[4] MDCT provides superior image quality by acquiring isotropic subcentimeter voxels, which allow 2-dimensional and 3-dimensional reconstructions in any orientation.[5]

This article reviews the spectrum of MDCT imaging findings in thoracic aortic diseases. Although discussion focuses on the thoracic aorta, initial examination of the aorta should include the entire aorta and iliac arteries; aortic diseases, such as aneurysm or dissection, frequently affect the whole aorta or may affect multiple regions of the aorta.

COMPUTED TOMOGRAPHY IMAGING PROTOCOL
Dose Reduction

Many patients undergoing evaluation of the aorta will require serial imaging follow-up over many years for monitoring of aneurysm size, extent of dissection, and postprocedural complications as outlined in the following sections. Several radiation dose reduction techniques have been introduced and should be used in this patient population when possible. Dual-energy CT has several potential advantages, including virtual noncontrast imaging, precluding the need for a separate precontrast acquisition, calcium subtraction, and iodine mapping for improved detection of extraluminal contrast. Iterative reconstruction algorithms allow for radiation dose reduction by improving signal-to-noise ratio at lower tube current levels. Tube current modulation and body mass index–based tube potential selection can further decrease radiation dose.

Noncontrast Computed Tomography

Inclusion of a noncontrast CT scan is imperative in aortic imaging for suspected acute aortic syndrome because aortic intramural hematomas are more evident without intra-arterial contrast. Calcification is best evaluated on noncontrast imaging because of high tissue contrast between calcium and unenhanced tissue. Moderate density calcification can be subtle on contrast-enhanced images because the density may be similar to enhanced tissue, even in very extensive cases, such as coral reef aorta, which can obstruct the distal thoracic aorta. Radiation dose is often reduced during this phase by increasing collimation, decreasing kilovolts peak, or increasing the noise index with concomitant reduction in effective milliampere-seconds (mAs).

Computed Tomography Angiography

Nongated thoracic aortic CT angiography is usually performed with a pitch of 1.0 to 1.5, a collimation of 0.5 to 1.0 mm, and reconstruction of 1.0- to 1.5-mm slices with spacing of 0.75 to 1.0 mm. The kilovolts peak is usually set at 120 kVp. A lower kilovolts peak (70–100 kVp) may be used in thin patients. Automated tube current modulation should be used when available, in conjunction with automatic tube potential selection (a relatively new technique not widely available).

With automatic tube current modulation, the tube current is automatically reduced when scanning regions of lower attenuation and increased for areas of higher attenuation.[6] A desired noise index is entered, defined as the standard deviation of Hounsfield units in the center of an image using soft tissue kernel reconstruction. A threshold-based bolus-tracking algorithm with a region of interest in the ascending aorta is typically used.

Contrast is injected at rates of 3 to 5 mL/s, and the overall contrast volume should be approximately the injection rate (in milliliters per second) multiplied by the scan duration in seconds plus 5 to 10 seconds; typical contrast volumes range from 60 to 120 mL. Adding 5 to 10 seconds to the contrast injection duration is necessary to compensate for the difference in position between the tracking position in the ascending aorta and the top of the chest. A small field of view can be selected to optimize spatial resolution. However, a full field-of-view series should be reconstructed to detect incidental findings. Initial examination of the thoracic aorta should include the abdominal aorta and iliac arteries because thoracic aortic pathology commonly involves these vessels.

Electrocardiogram (ECG) gating is not required for routine aortic angiography; but cardiac motion can result in significant artifact in the aortic root and ascending aorta, which can decrease the accuracy of measurement or even mimic aortic dissection. In cases whereby aortic root abnormality is suspected, such as prosthetic valve endocarditis, ECG gating can accurately evaluate for valve dehiscence, vegetations, para-valvular abscess, and pseudoaneurysm. **Fig. 1** and Video 1 demonstrate prosthetic valve endocarditis of

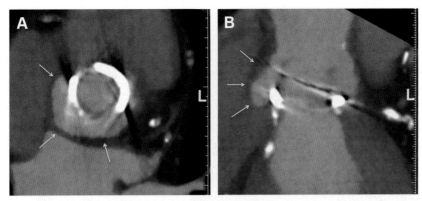

Fig. 1. (A) Left ventricular outflow tract short-axis and (B) long-axis multi-planar reformation of the aortic root on contrast-enhanced CT. Prosthetic valve endocarditis has resulted in a para-valvular pseudoaneurysm (arrows). Pseudoaneurysms fill with contrast, whereas para-valvular abscess remains unenhanced on CT angiography. ECG gating results in robust imaging of the aortic annulus and valve leaflets for detection of para-valvular leak and vegetations.

the aorta with para-valvular pseudoaneurysm. If ascending aortic dissection is suspected, ECG gating may also be a prudent option if technical expertise is available.

Delayed Scan

Delayed scans at 1 to 2 minutes after injection are obtained to assess for late filling of a false lumen in dissections, slow endoleaks in endovascular stent repair (more often used in the abdominal aorta), contrast extravasation from aortic rupture, or enhancement of inflammatory tissue in vasculitides and infection.

Postprocessing

Multi-planar maximum-intensity projections in the sagittal, sagittal-oblique (ie, candy cane), coronal, aortic short-axis, and aortic root long-axis planes are routinely acquired. Three-dimensional volume-rendered images at multiple viewing angles may also be created. However, the source data (axial images) and interactive multi-planar reformations are clinically more useful than are static postprocessed images.

NORMAL ANATOMY AND NORMAL VARIANTS

The thoracic aorta extends proximally from the aortic annulus to the diaphragmatic crura distally.[7] The thoracic aorta is subdivided into 3 parts: the ascending aorta, the arch, and the descending aorta (Fig. 2). The ascending thoracic aorta comprises the aortic root and the tubular ascending aorta. The aortic root lies between the aortic annulus and the sinotubular junction (Fig. 3). The sinuses of Valsalva arise from the aortic root. The tubular ascending aorta extends from the sinotubular junction to the brachiocephalic trunk. Approximately 3 cm of the proximal ascending aorta is within the pericardium. The coronary arteries are the only branches of the ascending aorta.

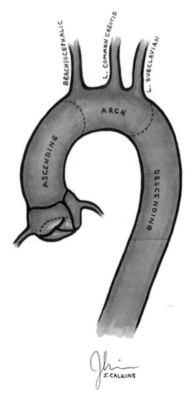

Fig. 2. The thoracic aorta demonstrating 3 main subdivisions: the ascending aorta, the aortic arch, and the descending thoracic aorta.

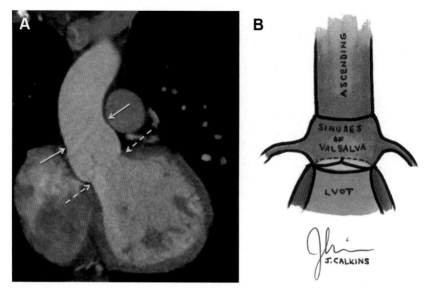

Fig. 3. (*A*) Normal thoracic aorta on coronal multi-planar reformation from contrast-enhanced CT. The aortic root extends from the aortic annulus (*dashed arrows*) to the sinotubular junction (*solid arrows*). (*B*) The aortic root. The coronary arteries—the only branches of the ascending aorta—arise from the aortic root. LVOT, left ventricle outflow tract.

The aortic arch extends from the brachiocephalic trunk to the origin of the left subclavian artery. The isthmus extends from the left subclavian artery to the ligamentum arteriosum. Three branches usually arise from the aortic arch: the brachiocephalic trunk (occasionally referred to as the *brachiocephalic artery* or *innominate artery*), the left common carotid artery, and the left subclavian artery. The brachiocephalic trunk divides into the right common carotid artery and the right subclavian artery.

Currently published normal measurements of the thoracic aorta are listed in **Table 1**. Most of currently accepted aortic dimensions are either based on other imaging modalities (which may measure the aorta differently) or on nongated MDCT (often derived from body axial [*x–y* plane] rather than from true aortic short-axis images). Therefore, some uncertainty exists as to the true normal size of the thoracic aorta. ECG-gated MDCT is poised to become the reference standard method for assessing the thoracic aorta, allowing

Table 1
Normal values for the thoracic aorta

Aorta	Normal Values
LVOT	20.3 ± 3.4 mm (2 SD)
Aortic annulus	25–37 mm (95% CI) (end-diastolic) 26.3 ± 2.8 mm (coronal) 23.5 ± 2.7 mm (sagittal)
Sinus of valsalva	34.2 ± 4.1 mm (2 SD) 36.9 ± 3.8 mm (2 SD) (end-diastolic, gated)
Sinotubular junction	29.7 ± 3.4 mm (2 SD)
Ascending aorta	32.7 ± 3.8 mm (2 SD) 33.6 ± 4.1 mm (2 SD) (male/intraluminal/end-systolic) 31.1 ± 3.9 mm (2 SD) (female/intraluminal/end-systolic) 21–35 mm (95% CI) (end-diastolic)
Descending thoracic aorta	17–26 mm (95% CI) (end-diastolic)

Abbreviations: CI, confidence interval; LVOT, left ventricular outlfow tract.
  Data from Refs.[8,100–103]

for reproducible measurements not reliant on operator skill. Furthermore, variations in the size of the aorta during different portions of the cardiac cycle could also be documented.[8]

In 6.6% of people, the left vertebral artery arises directly from the arch.[9] The bovine arch is another normal variant in which the left common carotid artery arises from the brachiocephalic trunk (**Fig. 4**) rather than the aorta, occurring in up to one-fourth of the population.[9] Although ingrained in the medical literature, the bovine arch is a misnomer for this aortic variant; cows actually have a single brachiocephalic trunk that splits into the bilateral subclavian arteries and a bicarotid trunk.[10] Another arch variant is the ductus diverticulum, a focal bulge along the inner aspect of the isthmus representing a remnant of the ductus arteriosus (**Fig. 5**). Traumatic aortic transection also occurs in this location and can occasionally be difficult to differentiate from a ductus diverticulum. However, the ductus diverticulum has smooth margins with obtuse angles relative to the adjacent aorta. Aortic transection has irregular margins with acute angles relative to the adjacent aorta.

The descending thoracic aorta extends from the isthmus to the diaphragmatic crura. In contrast to the ascending aorta, the descending thoracic

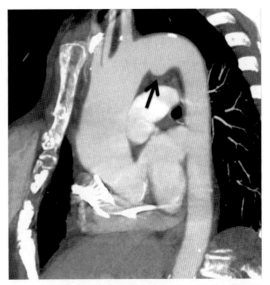

Fig. 5. Ductus diverticulum on contrast-enhanced CT. Oblique sagittal maximum intensity projection image of the aorta on contrast-enhanced CT shows a smooth protrusion (*arrow*) along the inferior inner aspect of the isthmus of the aorta with obtuse margins. This smooth protrusion is in contradistinction to traumatic transections of the aorta, which has abrupt acute transitions and irregular margins.

aorta has multiple branches, including the bronchial, intercostal, spinal, superior phrenic arteries, and various small mediastinal branches. Pseudocoarctation is a normal variant of the aortic arch and proximal descending aorta that occurs when the third to seventh embryonic dorsal segments fail to fuse appropriately; the resultant high proximal arch leads to pseudokinking of the redundant aorta where it is tethered to the pulmonary artery by the ligamentum arteriosum (**Fig. 6**).[11] No hemodynamically significant luminal aortic narrowing exists in pseudocoarctation.

ACUTE AORTIC SYNDROME

Acute aortic syndrome is a group of aortic pathologies that are acute emergencies. Underlying aortic diseases include penetrating atherosclerotic ulcer, intramural hematoma, aortic dissection, rupturing aneurysms, and traumatic aortic injury. MDCT is the preferred examination because of its rapid acquisition and excellent depiction of the aorta, its wall, and the end organs. ECG-gated CT is preferred, if readily available, especially if ascending aortic involvement is suspected. Nongated MDCT of the ascending aorta is limited by motion artifact, which can be misinterpreted as a dissection.[12] Motion artifact can be entirely eliminated by ECG gating the acquisition (**Fig. 7**, Video 2).

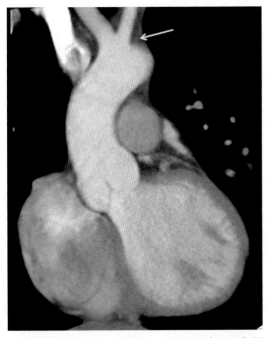

Fig. 4. Bovine aortic arch on contrast-enhanced CT. Coronal multi-planar reformation from CT angiography shows common origin of the brachiocephalic and left common carotid arteries (*arrow*) consistent with a bovine arch. Although thought to mirror normal cow anatomy, bovine arch is a misnomer.

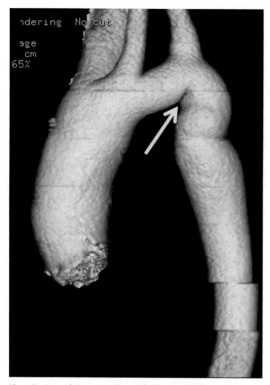

Fig. 6. Pseudocoarctation of the aorta on contrast-enhanced CT. Three-dimensional volume-rendered image of contrast-enhanced CT shows redundancy of the aortic arch resulting in a kinked appearance at the level of the ligamentum arteriosum (*arrow*). No significant collateral arteries are present, implying that the narrowing is not hemodynamically significant.

Aortic Dissection

Aortic dissection results from an intimal tear extending into the inner layer of the aortic media; an intimal flap separates the false and true lumens. The blood within the false lumen may be free flowing or thrombosed. Acute aortic dissection is potentially life threatening, with a reported incidence of 2.9 per 100,000 persons per year.[13] Risk factors for aortic dissection include preexisting thoracic aortic aneurysm, chronic hypertension, Marfan syndrome, bicuspid aortic valve, infection, and prior cardiovascular surgery. Dissections most commonly originate in the ascending aorta (approximately 65% of cases); 20% occur in the descending thoracic aorta, 10% in the aortic arch, and 5% in the abdominal aorta.[14] The dissected aorta can be dilated or normal in caliber.

Aortic dissections can be classified according to involvement of the ascending aorta or arch. This involvement implies a worse prognosis and usually requires surgical management.[15] The DeBakey and Stanford classification systems are the most commonly used systems to categorize aortic dissections and are based on location. In type I DeBakey dissections, the intimal flap involves both the ascending and descending thoracic aorta; in type II, the intimal flap involves the ascending aorta only; and in type III, the intimal flap is isolated to the descending thoracic aorta. In Stanford type A dissections, the intimal flap involves the ascending thoracic aorta (with or without extension into the descending aorta) (**Fig. 8**), whereas in type B, the flap does not involve the ascending thoracic aorta or arch (**Fig. 9**).

Dissections involving the ascending aorta (Stanford A; DeBakey I and II) are surgical emergencies because dissections in this area are prone to rupture or other critical complications, including development of hemopericardium, pericardial tamponade, and death. Other potential complications of ascending aortic dissections include aortic valve rupture, aortic insufficiency, coronary artery dissection, stroke, and myocardial infarction. Surgery in type B dissection is reserved for patients who have occlusion of major aortic branches, expansion or extension of the dissection, or aortic rupture and for patients with Marfan syndrome who have an acute distal dissection.[16] Mortality rates for untreated Stanford A dissection is 1% to 2% per hour during the first 24 hours and 80% during the first 2 weeks.[17]

MDCT is the most common modality to detect aortic dissections.[18] Its high sensitivity for detecting dissection, wide availability, and ability to identify alternative diagnoses for chest pain makes MDCT an excellent first choice in evaluating suspected dissection.[19–21] MDCT rapidly delineates extension of the intimal flap, allowing for efficient preoperative planning. It can also help identify the entry/reentry sites, relationships between the true and false lumens, flow in the aortic branches, perfusion of end organs, aortic insufficiency, and coronary artery involvement.

Other imaging modalities may also be used for analyzing aortic dissection. Catheter aortography was the traditional preferred modality for diagnosing aortic dissection (sensitivity, 77%–90%; specificity, 90%–100%).[22] However, the risks associated with catheter manipulation and high-flow contrast injection makes this modality less attractive.

Transesophageal echocardiogram (TEE) is currently the second most frequently used modality and can be considered an alternative that is especially useful in unstable patients. This modality has good accuracy, with a sensitivity of 90% to 100% and specificity of 77% to 100%.[23] However,

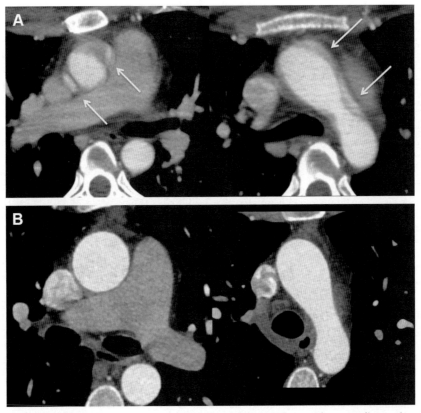

Fig. 7. (A) Transverse contrast-enhanced images of the aorta from CT chest without cardiac gating. Motion arti-fact is common on these studies and can mimic aortic dissection (arrows). (B) Matched images of the same patient from ECG-gated CT demonstrates normal aorta without dissection or motion artifact.

TEE is limited by reliance on operator skill, ultra-sound artifacts, and inconsistent visualization of the distal ascending aorta and proximal arch. Simi-larly, although MRI is highly accurate in detecting aortic dissections (sensitivity as high as 100%), widespread use of this modality has been hampered by long acquisition times, which is un-desirable in the emergent setting. Furthermore,

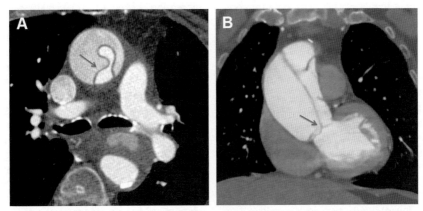

Fig. 8. (A) Type A aortic dissection on axial image from contrast-enhanced CT. Dissection flap (arrow) extends from the aortic root to the distal abdominal aorta. (B) Coronal multi-planar reformation from another patient with involvement of the aortic root (arrow) puts this patient at risk for rupture into the pericardial sac and resul-tant cardiac tamponade or aortic insufficiency as well as extension of the dissection flap into the coronary arteries.

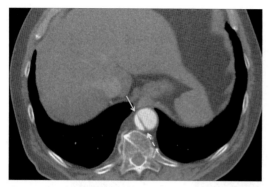

Fig. 9. Type B aortic dissection on axial contrast-enhanced CT. A dissection flap (*arrow*) is isolated to the descending thoracic aorta. Focal low-density thrombus is present in the beaked margin of the false lumen (*dashed arrow*), which helps delineate the false from the true lumen. As in most cases, the false lumen is larger than the true lumen.

many medical devices are ferromagnetic, which are contraindications to MRI.

Currently, no available data compare the utility of modern MDCT and MRI/TEE. Modern MDCT can image the entire aorta from supra-aortic branches to femoral arteries within a few seconds, can eliminate pulsation artifact with gating (which otherwise could mimic type A dissections), and can provide isovolumetric imaging, allowing reconstruction of images in any plane.[24] Furthermore, CT offers high-resolution images of the aortic wall.[25] However, MDCT should be used prudently, given its use of ionizing radiation. In addition, aortic evaluation on MDCT may suffer from streak artifacts, volume averaging with periaortic structures, and patient motion artifacts.[26]

The main MDCT finding in aortic dissection is the intimal flap, a thin linear filling defect that separates the true and false lumens. Differentiation of the false and true lumens is imperative in surgical repair and percutaneous treatment with endografts.

In most cases, the most reliable way to identify the true lumen is by determining continuity with the undissected portion of the aorta. If an undissected portion is not well visualized, there are several other signs that may be helpful. The true lumen often spirals through the aortic arch (anterior in the ascending aorta and medial in the descending aorta). The cross-sectional area of the false lumen is also often larger than that of the true lumen. The cobweb sign is insensitive but specific for the false lumen.[27] Thin linear areas of low attenuation are present in the false lumen, representing remnants of the media. Finally, the beak sign (see **Fig. 9**) is another helpful diagnostic sign

of the false lumen. It represents the section of hematoma that cleaves a space for the propagation of the false lumen.[27,28] Intimo-intimal intussusception is a rare type of aortic dissection characterized by circumferential dissection and invagination of the intimal layer, likened to a windsock.[29] Neurologic impairment from occlusion of the aorta or arch branches may be more common in this entity.[30]

The presence of identifiable flow in the false lumen and patency has prognostic implications and can be evaluated on MDCT. Slow flow in the false lumen eventually leads to thrombus formation.[28] A patent false lumen has a higher 3-year mortality rate (32%) compared with a partially thrombosed lumen (14%) among the survivors of type B dissection.[19]

Imaging follow-up of acute aortic dissections is appropriate to monitor for progression. For patients receiving medical treatment or treated with endovascular stent grafting, imaging is recommended at the time of discharge from the hospital, at 1, 3, and 6 months, and then yearly.[31] Following surgical repair of aortic root and ascending thoracic aortic dissection, follow-up is recommended at the time of discharge from the hospital and then yearly.[31]

Intramural Hematoma

Intramural hematoma (IMH) is hemorrhage localized to the aortic media in the absence of a visible intimal tear. IMH is considered equivalent to aortic dissection regarding prognostic and therapeutic implications because an IMH may progress to aortic dissection and rupture. IMH may develop secondary to spontaneous rupture of vasa vasorum of the medial aortic layer, penetrating aortic ulceration, or blunt trauma.[32] Hypertension is the most common predisposing risk factor.

Unenhanced CT is extremely valuable in identifying intramural hematomas. Typically, circumferential or crescent-shaped high-attenuation thickening of the aortic wall is present, representing hematoma within the medial wall of the aorta (**Fig. 10**), which sometimes narrows the aortic lumen.[33]

Several findings help differentiate IMH from a thrombosed false lumen of an aortic dissection: IMHs do not enhance; no intimal tear is seen; IMHs maintain a constant circumferential relationship with the aortic wall; the false lumen of a dissection has a longitudinal spiral geometry.[34] Involvement of the ascending aorta, pericardial or pleural effusion, and an aortic diameter of greater than 5 cm may predict progression of an IMH to a true dissection.[34,35]

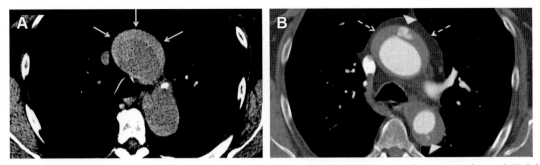

Fig. 10. Type B IMH from an ulcerated atherosclerotic plaque on axial noncontrast and contrast-enhanced CT. (*A*) Axial image from noncontrast CT shows a rind of hyperdense attenuation (*arrows*) around the ascending thoracic aorta. (*B*) Matched axial image from arterial phase shows focal ulcerations filling with contrast in the ascending and descending aorta (*arrowheads*). The hematoma remains unenhanced after the administration of contrast (*dashed arrows*).

Penetrating Aortic Ulcer

Penetrating aortic ulcer (PAU) represents an ulcerated atheroma disrupting the aortic intima.[36] PAU occurs when an atheromatous plaque ruptures, disrupting the elastic lamina, with variable extension into the media. Hypertension and advanced age are the most common risk factors. The descending aorta is most often affected.[37] CT commonly shows extensive aortic atherosclerosis. On CT, a discrete contrast-filled 'collar button' is often seen out-pouching beyond the expected confines of the aorta[36] (**Fig. 11**). PAUs are often multifocal, which is not surprising considering the diffuse nature of atherosclerosis.

PAU can be difficult to differentiate from simple ulcerated atherosclerotic plaque. The presence of contour deformity of the vessel is highly suggestive of PAU. Extension of the aortic ulcer into the medial layer can result in an IMH, localized aortic dissection, saccular pseudoaneurysm, or mediastinal hematoma.[38] Invasive intervention (surgery or endovascular repair) should be considered in patients with pain, hemodynamic instability, or signs of aortic expansion.[39] Asymptomatic patients can be followed closely with optimization of medical management.

If treated medically, imaging follow-up for both IMH and PAU is recommended at the time of discharge from the hospital, at 1, 3, and 6 months, and then yearly.[31]

Traumatic Aortic Transection

Traumatic aortic transection is a tear involving all layers of the aortic wall, usually caused by rapid deceleration (high-speed motor vehicle accident or fall from significant height). The mortality rate

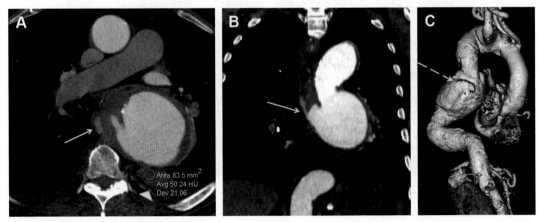

Fig. 11. Ruptured penetrating aortic ulceration on contrast-enhanced CT. (*A*) Axial image and (*B*) coronal multiplanar reformation from contrast-enhanced CT shows irregular out-pouching of contrast (*arrows*) along the right lateral aspect of the aorta, consistent with penetrating aortic ulcer. The adjacent right pleural effusion is high density (*arrowhead*), concerning for hemothorax secondary to aortic rupture. (*C*) Three-dimensional reformat from the same study demonstrates the irregularity of the ruptured aortic ulcerations (*dashed arrow*).

is high, with most patients dying in the field.[40,41] Survival is highest for tears at the aortic isthmus. Aortic injury also occurs at the aortic root and at the diaphragmatic hiatus. Proposed mechanisms for aortic injury include shearing and hydrostatic forces secondary to rapid deceleration and osseous pinching. Given its accuracy, rapid acquisition, and wide availability, CT is usually the preferred imaging modality for suspected aortic transection.

MDCT imaging findings include small, contained periaortic hematomas, traumatic pseudoaneurysm, mediastinal hematoma, focal contour abnormality, abrupt change in aortic caliber, or an intraluminal ridge, flap, or thrombus (**Fig. 12**, Video 3).[42] A residual ductus diverticulum can mimic traumatic pseudoaneurysm. Absence of mediastinal hemorrhage, smooth contours, and obtuse margins with the adjacent aorta are more suggestive of a ductus diverticulum (see **Fig. 5**) than an acute injury.

THORACIC AORTIC ANEURYSM

A true aortic aneurysm represents greater than 50% dilation of the aorta; the wall of a true

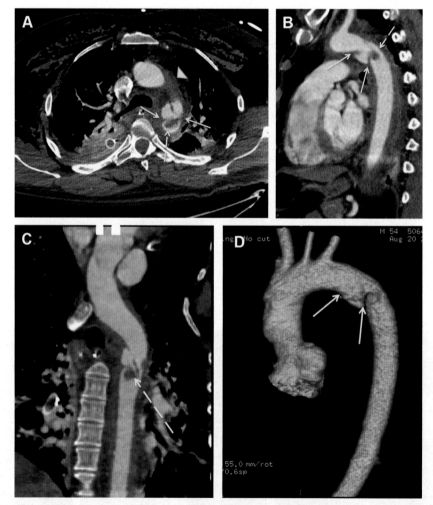

Fig. 12. Traumatic aortic pseudoaneurysm on contrast-enhanced CT. Axial image (*A*), oblique sagittal multiplanar reformation (MPR) (*B*), curved MPR (*C*), and 3-dimensional volume-rendered (*D*) images from contrast-enhanced CT shows irregular focal outpouching of the isthmic aorta with a narrow neck (*arrows*), consistent with partial aortic transection and pseudoaneurysm formation in this patient who has a history of a high-speed motor vehicle collision. There is intraluminal thrombus associated with the intimal injury (*dashed arrows*). High density left of the aorta is consistent with mediastinal hematoma (*arrowhead*). This site is the most common location of traumatic aortic injury identified by imaging; individuals with injuries in other regions of the thoracic aorta, such as the aortic root, seldom survive to receive medical attention.

aneurysm comprises the intima, media, and adventitia.[43] Aortic aneurysms are the 13th most common cause of death in the United States. The incidence and prevalence of aortic aneurysms have increased concomitantly with life expectancy. The incidence of thoracic aortic aneurysms is currently 10.4 cases per 100,000 persons per year.[44] Affected individuals are most often in their 60s, and men are affected 2 to 4 times more often than women. Hypertension is present in 60% of cases. Thoracic aortic aneurysms are less common than abdominal aortic aneurysms. Up to 25% of patients with thoracic aneurysm will also have an abdominal aortic aneurysm.[45]

The aortic root and ascending aorta (aortic valve to innominate artery) are affected in 60% of patients with thoracic aneurysm (**Fig. 13**), the arch in 10%, the descending thoracic aorta (distal to left subclavian artery) in 40%, and the thoracoabdominal aorta in 10%.[46] The extent, location, and size of the aneurysm should be documented on MDCT. Size should be reported in the aortic short axis (orthogonal to the aortic segment long axis). In addition to evaluating aortic aneurysm morphology, MDCT can accurately detect the presence of complications, such as rupture, infection, and fistulas. MDCT is ideal for postsurgical surveillance and surveillance in patients being treated medically. Furthermore, CT can detect involvement of aortic branches, which is essential for preoperative surgical evaluation.[47]

Thoracic aortic aneurysms can be classified based on extent or morphology. The Crawford classification includes 4 types of thoracoabdominal aneurysms.[48] Type I aneurysms extend from the left subclavian artery to the renal artery. Type II aneurysms extend from the left subclavian artery to the aortic bifurcation; these have the worst postsurgical outcome. Type III aneurysms extend from the midthorax to the aortic bifurcation, and type IV aneurysms extend from the diaphragm to the aortic bifurcation. Morphologically, thoracic aneurysms are divided into fusiform (dilation of the entire circumference of the aorta usually involving several centimeters of length), saccular (localized outpouching of the aorta), and pseudoaneurysm (contained rupture of the aortic wall with disruption of the intima and media, with usually a narrow mouth).

Size is the only established risk factor predicting aortic rupture. No significant risk for aortic rupture is associated with aneurysms smaller than 4.0 cm. The risk for aortic rupture increases incrementally with aneurysm size; aneurysms 4.0 to 5.9 cm have a 16% risk for rupture, and those greater than 6.0 cm have a 31% risk for rupture.[44] The average growth rate of thoracic aortic aneurysms is 1.0 mm per year.[49] Descending midaortic aneurysms have the fastest growth rate, and ascending aneurysms have the slowest despite larger initial diameter.[49] In general, larger aneurysms grow faster. Aneurysms larger than 5.0 cm in diameter grow on average 7.9 mm per year versus 1.7 mm per year for smaller aneurysms.[50] Higher rates are also observed in familial thoracic aortic aneurysm, Marfan syndrome, Ehlers-Danlos, bicuspid aortic valve, and, most notably, Loeys-Dietz syndrome whereby the growth rate can reach 10 mm per year.[51,52]

Risk for dissection is also related to the size of the aneurysm. The dissection risk per year is 2% for aneurysms smaller than 5.0 cm and 3% for aneurysms 5.0 to 5.9 cm. Aneurysms larger than 6.0 cm in diameter have a dissection risk of more than 7% per year, and these patients have a 5-year survival rate of only 54% without surgery.[53]

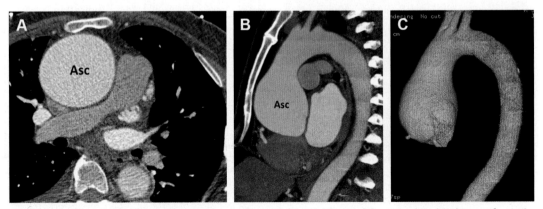

Fig. 13. Ascending aortic aneurysm on contrast-enhanced CT. Axial image (*A*), coronal multi-planar reformation (*B*), and 3-dimensional volume-rendered (*C*) images from contrast-enhanced CT show a large aneurysm of the aortic root and ascending aorta (Asc). The sinotubular junction is effaced and dilated creating the classic tulip-bulb appearance.

In patients with Marfan syndrome and Ehlers-Danlos syndrome, aortic root aneurysms may efface the sinotubular junction (annuloaortic ectasia), resulting in a classic tulip bulb configuration (see **Fig. 13; Fig. 14**).[54]

Aortic root aneurysms may also occur in the setting of bicuspid aortic valves and familial thoracic aortic aneurysm syndrome (FTAAS). Most aneurysms of the tubular ascending aorta are idiopathic but may also occur with bicuspid aortic valve, FTAAS, giant cell arteritis, and syphilis. Nineteen percent of patients with thoracic aneurysms have a family history independent of Marfan or Ehlers-Danlos syndromes.[55–58] Bicuspid aortic valve is known to be an independent predictor of ascending aortic aneurysm formation after surgical correction of coarctation.[56] Furthermore, normally functioning bicuspid aortic valves have been associated with enlargement of the aortic root or ascending aorta in 52% of patients.[55]

Aneurysms of the ascending aorta or the aortic arch may cause hoarseness from left vagus or left recurrent laryngeal nerve compression, hemidiaphragmatic paralysis from phrenic nerve compression, asthmalike symptoms from tracheobronchial compression, dysphasia from esophageal compression, and facial swelling from superior vena cava compression. Thoracic aortic aneurysms also predispose patients to thromboembolism, aortoesophageal fistula, and aortic dissection.

Surgery is usually recommended for thoracic aortic aneurysms 5.5 cm or greater.[31,59] Lower thresholds are used in patients with bicuspid aortic valve and genetic and syndromic conditions predisposing to aortic aneurysms.[31,60–63] Surgery may be recommended for aneurysms of 5.0 cm or greater or a growth rate greater than 3 mm/y in Marfan syndrome, Turner syndrome, Loeys-Dietz, Ehlers-Danlos, and bicuspid aortic valve or 4.5 cm or greater in the these patients when additional risk factors are present, including family history of aortic dissection, severe aortic regurgitation, or desire for pregnancy.[64–66] Aortic size index (ratio of aortic diameter over body surface area in square meters) greater than 2.75 cm/m^2 is a useful threshold in patients of small stature or in Turner syndrome,[67] as is accelerated growth (>10 mm/y growth in aneurysms <5 cm).[68] Aortic regurgitation, in conjunction with an aortic root or ascending aortic aneurysm, requires aortic valve replacement plus aortic root repair if the aneurysm is 5 cm or greater (**Table 2**).[69,70] Furthermore, in functional bicuspid aortic valves, aortic root repair or replacement of the ascending aorta is indicated if the root or ascending aorta is greater than 5.0 cm in diameter or is growing faster than 0.5 cm/y (see **Table 2**).[70]

CT angiography is suitable for surveillance of thoracic aortic aneurysm (TAA). Initial follow-up at 6 months in degenerative TAA or 3 months in syndromic or familial cases can be performed to establish the growth rate followed by a size-adjusted surveillance schedule as per **Table 3**.[31,46]

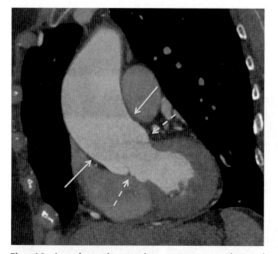

Fig. 14. Annuloaortic ectasia on contrast-enhanced CT. Long-axis multi-planar reformation of the aortic root shows aortic root aneurysm with effacement and dilatation of the sinotubular junction (*solid arrows*), and widening of the aortic annulus (*dashed arrows*), indicating annuloaortic ectasia in this patient with Marfan syndrome.

Table 2
Threshold for surgical intervention in thoracic aortic aneurysm

	Indication
Degenerative	Size ≥5.5 cm Growth ≥0.5 cm/y
Syndromic/familial[a]	Size ≥5.0 cm or 2.75 cm/m^{2}[b] Growth ≥0.5 cm/y
Syndromic/Familial with Risk Factors[c]	Size ≥4.5 cm
Requiring other cardiac Surgery[d]	Size ≥4.5 cm

[a] Bicuspid aortic valve, Marfan, Turner, Loeys-Dietz, Ehlers-Danlos, and familial aortic aneurysm.
[b] Aortic diameter divided by body surface area.
[c] Family history of aortic dissection, severe aortic regurgitation, desire for pregnancy.
[d] Coronary artery bypass grafting or aortic valve replacement.
Data from Refs.[59,64–67,104]

Table 3
Recommended follow-up schedule for TAA and postsurgical thoracic aorta

	Size (cm)	Initial	Surveillance
Degenerative	3.5–4.4	6 mo	Yearly
	4.5–5.4	6 mo	6 mo
Familial and syndromic[a]	3.5–4.4	3–6 mo	Yearly
	4.5–5.0	3 mo	6 mo
Acute dissection	—	Discharge from hospital	1, 3, and 6 mo, then yearly
TEVAR	—	Discharge from hospital	1, 3, and 6 mo, then yearly
Surgical repair	—	Discharge from hospital	Yearly[b]

Abbreviation: TEVAR, thoracic endovascular repair.
  [a] Bicuspid aortic valve, Marfan, Turner, Loeys-Dietz, Ehlers-Danlos, and familial aortic aneurysm.
  [b] Two to 3 years if initially stable.
  Data from Hiratzka LF, Bakris GL, Beckman JA, et al. 2010 ACCF/AHA/AATS/ACR/ASA/SCA/SCAI/SIR/STS/SVM guidelines for the diagnosis and management of patients with thoracic aortic disease: a report of the American College of Cardiology Foundation/American Heart Association Task Force on Practice Guidelines, American Association for Thoracic Surgery, American College of Radiology, American Stroke Association, Society of Cardiovascular Anesthesiologists, Society for Cardiovascular Angiography and Interventions, Society of Interventional Radiology, Society of Thoracic Surgeons, and Society for Vascular Medicine. Circulation 2010;121:e266–369.

Sinus of Valsalva Aneurysm

Sinus of Valsalva aneurysms are rare congenital anomalies resulting from failure of proper development of elastic components in the aortic media. The right coronary sinus of Valsalva is most commonly affected, followed by the noncoronary sinus.[71] These aneurysms usually rupture into the right heart (right atrium or ventricle), causing left to right shunting. Rupture into the pericardial sac can lead to cardiac tamponade.

Sinus of Valsalva aneurysms may protrude into or obstruct the right ventricular outflow tract. Ventricular septal defect, aortic insufficiency, aortic coarctation, and bicuspid aortic valve are all associated with sinus of Valsalva aneurysms.[72] CT will show asymmetric dilatation of one or more of the sinuses of Valsalva (**Fig. 15**). Progressive increases in size rather than absolute size is more frequently used when determining proper surgical timing in asymptomatic patients.[73]

Pseudoaneurysms are commonly secondary to blunt trauma and iatrogenic injury and less commonly infection. Growth rates are less predictable; serious complications include rupture, fistula formation, and erosion of adjacent structures. Endovascular treatment or surgical repair is indicated regardless of size, if feasible.[66]

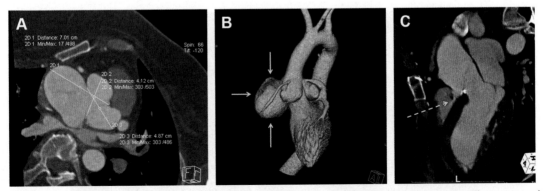

Fig. 15. Sinus of Valsalva (SOV) aneurysm on contrast-enhanced CT. (*A*) Axial image shows asymmetric aneurysmal enlargement of the noncoronary SOV. Accurate measurements of the SOVs are taken from the commissure between 2 valve leaflets to the farthest point of the opposing sinus. In this case, the diameter from the commissure between right and left coronary cusps to the noncoronary SOV is 7.0 cm. (*B*) Three-dimensional volume-rendered images demonstrates the SOV aneurysm (*arrows*). (*C*) Three-chamber view multi-planar reformation from CT angiography in another patient demonstrates right SOV aneurysm complicated by fistula to the right ventricle (*dashed arrow*).

AORTIC COARCTATION

Aortic coarctation is focal narrowing of the thoracic aorta, which can occur anywhere in the aorta, although it is most common at the isthmus. Aortic coarctation is a common malformation, affecting men 2 to 5 times more often than women.[74] Aortic coarctation has 3 major subtypes: focal (aortic coarctation), diffuse (hypoplastic isthmus), and complete (aortic arch interruption). The narrowing in aortic coarctation is caused by a fibrous ridge, arising from abnormal hyperplasia of the tunica media. Hemodynamic compromise leads to the development of collaterals to bypass the narrowed aorta (**Fig. 16**). The extent of collaterals depends on the severity of stenosis. Collaterals may compress the spinal cord or may rupture.[75]

Most aortic coarctation classifications are based on anatomy. Aortic coarctations have been traditionally divided into preductal (infantile) and postductal (adult) subtypes; however, this classification system can be misleading. The contemporary approach is to use left subclavian artery as a landmark for distinguishing between the more common distal (juxtaductal) and less common proximal subtypes.[74]

Aortic coarctations are associated with multiple other abnormalities. Among patients with aortic coarctation, 30% to 40% will also have a bicuspid aortic valve.[76] Patients with Turner syndrome have a higher prevalence of aortic coarctation. Other abnormalities associated with aortic coarctation include ventricular septal defect, patent ductus arteriosus, aortic stenosis, and mitral stenosis.[77] Patients with aortic coarctation must also be evaluated for intracerebral berry aneurysms.

Intracerebral aneurysms can rupture, leading to subarachnoid or intracerebral hemorrhage, even long after successful coarctation repair.[78]

Rare cases of acquired aortic narrowing have also been reported. Inflammatory aortitis (Takayasu aortitis) is a well-described cause of acquired aortic stenosis and usually involves the midthoracic or abdominal aorta.[79] Takayasu aortitis predominantly affects young women of Asian descent, with a mean age of 35 years at diagnosis.[80] Imaging findings suggesting Takayasu aortitis include thickening of the walls of the aorta and its branches (**Fig. 17**), stenosis of the aorta and arch vessels, aneurysmal dilation of the aorta and its major branches, and aortic regurgitation from aortic root dilation.

Treatment of congenital aortic coarctation largely depends on age, clinical presentation, and severity. Early repair is important to prevent long-standing hypertension. Indications for repair include arterial hypertension, congestive heart failure, and pressure gradient greater than 30 mm Hg (though resting pressure gradient in isolation is an unreliable indicator of severity in the presence of extensive collaterals).[81] Multiple surgical techniques are available, including resection with end-to-end anastomosis, subclavian flap aortoplasty in infants with long-segment coarctation, prosthetic patch (now rarely used because of increased risk for postoperative aneurysms and ruptures), and bypass grafting across the coarctation.[82] Balloon angioplasty is a viable alternative to surgery and can be used in patients with native coarctation or those who develop restenosis after surgery.[83,84] Postprocedural surveillance of these patients is mandatory to monitor for residual

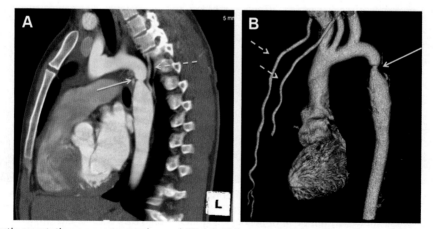

Fig. 16. Aortic coarctation on contrast-enhanced CT. (*A*) Oblique sagittal (candy cane) multi-planar reformation and (*B*) 3-dimensional volume-rendered reformatted images of the thoracic aorta shows narrowing (*arrow*) of the proximal descending aorta. Multiple enlarged collateral arteries are present (*dashed arrows*), including internal mammary arteries, which bypass the stenotic portion of the aorta and provide blood flow to the lower body.

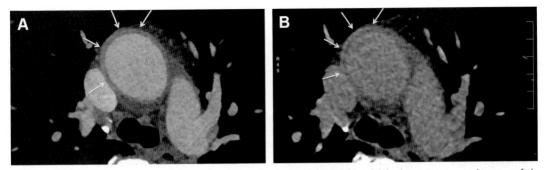

Fig. 17. Takayasu aortitis on contrast-enhanced CT. Arterial (*A*) and delayed (*B*) phase transverse images of the aorta shows diffuse thickening of the aortic wall (*arrows* in *A*) and mural enhancement (*arrows* in *B*). As opposed to cases of atherosclerosis, the aortic wall shows a general paucity of calcification.

coarctation (most common with resection and end-to-end anastomosis), aortic arch hypoplasia, aneurysm formation at the site of repair, restenosis, aortic dissection, and pseudoaneurysm formation (most common with balloon angioplasty).[85]

Pseudocoarctation should not be misdiagnosed as true aortic coarctation. In pseudocoarctation, the aortic arch is elongated and has a kinked appearance from fixation of the proximal descending aorta by the ligamentum arteriosum. Chest wall collaterals, fibrous ridge, and pressure gradient are absent. Over time, progressive dilation and aortic dissection may complicate pseudocoarctation (see **Fig. 6**).[86,87]

POSTPROCEDURAL EVALUATION OF THE AORTA
Evaluation after Repair of Aortic Dissection and Aneurysm

After surgical repair, patients require regular screening to exclude signs of impending aortic rupture or other complications, including endoleak, prosthetic graft degeneration, infection, malfunction of aortic valve prosthesis, and aneurysm formation in other portions of the aorta. Aortic rupture is usually preceded by rapid expansion. Therefore, early detection of aortic enlargement is imperative. Follow-up after thoracic endovascular repair is recommended at discharge, at 1, 3, and 6 months, and then yearly. Follow-up after surgical repair is recommended at discharge and then yearly but can be extended to 2 to 3 years if there is stability for the first year.[31,66] If a metachronous untreated aneurysm is present in an untreated segment of the aorta, aneurysm size should dictate the follow-up interval (ie, annually if 40–45 mm or semiannually if $\geq$45 mm and <55 mm [see **Table 2**]).[66,88] The normal postoperative appearance of the aorta includes a high-attenuation surgical pledget in the extraluminal space at the site of graft anastomosis and oversewn cannulation sites, which should not be confused for dehiscence or graft failure (**Fig. 18**).

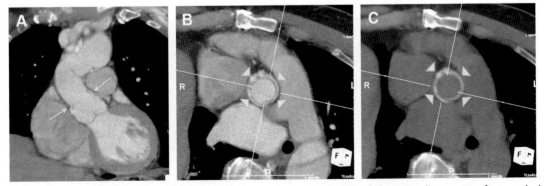

Fig. 18. (*A*) Contrast-enhanced coronal multi-planar reformation (MPR) of the ascending aorta after surgical replacement of the ascending aorta. There is high-density pledget material (*arrows*) at the surgical anastomosis. In distinction to contrast extravasation, the dense pledget material forms a complete ring around the aorta (*arrowheads*) as seen on short-axis MPR of the aorta (*B*) and is also present on corresponding noncontrast MPR images (*C*) (*arrowheads*).

Elephant Trunk and Staged Thoracic Aortic Repair

Aneurysms involving the distal aortic arch or proximal descending thoracic aorta with extension in the descending aorta present special challenges to the surgeon requiring both sternotomy and thoracotomy with long procedure times. These complex procedures can be performed contemporaneously but confer high morbidity, including increased blood loss and higher rates of cerebrovascular accident and spinal cord ischemia.[89,90] A staged procedure whereby the arch is repaired via sternotomy and the descending aortic repair is completed after a brief recovery period, usually approximately 6 weeks, results in decreased morbidity.[91] There are many variations on this approach depending on the anatomy pathology of each patient: if the ascending aorta or root are involved in the aneurysm, the surgical repair in the first stage will include these segments; if the distal aneurysm involves the thoracoabdominal aorta, the second stage repair will include these segments. Borst and colleagues[92] first developed the elephant trunk technique in 1983 to overcome the difficulty of performing the proximal graft-graft anastomosis of the second, descending thoracic, stage of repair. The elephant trunk refers to a distal segment of the aortic arch graft that projects into and floats freely in the descending aortic lumen (**Fig. 19**). During the second stage of repair, the elephant trunk is more easily accessible for end-end graft anastomosis in open repair or provides an ideal proximal landing zone in endovascular repair.[90] Endovascular stent grafting of the descending thoracic aorta with the proximal landing zone in the surgically placed elephant trunk graft constitutes hybrid elephant trunk repair. Familiarity

with the normal appearance of the elephant trunk graft after stage 1 repair is important. The appearance of contrast surrounding the free-floating portion of the graft should not be mistaken for dehiscence or graft failure. Although the elephant trunk is commonly imaged during reevaluation of the descending aortic aneurysm before completion of repair, 32% to 60% of patients do not undergo the second stage, usually secondary to comorbidities associated with the first surgery or refusal of additional surgery.[91,93] It is also common to observe significant enlargement of the descending thoracic aneurysm following elephant trunk repair; therefore, familiarity with the normal graft appearance and comparison with preoperative imaging is important.[90]

Elephant trunk repair is also used in the treatment of aortic dissection, although less commonly. In this setting, an incomplete repair may demonstrate the free-floating elephant trunk graft extending into the true lumen of a residual Stanford type B dissection.

PREPROCEDURAL EVALUATION FOR TRANSCATHETER AORTIC VALVE REPLACEMENT

Severe and symptomatic aortic stenosis is associated with high morbidity and mortality and often occurs in an aging population with comorbidities precluding the possibility of surgical valve replacement. In these patients, transcatheter aortic valve replacement (TAVR) can decrease mortality and hospitalization rates in the short-term.[94,95] CT angiography plays an important role in preprocedural selection and planning. Evaluation of the aortic annulus and thoracic aortic anatomy is key in the selection of appropriate prosthesis size

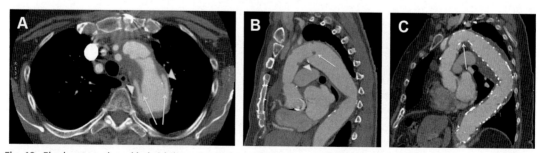

Fig. 19. Elephant trunk and hybrid thoracic aortic repair on contrast-enhanced CT. (*A*) Axial image and (*B*) sagittal oblique multi-planar reformation (MPR) of the aortic arch shows a tubular graft material extending into the descending aorta (*arrows*) with contrast extending between the graft (elephant trunk) and the native aortic wall (*arrowheads*). This appearance is the normal appearance after the first stage of elephant trunk repair. (*C*) Sagittal oblique MPR of the aorta following completion of the staged hybrid elephant trunk repair shows an endovascular graft with proximal attachment in the elephant trunk (*arrow*). The descending thoracic aneurysm no longer enhances with contrast.

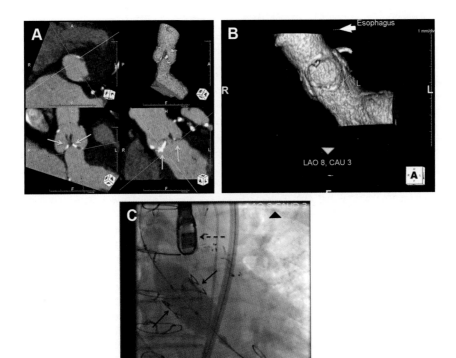

Fig. 20. Preoperative TAVR CT angiography study. (*A*) Multi-planar reformation of the aortic root from ECG-gated, contrast-enhanced CT. The annular area and circumference can be accurately measured in the double-oblique short-axis view (*upper left panel*). Measurement is performed during systole when the annulus is largest to avoid undersizing the prosthesis, which can result in para-valvular leak. Extensive thickening and calcification of the valve leaflets (*arrows*) with restricted opening are consistent with severe aortic stenosis. (*B*) Three-dimensional volume-rendered image of the aorta shows the true plane of the annulus where the nadir of each aortic cusp is aligned on a single plane. The cusps are marked *L* (left coronary cusp), *R* (right coronary cusp), and *N* (noncoronary cusp). Coordinates for the expected c-arm location during the procedure are displayed (*arrowhead*). The esophagus marker corresponds to the expected location of the transesophageal echocardiography probe that will be in place during the valve replacement procedure. This marker helps predict the optimal view of the valve without obscuration by the esophageal probe. (*C*) Intraoperative fluoroscopic image shows the valve (*arrows*) being deployed over a balloon. The c-arm coordinates (*arrowhead*) and esophageal probe (*dashed arrow*) match the CT image in (*B*). LAO, left anterior oblique; CAU, Caudal.

and identification of important prognostic and contraindicating features. An ECG-gated acquisition of the aortic root is required for evaluation of annular area and circumference, preferably during ventricular systole because the annular size varies through the cardiac cycle with the largest size in midsystole.[96–98] Annular measurement and evaluation are performed at the basal ring of the aortic root, defined by the lowest points of the 3 aortic valve leaflets (**Fig. 20**, Video 4). Other important features include annular calcification, which increases the risk of para-valvular leak; the degree of aortic valve calcification and coronary ostial height above the annulus, which predicts coronary obstruction at the time of procedure; presence of aortic or iliofemoral artery dissection, narrowing, tortuosity, mural thrombus, or ulcerated plaque, which may preclude catheter-based delivery of the prosthetic valve.[96,99]

SUMMARY

This article reviews the MDCT imaging appearance of common entities that are part of the wide spectrum of diseases involving the thoracic aorta. ECG-gated MDCT is poised to become the reference standard method in assessing the thoracic aorta. Reproducible images of the aorta can be acquired independent of operator skill.

SUPPLEMENTARY DATA

Supplementary data related to this article can be found online at http://dx.doi.org/10.1016/j.rcl. 2015.08.004.

REFERENCES

1. Kaatee R, Van Leeuwen MS, De Lange EE, et al. Spiral CT angiography of the renal arteries: should

a scan delay based on a test bolus injection or a fixed scan delay be used to obtain maximum enhancement of the vessels? J Comput Assist Tomogr 1998;22(4):541–7.

2. Van Hoe L, Baert AL, Gryspeerdt S, et al. Supra- and juxtarenal aneurysms of the abdominal aorta: preoperative assessment with thin-section spiral CT. Radiology 1996;198(2):443–8.

3. Armerding MD, Rubin GD, Beaulieu CF, et al. Aortic aneurysmal disease: assessment of stent-graft treatment—CT versus conventional angiography1. Radiology 2000;215(1):138–46.

4. Katz DS, Jorgensen MJ, Rubin GD. Detection and follow-up of important extra-arterial lesions with helical CT angiography. Clin Radiol 1999;54(5):294–300.

5. Rubin GD. MDCT imaging of the aorta and peripheral vessels. Eur J Radiol 2003;45:S42–9.

6. Lee AM, Engel L-C, Shah B, et al. Coronary computed tomography angiography during arrhythmia: radiation dose reduction with prospectively ECG-triggered axial and retrospectively ECG-gated helical 128-slice dual-source CT. J Cardiovasc Comput Tomogr 2012;6(3):172–83.e2.

7. Abbara S, Kalva S, Cury RC, et al. Thoracic aortic disease: spectrum of multidetector computed tomography imaging findings. J Cardiovasc Comput Tomogr 2007;1(1):40–54.

8. Mao SS, Ahmadi N, Shah B, et al. Normal thoracic aorta diameter on cardiac computed tomography in healthy asymptomatic adults: impact of age and gender. Acad Radiol 2008;15(7):827–34.

9. Berko NS, Jain VR, Godelman A, et al. Variants and anomalies of thoracic vasculature on computed tomographic angiography in adults. J Comput Assist Tomogr 2009;33(4):523–8.

10. Layton KF, Kallmes DF, Cloft HJ, et al. Bovine aortic arch variant in humans: clarification of a common misnomer. AJNR Am J Neuroradiol 2006;27(7):1541–2.

11. Murillo H, Lane MJ, Punn R, et al. Imaging of the aorta: embryology and anatomy. Seminars in ultrasound. Semin Ultrasound CT MR 2012;33(3):169–90.

12. Roos JE, Willmann JK, Weishaupt D, et al. Thoracic aorta: motion artifact reduction with retrospective and prospective electrocardiography-assisted multi–detector row CT1. Radiology 2002;222(1):271–7.

13. Mészáros I, Mórocz J, Szlávi J, et al. Epidemiology and clinicopathology of aortic dissection: a population-based longitudinal study over 27 years. Chest 2000;117(5):1271–8.

14. Isselbacher EM. Diseases of the aorta: aortic dissection. In: Braunwald's heart disease: a textbook of cardiovascular medicine. 7th edition. Philadelphia: Saunders; 2005.

15. Rojas CA, Restrepo CS. . Mediastinal hematomas: aortic injury and beyond. J Comput Assist Tomogr 2009;33(2):218–24.

16. DeSanctis RW, Doroghazi RM, Austen WG, et al. Aortic dissection. N Engl J Med 1987;317(17):1060–7.

17. Coady MA, Rizzo JA, Goldstein LJ, et al. Natural history, pathogenesis, and etiology of thoracic aortic aneurysms and dissections. Cardiol Clin 1999;17(4):615–35.

18. Hagan PG, Nienaber CA, Isselbacher EM, et al. The International Registry of Acute Aortic Dissection (IRAD): new insights into an old disease. JAMA 2000;283(7):897–903.

19. Moore AG, Eagle KA, Bruckman D, et al. Choice of computed tomography, transesophageal echocardiography, magnetic resonance imaging, and aortography in acute aortic dissection: International Registry of Acute Aortic Dissection (IRAD). Am J Cardiol 2002;89(10):1235–8.

20. Cigarroa JE, Isselbacher EM, DeSanctis RW, et al. Diagnostic imaging in the evaluation of suspected aortic dissection. Old standards and new directions. N Engl J Med 1993;328(1):35–43.

21. Nienaber CA, Kodolitsch von Y, Nicolas V, et al. The diagnosis of thoracic aortic dissection by noninvasive imaging procedures. N Engl J Med 1993;328(1):1–9.

22. Bansal RC, Chandrasekaran K, Ayala K, et al. Frequency and explanation of false negative diagnosis of aortic dissection by aortography and transesophageal echocardiography. J Am Coll Cardiol 1995;25(6):1393–401.

23. Mammen L, Yucel EK, Khan A. Expert panel on cardiac imaging. Criteria® acute chest pain. 2008.

24. Morgan-Hughes GJ, Marshall AJ, Roobottom CA. Refined computed tomography of the thoracic aorta: the impact of electrocardiographic assistance. Clin Radiol 2003;58(8):581–8.

25. Greenberg RK, Secor JL, Painter T. Computed tomography assessment of thoracic aortic pathology. Semin Vasc Surg 2004;17(2):166–72.

26. Batra P, Bigoni B, Manning J, et al. Pitfalls in the diagnosis of thoracic aortic dissection at CT angiography. Radiographics 2000;20(2):309–20.

27. LePage MA, Quint LE, Sonnad SS, et al. Aortic dissection: CT features that distinguish true lumen from false lumen. Am J Roentgenol.

28. Williams MP, Farrow R. Atypical patterns in the CT diagnosis of aortic dissection. Clin Radiol 1994;49(10):686–9.

29. Nelsen KM, Spizarny DL, Kastan DJ. Intimointimal intussusception in aortic dissection: CT diagnosis. AJR Am J Roentgenol 1994;162(4):813–4.

30. Fan ZM, Zhang ZQ, Ma XH, et al. Acute aortic dissection with intimal intussusception: MRI appearances. Am J Roentgenol 2006;186(3):841–3.

31. Hiratzka LF, Bakris GL, Beckman JA, et al. 2010 ACCF/AHA/AATS/ACR/ASA/SCA/SCAI/SIR/STS/SVM guidelines for the diagnosis and management of patients with thoracic aortic disease n.d.Circulation 2010;121: e266–e369.

32. Fattori R, Bertaccini P, Celletti F, et al. Intramural posttraumatic hematoma of the ascending aorta in a patient with a double aortic arch. Eur Radiol 1997;7(1):51–3.

33. Nienaber CA, Kodolitsch von Y, Petersen B, et al. Intramural hemorrhage of the thoracic aorta. Diagnostic and therapeutic implications. Circulation 1995;92(6):1465–72.

34. von Kodolitsch Y, Nienaber CA. Intramural hemorrhage of the thoracic aorta: diagnosis, therapy and prognosis of 209 in vivo diagnosed cases. Z Kardiol 1998;87(10):797–807.

35. Kaji S, Nishigami K, Akasaka T, et al. Prediction of progression or regression of type A aortic intramural hematoma by computed tomography. Circulation 1999;100(Suppl 19):II281–6.

36. Quint LE, Williams DM, Francis IR, et al. Ulcerlike lesions of the aorta: imaging features and natural history. Radiology 2001;218(3):719–23.

37. Hayashi H, Matsuoka Y, Sakamoto I, et al. Penetrating atherosclerotic ulcer of the aorta: imaging features and disease concept. Radiographics 2000;20(4):995–1005.

38. Kazerooni EA, Bree RL, Williams DM. Penetrating atherosclerotic ulcers of the descending thoracic aorta: evaluation with CT and distinction from aortic dissection. Radiology 1992;183(3):759–65.

39. Stanson AW, Kazmier FJ, Hollier LH, et al. Penetrating atherosclerotic ulcers of the thoracic aorta: natural history and clinicopathologic correlations. Ann Vasc Surg 1986;1(1):15–23.

40. Feczko JD, Lynch L, Pless JE, et al. An autopsy case review of 142 nonpenetrating (blunt) injuries of the aorta. J Trauma 1992;33(6):846–9.

41. Burkhart HM, Gomez GA, Jacobson LE, et al. Fatal blunt aortic injuries: a review of 242 autopsy cases. J Trauma 2001;50(1):113–5.

42. Steenburg SD, Ravenel JG, Ikonomidis JS, et al. Acute traumatic aortic injury: imaging evaluation and management. Radiology 2008;248(3):748–62.

43. Johnston KW, Rutherford RB, Tilson MD, et al. Suggested standards for reporting on arterial aneurysms. Subcommittee on Reporting Standards for Arterial Aneurysms, Ad Hoc Committee on Reporting Standards, Society for Vascular Surgery and North American Chapter, International Society for Cardiovascular Surgery. J Vasc Surg 1991;13(3): 452–8.

44. Clouse WD, Hallett JW, Schaff HV, et al. Improved prognosis of thoracic aortic aneurysms: a population-based study. JAMA 1998;280(22): 1926–9.

45. Crawford ES, Cohen ES. Aortic aneurysm: a multifocal disease. Presidential address. Arch Surg 1982;117(11):1393–400.

46. Isselbacher EM. Thoracic and abdominal aortic aneurysms. Circulation 2005;111(6):816–28.

47. Quint LE, Francis IR, Williams DM, et al. Evaluation of thoracic aortic disease with the use of helical CT and multiplanar reconstructions: comparison with surgical findings. Radiology 1996;201(1):37–41.

48. Svensson LG, Crawford ES, Hess KR, et al. Experience with 1509 patients undergoing thoracoabdominal aortic operations. J Vasc 1993; 17(2):357–68.

49. Bonser RS, Pagano D, Lewis ME, et al. Clinical and patho-anatomical factors affecting expansion of thoracic aortic aneurysms. Heart 2000;84(3): 277–83.

50. Dapunt OE, Galla JD, Sadeghi AM, et al. The natural history of thoracic aortic aneurysms. J Thorac Cardiovasc Surg 1994;107(5):1323–32 [discussion: 1332–3].

51. Kuzmik GA, Sang AX, Elefteriades JA. Natural history of thoracic aortic aneurysms. J Vasc Surg 2012;56(2):565–71.

52. Detaint D, Michelena HI, Nkomo VT, et al. Aortic dilatation patterns and rates in adults with bicuspid aortic valves: a comparative study with Marfan syndrome and degenerative aortopathy. Heart 2014; 100(2):126–34.

53. Davies RR, Goldstein LJ, Coady MA, et al. Yearly rupture or dissection rates for thoracic aortic aneurysms: simple prediction based on size. Ann Thorac Surg 2002;73(1):17–27.

54. Adams JN, Trent RJ. Aortic complications of Marfan's syndrome. Lancet 1998;352(9142): 1722–3.

55. Nistri S, Sorbo MD, Marin M, et al. Aortic root dilatation in young men with normally functioning bicuspid aortic valves. Heart 1999;82(1):19–22.

56. Kodolitsch von Y, Aydin MA, Koschyk DH, et al. Predictors of aneurysmal formation after surgical correction of aortic coarctation. J Am Coll Cardiol 2002;39(4):617–24.

57. Coady MA, Davies RR, Roberts M. Familial patterns of thoracic aortic aneurysms. Arch Surg 1999;134(4):361–7.

58. Nuenninghoff DM, Hunder GG, Christianson TJ, et al. Incidence and predictors of large-artery complication (aortic aneurysm, aortic dissection, and/or large-artery stenosis) in patients with giant cell arteritis: a population-based study over 50 years. Arthritis Rheum 2003;48(12):3522–31.

59. Coady MA, Rizzo JA, Hammond GL, et al. Surgical intervention criteria for thoracic aortic aneurysms: a study of growth rates and complications. Ann Thorac Surg 1999;67(6):1922–6 [discussion: 1953–8].

60. Svensson LG, Kouchoukos NT, Miller DC, et al. Expert consensus document on the treatment of descending thoracic aortic disease using endovascular stent-grafts. Ann Thorac Surg 2008; 85(1):S1–41.
61. Kouchoukos NT, Dougenis D. Surgery of the thoracic aorta. N Engl J Med 1997;336(26): 1876–89.
62. Elefteriades JA. Natural history of thoracic aortic aneurysms: indications for surgery, and surgical versus nonsurgical risks. Ann Thorac Surg 2002; 74(5):S1877–80.
63. Vallely MP, Semsarian C, Bannon PG. Management of the ascending aorta in patients with bicuspid aortic valve disease. Heart Lung Circ 2008;17(5): 357–63.
64. Jondeau G, Detaint D, Tubach F, et al. Aortic event rate in the marfan population: a cohort study. Circulation 2012;125(2):226–32.
65. Attias D, Stheneur C, Roy C, et al. Comparison of clinical presentations and outcomes between patients with TGFBR2 and FBN1 mutations in Marfan syndrome and related disorders. Circulation 2009; 120(25):2541–9.
66. Erbel R, Aboyans V, Boileau C, et al. 2014 ESC Guidelines on the diagnosis and treatment of aortic diseases: document covering acute and chronic aortic diseases of the thoracic and abdominal aorta of the adult. The task force for the diagnosis and treatment of aortic diseases of the European Society of Cardiology (ESC). Eur Heart J 2014; 35(41):2873–926.
67. Davies RR, Gallo A, Coady MA, et al. Novel measurement of relative aortic size predicts rupture of thoracic aortic aneurysms. Ann Thorac Surg 2006;81(1):169–77.
68. Lobato AC, Puech-Leao P. Predictive factors for rupture of thoracoabdominal aortic aneurysm. J Vasc Surg 1998;27(3):446–53.
69. Gott VL, Pyeritz RE, Magovern GJ Jr, et al. Surgical treatment of aneurysms of the ascending aorta in the Marfan syndrome. Results of composite-graft repair in 50 patients. N Engl J Med 1986;314(17): 1070–4.
70. American College of Cardiology/American Heart Association Task Force on Practice Guidelines, Society of Cardiovascular Anesthesiologists, Society for Cardiovascular Angiography and Interventions, et al. ACC/AHA 2006 guidelines for the management of patients with valvular heart disease: a report of the American College of Cardiology/American Heart Association Task Force on Practice Guidelines (writing committee to revise the 1998 guidelines for the management of patients with valvular heart disease): developed in collaboration with the Society of Cardiovascular Anesthesiologists: endorsed by the Society for Cardiovascular Angiography and Interventions and the Society of Thoracic Surgeons. Circulation 2006;114(5):e84–231.
71. Meier JH, Seward JB, Miller FA, et al. Aneurysms in the left ventricular outflow tract: clinical presentation, causes, and echocardiographic features. J Am Soc Echocardiogr 1998;11(7):729–45.
72. Takach TJ, Reul GJ, Duncan JM, et al. Sinus of Valsalva aneurysm or fistula: management and outcome. Ann Thorac Surg 1999;68(5):1573–7.
73. GDSJ Webb, Therrier J. Congenital heart disease. In: Braunwald E, Zipes DP, Libby PL, et al, editors. Braunwalds heart disease. 7th edition. Philadelphia: Elsevier Health Sciences; 2005. p. 1535–6.
74. Brickner ME, Hillis LD, Lange RA. Congenital heart disease in adults. N Engl J Med 2000; 342(4):256–63.
75. Watson AB. Spinal subarachnoid haemorrhage in patient with coarctation of aorta. Br Med J 1967; 4(5574):278–9.
76. Nihoyannopoulos P, Karas S, Sapsford RN, et al. Accuracy of two-dimensional echocardiography in the diagnosis of aortic arch obstruction. J Am Coll Cardiol 1987;10(5):1072–7.
77. Levine JC, Sanders SP, Colan SD, et al. The risk of having additional obstructive lesions in neonatal coarctation of the aorta. Cardiol Young 2001; 11(1):44–53.
78. Hodes HL, Steinfeld L, Blumenthal S. Congenital cerebral aneurysms and coarctation of the aorta. Arch Pediatr 1959;76(1):28–43.
79. Pagni S, Denatale RW, Boltax RS. Takayasu's arteritis: the middle aortic syndrome. Am Surg 1996; 62(5):409–12.
80. Maksimowicz-McKinnon K, Hoffman GS. Takayasu arteritis: what is the long-term prognosis? Rheum Dis Clin North Am 2007;33(4):777–86.
81. Attenhofer Jost CH, Schaff HV, Connolly HM, et al. Spectrum of reoperations after repair of aortic coarctation: importance of an individualized approach because of coexistent cardiovascular disease. Mayo Clin Proc 2002;77(7):646–53.
82. Parikh SR, Hurwitz RA, Hubbard JE, et al. Preoperative and postoperative "aneurysm" associated with coarctation of the aorta. J Am Coll Cardiol 1991;17(6):1367–72.
83. Fawzy ME, Awad M, Hassan W, et al. Long-term outcome (up to 15 years) of balloon angioplasty of discrete native coarctation of the aorta in adolescents and adults. J Am Coll Cardiol 2004;43(6): 1062–7.
84. Hellenbrand WE, Allen HD, Golinko RJ, et al. Balloon angioplasty for aortic recoarctation: results of Valvuloplasty and Angioplasty of Congenital Anomalies Registry. Am J Cardiol 1990;65(11):793–7.
85. Therrien J, Thorne SA, Wright A, et al. Repaired coarctation: a "cost-effective" approach to identify

complications in adults. J Am Coll Cardiol 2000; 35(4):997–1002.

86. Safir J, Kerr A, Morehouse H, et al. Magnetic resonance imaging of dissection in pseudocoarctation of the aorta. Cardiovasc Intervent Radiol 1993; 6(3):180–2.

87. Sebastià C, Quiroga S, Boyé R, et al. Aortic stenosis: spectrum of diseases depicted at multisection CT 1. Radiographics 2003;23(Spec No):S79–91.

88. Heinemann M, Laas J, Karck M, et al. Thoracic aortic aneurysms after acute type A aortic dissection: necessity for follow-up. Ann Thorac Surg 1990;49(4):580–4.

89. Massimo CG, Perna AM, Cruz Quadron EA, et al. Extended and total simultaneous aortic replacement: latest technical modifications and improved results with thirty-four patients. J Card Surg 1997; 12(4):261–9.

90. Castrovinci S, Murana G, de Maat GE, et al. The classic elephant trunk technique for staged thoracic and thoracoabdominal aortic repair: long-term results. J Thorac Cardiovasc Surg 2015;149(2):416–22.

91. Safi HJ, Miller CC, Estrera AL, et al. Optimization of aortic arch replacement: two-stage approach. Ann Thorac Surg 2007;83(2):S815–8 [discussion: S824–31].

92. Borst HG, Walterbusch G, Schaps D. Extensive aortic replacement using "elephant trunk" prosthesis. Thorac Cardiovasc Surg 1983;31(1):37–40.

93. Di Bartolomeo R, Pacini D, Savini C, et al. Complex thoracic aortic disease: single-stage procedure with the frozen elephant trunk technique. J Thorac Cardiovasc Surg 2010;140(Suppl 6): S81–5 [discussion: S86–91].

94. Leon MB, Smith CR, Mack M, et al. Transcatheter aortic-valve implantation for aortic stenosis in patients who cannot undergo surgery. N Engl J Med 2010;363(17):1597–607.

95. Makkar RR, Fontana GP, Jilaihawi H, et al. Transcatheter aortic-valve replacement for inoperable severe aortic stenosis. N Engl J Med 2012; 366(18):1696–704.

96. Achenbach S, Delgado V, Hausleiter J, et al. SCCT expert consensus document on computed tomography imaging before transcatheter aortic valve implantation (TAVI)/transcatheter aortic valve replacement (TAVR). J Cardiovasc Comput Tomogr 2012;6(6):366–80.

97. Leipsic J, Gurvitch R, LaBounty TM, et al. Multidetector computed tomography in transcatheter aortic valve implantation. JACC Cardiovasc Imaging 2011;4(4):416–29.

98. Bloomfield GS, Gillam LD, Hahn RT, et al. A practical guide to multimodality imaging of transcatheter aortic valve replacement. JACC Cardiovasc Imaging 2012;5(4):441–55.

99. Willson AB, Webb JG, LaBounty TM, et al. 3-Dimensional aortic annular assessment by multidetector computed tomography predicts moderate or severe paravalvular regurgitation after transcatheter aortic valve replacement: a multicenter retrospective analysis. J Am Coll Cardiol 2012; 59(14):1287–94.

100. Lu T, Huber CH, Rizzo E, et al. Ascending aorta measurements as assessed by ECG-gated multidetector computed tomography: a pilot study to establish normative values for transcatheter therapies. Eur Radiol 2009;19(3):664–9.

101. Lin FY, Devereux RB, Roman MJ, et al. Assessment of the thoracic aorta by multidetector computed tomography: age-and sex-specific reference values in adults without evident cardiovascular disease. J Cardiovasc Comput Tomogr 2008;2(5):298–308.

102. Tops LF, Wood DA, Delgado V, et al. Noninvasive evaluation of the aortic root with multislice computed tomography: implications for transcatheter aortic valve replacement. J Am Coll Cardiol Img 2008;1(3):321–30.

103. Ocak I, Lacomis JM, Deible CR, et al. The aortic root: comparison of measurements from ECG-gated CT angiography with transthoracic echocardiography. J Thorac Imaging 2009;24(3):223–6.

104. Hiratzka LF, Bakris GL, Beckman JA, et al. ACCF/ AHA/AATS/ACR/ASA/SCA/SCAI/SIR/STS/SVM guidelines for the diagnosis and management of patients with thoracic aortic disease: a report of the American College of Cardiology Foundation/American Heart Association Task Force on Practice Guidelines, American Association for Thoracic Surgery, American College of Radiology, American Stroke Association, Society of Cardiovascular Anesthesiologists, Society for Cardiovascular Angiography and Interventions, Society of Interventional Radiology, Society of Thoracic Surgeons, and Society for Vascular Medicine. Circulation 2010; 121(13):e266–369.

Computed Tomographic Angiography of the Abdominal Aorta

Neil J. Hansen, MD

KEYWORDS

- Computed tomographic angiography • Aorta • Aneurysm • Aortitis • Abdominal aortic aneurysm
- Aortic dissection

KEY POINTS

- CT angiography has become the preferred imaging method for planning aortic aneurysm repair, monitoring complications, and routine follow-up.
- CT angiography is widely available, using thin slice isotropic imaging, rapid bolus contrast injection, and fast multidetector CT technology.
- Acute aortic syndromes, aortitis/inflammatory vasculitides, and chronic atherosclerotic changes have characteristic CT angiographic manifestations that allow radiologists to provide accurate diagnoses and guide management.
- In development are new CT angiographic techniques that will enable aortic evaluation with lower contrast and radiation doses.

INTRODUCTION

Computed tomographic angiography (CTA) of the abdominal aorta has replaced angiography as the initial imaging test of choice for acute aortic disease, occlusive atherosclerotic disease, inflammatory vasculitis workups, and preintervention/postintervention imaging of abdominal aortic aneurysms (AAA) at most centers. For many years after its arrival in 1971, CT was too slow for optimal imaging of the cardiovascular system. With the introduction of slip ring technology and the change from single to multiple detector CT (MDCT), the temporal capabilities of CT became adequate for assessing the vascular system.[1] With the widespread availability of state-of-the-art multidetector technology, CT can provide submillimeter resolution along the z-axis, allowing for isotropic volumetric data sets. This technology offers exquisite detailed anatomic information that guides operative procedures for AAA. In addition, it rapidly dictates patient management in the acute and chronic settings for most aortic diseases. In this article, basic abdominal aortic anatomy is reviewed, technical aspects of CTA image acquisition and the latest advances in technology are outlined, and diagnoses of various acute and chronic aortic diseases in the abdomen are discussed.

ANATOMY

Normal Anatomy

The abdominal aorta begins at the level of the diaphragmatic hiatus, which is usually at approximately the T12 vertebral body level (Fig. 1). The abdominal aorta gives off several major and minor branches in the anterior, lateral, and posterior directions before it terminates at the L4 vertebral body level into bilateral common iliac arteries (CIAs). Unpaired anterior branches supply the gastrointestinal tract; the celiac axis (CA), superior mesenteric artery (SMA), and the inferior

Disclosure Statement: The author and his immediate family members have no relevant financial disclosures.
Department of Radiology, University of Nebraska Medical Center, 981045 Nebraska Medical Center, Omaha, NE 68198-1045, USA
E-mail address: njhansen@unmc.edu

Radiol Clin N Am 54 (2016) 35–54
http://dx.doi.org/10.1016/j.rcl.2015.08.005

radiologic.theclinics.com

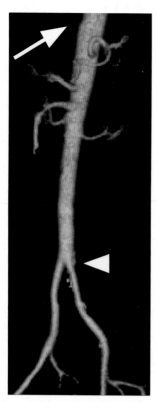

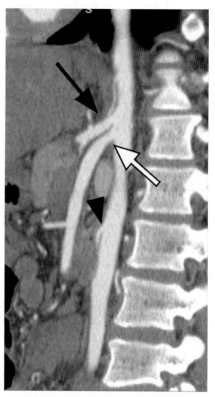

Fig. 1. Oblique coronal three-dimensional volume-rendered image of the abdominal aorta in a normal 19-year-old man. The abdominal aorta originates at the diaphragmatic hiatus (T12 level [*arrow*]) and extends until the bifurcation into the CIAs (*arrowhead*).

Fig. 2. Sagittal CTA image of the abdominal aorta well shows the origins of the CA (*black arrow*), SMA (*white arrow*), and IMA (*black arrowhead*).

mesenteric artery (IMA) are often best visualized in the sagittal plane (**Fig. 2**). Paired arteries in the lateral plane arise off the aorta to supply the genitourinary and endocrine organs: the renal, adrenal, and gonadal (ovarian or testicular) arteries (**Fig. 3**), often best seen in the coronal plane. In the posterior plane, paired inferior phrenic and lumbar arteries arise from the aorta to supply the diaphragm and body wall musculature (**Fig. 4**). The artery of Adamkiewicz provides collateral supply to the lower spinal cord, arising variably from a lumbar artery or a posterior intercostal artery near the level of the thoracolumbar junction.[2] The middle sacral artery is an unpaired posterior branch of the aorta near the bifurcation that supplies the rectum.

The paired CIAs arise from the aortic bifurcation to then bifurcate at the pelvic brim into the external iliac artery (EIA) and internal iliac artery (IIA, also called hypogastric artery). The EIAs then supply the lower extremities, whereas the IIA bifurcates into anterior and posterior divisions (**Fig. 5**). Anterior division branches include obturator, inferior gluteal, umbilical, uterine and vaginal (females),

inferior vesicular, internal pudendal, and middle rectal arteries. Posterior division branches include iliolumbar, lateral sacral, and superior gluteal branches. Anatomic variations of these divisions are common, and numerous classification schemes are used for interventional purposes.[3]

Variant Anatomy

Anatomic variation of the visceral branches arising off the aorta is commonly encountered. The most common branching variant is that of accessory renal arteries, with many patients having 3 or more renal arteries arising off the aorta (**Fig. 6**). CTA has proved to have excellent correlation with surgical findings in the evaluation of variant renal arterial supply in the renal donor population.[4] Similarly, the branching pattern of the CA frequently shows variation (**Fig. 7**).[5–7] The most common variants involve the hepatic arteries, with the right hepatic artery being replaced off the SMA in up to 17.7% of individuals and the left hepatic artery arising off the left gastric artery in up to 5.5% of people.[5,7] With

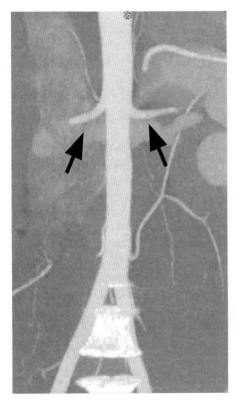

Fig. 3. Oblique coronal maximum intensity projection image of the abdominal aorta shows paired single bilateral renal arteries (*arrows*).

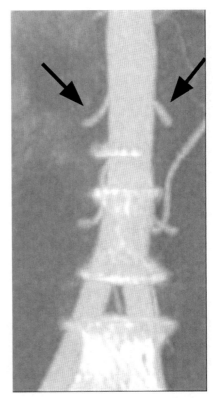

Fig. 4. Oblique coronal maximum intensity projection image showing paired lumbar arteries (*arrows*) arising off the aorta posteriorly.

increasing use of transarterial chemoembolization procedures for hepatocellular carcinoma and liver metastases, these variants can be clinically significant to the angiographer. More rare aortic branching variants include a common trunk of the CA and the SMA, and a persistent sciatic artery that is a vestigial artery coursing along the sciatic nerve, replacing the ipsilateral common and EIAs and exiting the pelvis through the sciatic notch.[7,8] All of these variants are easily detected at CTA.

IMAGE ACQUISITION TECHNIQUE AND POSTPROCESSING

Before image interpretation, it is essential to optimize technical factors to obtain adequate arterial phase images for accurate diagnosis (**Table 1**). The history, evolution, and current technical standards of aorta CTA have been thoroughly outlined in numerous articles.[1,9–12] Critical parameters include scanner setup, contrast injection technique, and specific prescribed protocol for the imaging task at hand. Postprocessing can be essential for surgical colleagues, and as is always the case with CT, patient dose/radiation exposure deserves special mention.

Scanner Setup

MDCT is widely available at large tertiary medical centers as well as small community hospitals and outpatient clinics. State-of-the-art CTA is performed on MDCT. A minimum of 16 detector rows provides adequate temporal capability, with a preference for 64 detector rows or greater. MDCT allows for rapid data acquisition with isotropic or near isotropic voxels, which are necessary for generating adequate three-dimensional (3D) and multiplanar reformations.[13,14] Pixel spacing for modern CTA is submillimeter (0.5–0.75 mm) with a typically used slice thickness of around 1 mm depending on scanner type/manufacturer. Images are routinely reconstructed at a thicker slice thickness (3–5 mm) to decrease noise for optimal clinical evaluation of parenchymal organs. Many current setups use low pitch values (near to or <1) for sufficient sampling/overlap, although newer scanners and dual source technology allow for adequate higher pitch use with associated radiation dose reduction.[15–17] Typically used kVp settings for abdominal CTA range from 100 to 120 kVp. Many centers prescribe energy levels to optimize imaging based on patient body habitus, with lower kVp (eg, 80–100)

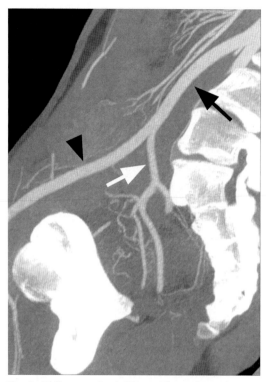

Fig. 5. Oblique sagittal CTA maximum intensity projection image of the right pelvis showing the iliac vasculature. The right CIA (*black arrow*) bifurcates into the EIA (*black arrowhead*) and the IIA (*white arrow*). The IIA can then be seen to bifurcate into its anterior and posterior divisions.

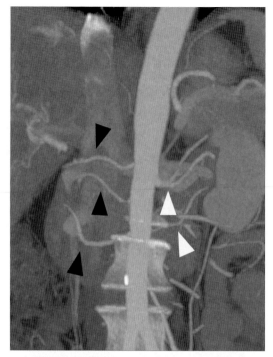

Fig. 6. Oblique coronal CTA maximum intensity projection image shows anatomic variant branching of the renal arterial system. Three right renal arteries supply the right kidney (*black arrowheads*), whereas 2 left renal arteries are present (*white arrowheads*). The upper left renal artery bifurcates shortly after its origin.

for patients with a lower body mass index (BMI, calculated as weight in kilograms divided by the square of height in meters), reserving higher kVps (eg, 120) for obese (BMI >30) and morbidly obese patients, respectively. Automatic tube current modulation is a standard feature of modern CT systems.

Contrast Injection Technique

The general principles of abdominal aorta CTA are to deliver the optimal amount of iodine in a concentrated uniform manner with subsequent imaging during the time of peak aortic enhancement. Ideally, CTA should provide aortic opacification greater than the 250-HU range at minimum, with greater than 300 HU uniformly being ideal.[9] How individual institutions achieve this goal is highly variable, but in general, fast injection rates and high concentrations of iodine are ubiquitous. A total of 60 to 140 mL of nonionic iodinated contrast is injected at a rate of 4 to 6 mL/s. This high injection rate necessitates a power injector, preferably with an 18-gauge intravenous (IV) line, usually in the antecubital fossa. Power injection

compatible central venous access devices are also acceptable. Many institutions opt for a standardized approach that is generally acceptable for a wide patient population (eg, 100 mL of 370 mg iodine/mL contrast media at 4 mL/s); however, given the extreme variations in patient body habitus encountered in daily practice in addition to variable cardiac output, a more tailored approach may be beneficial. Many institutions tailor examinations based on body habitus, gradually increasing the injected volume (72–100 mL+) and flow rate velocity (4–6 mL/s) based on patient size.[10,18–21] Contrast injection is commonly followed by a 20-mL to 30-mL saline flush to further increase arterial opacification and decrease concentration of contrast present in the ipsilateral central venous system.

Postcontrast imaging is generally timed by 1 of 2 methods: either automatic scan triggering by bolus tracking software (**Fig. 8**) or the use of a test bolus.[9,10,22–24] Bolus tracking software in general places a region of interest (ROI) in the aorta at a specific level (commonly the CA in abdominal CTA) and then acquires a series of low-dose scans at this level during the initial contrast administration. Once an arbitrary threshold is reached

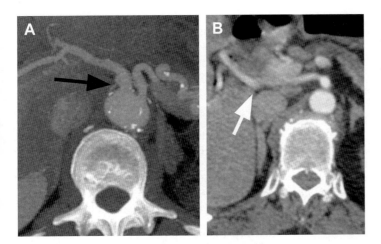

Fig. 7. Axial CTA maximum intensity projection image (A) shows anatomic variant branching of the CA, with a separate origin of the hepatic artery and splenic artery off the aorta (black arrow). In a different patient, another common anatomic variant is present (B), with replacement of the right hepatic artery off the SMA (white arrow) on this axial CTA.

Table 1		
Key technical parameters for CTA image acquisition		
Scanner	Minimum of 16 detector rows, preferably 64+	
Slice thickness	~1 mm	
Reconstructions	3–5 mm in axial, coronal, sagittal planes	
Pitch	~1	
kVp	100–120 kVp typically	
Contrast dose and delivery	60–140 mL of iodine contrast agent with 300–370 mg iodine/mL concentration, power injected at 4–6 mL/min followed by saline flush	
Arterial phase timing	Ideally performed with either bolus tracking software or a test bolus because of patient variability	

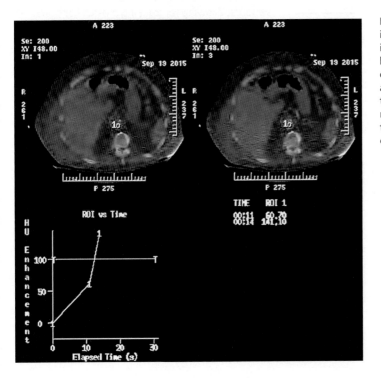

Fig. 8. Image obtained from abdominal CTA where arterial phase imaging was accomplished via SmartPrep bolus tracking software. A region of interest (ROI) is placed into the abdominal aorta, and during the contrast injection, density/HU measurements are taken. Once a threshold is reached (150 HU in this case), then, the scan is triggered.

(commonly 100–150 HU), then, the scan is triggered after a set delay. Given the rapid imaging speed of modern MDCT systems, most setups necessitate a built-in delay of 2 to 10 seconds or more depending on scanner type, table speed, pitch, and so forth. Benefits of bolus tracking include a decrease in the overall contrast needed and no opacification of parenchymal organs from a test bolus.[10] In distinction, a test bolus uses a small contrast injection (15–20 mL) followed by obtaining a limited low-dose dynamic set of images over the ROI (aorta). Using HU information obtained, the contrast media transit time can be calculated. This method is a robust way to account for differences in individual transit times (highly individually variable, especially in vasculopaths with poor cardiac output). The main limitations to a test bolus are the need for additional contrast administration and the additional time needed to perform this.

Much of the current investigative work in CTA is being performed to achieve acceptable images with the use of lower contrast volumes (usually for renal protective purposes). Numerous techniques are being investigated, including preferential iodine attenuation by use of fast MDCT scanners with lower tube voltages (eg, 70–100 kVp)[25,26] and the use of dual energy and iterative reconstruction techniques for enhanced iodine conspicuity.[27–32]

Abdominal Aorta Computed Tomographic Angiography Protocols

Single arterial phase studies are generally sufficient for preoperative planning (either open or endograft AAA repair). When there is clinical suspicion of acute abdominal aortic disease (eg, acute abdominal pain), a noncontrast series is necessary to evaluate for intramural hematoma (IMH), which can be difficult to diagnose on arterial phase imaging alone. If there is a history of previous endograft

AAA repair, a noncontrast series is also useful to evaluate calcifications and postoperative material, which can simulate endoleak (**Fig. 9**). In addition, most institutions obtain a delayed set of postcontrast images (90–120 s delay) in the setting of previous endograft repair to assess for endoleak. If there is a need for imaging in the setting of suspected AAA rupture, noncontrast CT may be sufficient for diagnosis before immediate operative intervention. Historically, there has not been a need for contrast-enhanced imaging in this setting, although some surgeons advocate for arterial phase imaging as a result of increasing use of endograft repair in the acute setting.

Postprocessing

The most commonly used postprocessing tools are summarized in **Table 2**. CTA lends itself to several postprocessing methods related to its inherent intraluminal high-attenuation material. Isotropic imaging allows for generation of multiplanar reformatted (MPR) images, which are obliquely angled two-dimensional images created from a 3D data set (**Fig. 10**). A double oblique technique allows for accurate delineation of cross-sectional measurements in tortuous vessels, and curved planar reformats (CPRs) allow for a tortuous atherosclerotic aorta to be shown on 1 image in a contiguous fashion. This technique assists the surgeon in planning complex repairs, such as endovascular aortic aneurysm repair.[33] Centerline analysis is available from numerous commercial vendors, allowing for tracking a vessel or branches along an automated or semiautomated central axis (**Fig. 11**). Similar to MPR, this technology allows for visualization of tortuous vessels on a single image and provides more accurate determination of cross-sectional diameter. These postprocessing techniques have been associated with decreased interobserver variation in terms of aneurysm measurement and preprocedural

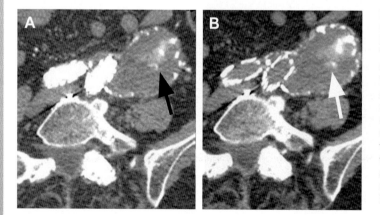

Fig. 9. Axial CT images in a 60-year-old man, status after previous aortobiliac endograft repair of aneurysm. The arterial phase images (*A*) showed focal high-density material in the excluded aneurysm sac (*black arrow*). This material could be an endoleak or could just be partially calcified thrombus. Noncontrast images (*B*) are beneficial in this situation (*white arrow*), because the finding was present before contrast administration and is therefore merely calcified thrombus. No endoleak was present.

Table 2 Commonly used CTA postprocessing techniques	
Technique	**Advantages**
Multiplanar reformats/ double obliques	More accurate diameter measurement for tortuous and unwound aortas
Centerline analysis and CPRs	Less interreader variation in stenotic severity assessment
Volume rendering	Big picture display of complex aneurysms requiring hybrid or staged repairs
Maximum projection intensity	Preferential display of high-density voxels for optimal evaluation of small vessels

planning.[34,35] Both techniques may be limited if there are complex aortic dissections or large amounts of intraluminal thrombus.

Volume-rendered (VR) CTA images are created by software programs that make 3D image renderings by using predetermined density threshold values to preferentially show intraluminal contrast and higher density material such as stent grafts (**Fig. 12**A). Automatic features such as bone subtraction are widely available. These images assist in visualizing complex diseases and postoperative anatomy. They are also useful for patient education, because these 3D images tend to be easier for nonmedical personnel to understand. Maximum intensity projection (MIP) images represent preferential display of only the highest-density voxels from a data set onto a predefined single image plane (see **Fig. 12**B). These images can be created at variable slice thickness and are useful for evaluating high-density material like stent grafts, calcifications, and contrast.

Computed Tomographic Angiography Radiation Dose Considerations

Given the attention directed toward iatrogenic medical radiation exposure in both the medical literature and the lay press, it is understandable that much of the recent work for abdominal aortic CTA, and CT in general, has been directed toward dose reduction (**Table 3**). In general, many of the new techniques for radiation dose reduction are the same as those used to reduce iodine load. Much recent investigation has focused on the use of low kVp to reduce dose.[17,25,30,36,37] In addition, the use of a dual energy CT technique to improve iodine visualization or create virtual non-contrast images to eliminate the need for multiphasic studies is also being investigated.[38–42] Most of the improvements in the near future for CTA dose reduction will come from technological advancements in image reconstruction. Improved computational abilities have allowed partial and full iterative reconstructive techniques to enable dose reductions of more than 70%.[17,41,43–45]

PATHOLOGIC CONDITIONS OF THE ABDOMINAL AORTA
Abdominal Aortic Aneurysm

Clinical presentation and pathophysiology

- Primary risk factors for AAA development include age, smoking, family history, and atherosclerotic vascular disease. AAA has negative associations with female gender, African American race, and diabetes.[46]
- Most nonruptured aneurysms are not symptomatic and are frequently diagnosed by screening programs.[47] Variably, nonspecific symptoms such as back pain, constipation, and abdominal pain have been ascribed to AAA.
- Ruptured AAA tends to present as acute abdominal pain, hypotension, and a pulsatile abdominal mass. Rupture has high mortality

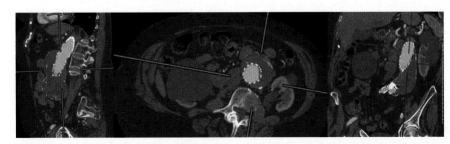

Fig. 10. Three images show the use of double oblique MPR to evaluate the abdominal aorta. Especially in tortuous atherosclerotic aortas, double oblique manipulation can provide more accurate measurements than a true axial plane.

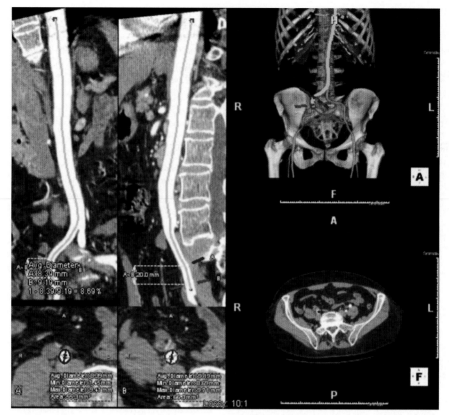

Fig. 11. Representative image of aortic evaluation using centerline technique. Postprocessing software is used to create a centerline down the dense contrast column on this arterial phase CT. In many cases, centerline analysis allows for optimal diameter measurements and stenosis evaluation and decreases interreader variability.

(85%–90%), with patients often critically ill when they reach the hospital.[48]

- Although traditionally viewed as a result of hypertension and atherosclerotic processes, AAA development is now known to be multifactorial with involvement of polygenetic predisposition, numerous extracellular signaling and inflammatory processes, and alterations in the extracellular matrix involving matrix metalloproteinases and various other enzymes.[49]

Imaging and differential diagnosis

- AAA is generally defined as a 50% or more increase in anteroposterior (AP) diameter of the aorta (diaphragm to iliac bifurcation), generally 3 cm or greater in the average adult.
- More than 85% of AAA are infrarenal (>1 cm below the lowest renal artery), most being diagnosed before the threshold for intervention (5–5.5 cm)[47] (**Fig. 13**).
- Less commonly, an AAA can be juxtarenal (**Fig. 14**A) (involving the renal arteries or with 1 cm of them) or suprarenal (**Fig. 14**B)

(involving the aorta and visceral branches above the renal arteries).[50,51] More cephalad aneurysm extension is associated with a more complex repair.

- AAA is usually a fusiform or a saccular configuration, can be bilobed, and often extends into the CIAs, necessitating changes in repair planning (**Fig. 15**).
- The main differential encountered in practice is whether or not an AAA is ruptured. Rupture (**Fig. 16**) is most frequently into the retroperitoneum along the posterolateral wall.[52,53] Disrupted intimal calcium, frank aortic wall discontinuity, and extravasated IV contrast are all specific signs of rupture (**Fig. 17**).
- Additional CT signs for rupture include the crescent sign and the drape sign (see **Fig. 17**). The crescent sign is a high-attenuation (higher than psoas muscle) crescent-shaped abnormality that is associated with the aneurysm mural thrombus/aortic wall.[54,55] The drape sign occurs when the posterior aortic wall lacks a sharp margin and distinct fat plane with the adjacent vertebral body (drapes over it).[56]

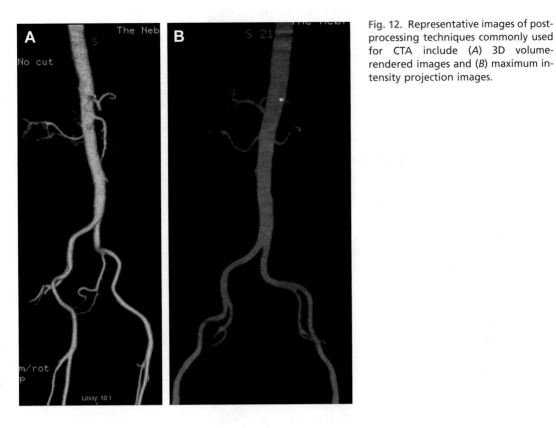

Fig. 12. Representative images of post-processing techniques commonly used for CTA include (*A*) 3D volume-rendered images and (*B*) maximum intensity projection images.

- Mycotic/infected AAAs are more prone to rupture (**Fig. 18**).

Pearls and pitfalls

- Inappropriate measurement of an oblique tortuous aorta on axial images can create a falsely high aneurysm measurement (**Fig. 19**).
- Coexistent AAA and retroperitoneal hemorrhage from other sources (anticoagulation, recent catheterization) can mimic AAA rupture (**Fig. 20**). Keys to differentiation include assessing stability with previous imaging, assessing intimal calcium for displacement, and assessing crescent and drape signs.
- Inflammatory AAAs (**Fig. 21**) can mimic rupture and may respond to steroids.[57]

What the referring physician needs to know
Table 4 highlights essential information needed for evaluating an AAA. Most is directed toward whether therapy is needed or not and toward procedural planning if intervention is indicated. Key items to report include maximal AP diameter and change from previous imaging, distance from lowest renal artery to start of aneurysm, configuration in relation to the renal arteries, total

Table 3
Commonly used aortic CTA strategies for radiation dose reduction

Technique	Advantage	Disadvantage
Low kVp	Readily available, takes advantage of inherent high-contrast study	Of limited usefulness in obese patients
Dual energy	Allows for virtual noncontrast images, decreasing number of phases needed	Need for special equipment and postprocessing time
Iterative reconstruction	Allows for imaging at lower dose because of improved noise reduction	Need for special equipment/software. Full iterative reconstruction can be time consuming

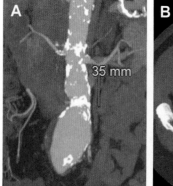

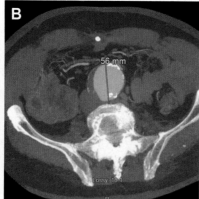

Fig. 13. Typical appearance of a common infrarenal AAA. (A) The beginning of the aneurysm is more than 1 cm inferior to the left renal artery on this coronal MIP image. (B) Axial CTA shows an AP dimension of 5.6 cm. This patient subsequently underwent endograft repair.

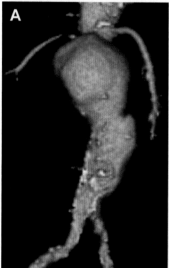

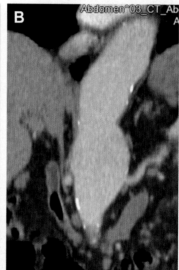

Fig. 14. (A) VR image of a 65-year-old woman from CTA shows a juxtarenal AAA. The aneurysm arises within 1 cm of the renal arteries. Options for repair include open surgery and the use of fenestrated stent grafts. (B) Coronal CTA images in a different patient show a suprarenal AAA, with the aneurysmal dilation extending well above the renal arteries. Repair becomes increasingly complex with more cephalad extension, often requiring jump grafts to visceral branch vessels or hybrid open/endovascular repairs.

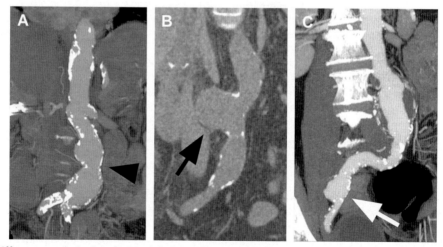

Fig. 15. Different morphologies of AAAs. (A) Coronal oblique MIP from CTA image shows a bilobed infrarenal AAA (*black arrowhead*) with extension to the iliac bifurcation. (B) Coronal MIP from noncontrast CT shows a saccular type of AAA (*black arrow*). (C) Oblique coronal MIP from CTA image shows an infrarenal AAA with nonocclusive intraluminal thrombus. There is extension of the aneurysm into the right CIA, with more focal aneurysmal dilatation at the right iliac bifurcation (*white arrow*). This situation affects the strategy for endovascular repair.

EVALUATING REPAIR OF ABDOMINAL AORTIC ANEURYSM
Clinical Presentation and Pathophysiology

- AAA that have rapidly enlarged, meet size criteria, have ruptured, or are believed to be symptomatic are generally repaired.
- Endovascular repair has become the preferred choice for AAA repair, even in the setting of rupture secondary to improved perioperative mortalities.[58] Advancements in graft technology (eg, fenestrated grafts) allow for increased use of endografts in even the most complex juxtarenal aneurysms.
- Hybrid surgical and endovascular repairs are being increasingly used for fixing complex suprarenal aneurysms that involve visceral branches.

Imaging and Differential Diagnosis

- Surveillance imaging of endovascular repair typically includes reporting excluded aneurysm sac size and evaluating for endoleak (**Fig. 22, Table 5**).
- Open repairs are most often complicated by the typical vascular surgery complications, including pseudoaneurysm formation and infection.
- Aortoenteric fistulas can occur after repair, often in the setting of graft infection, and

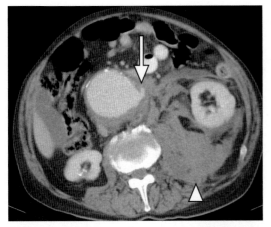

Fig. 16. Axial CT image of a ruptured AAA. There is a large amount of retroperitoneal hemorrhage on the left (*arrowhead*), with a focal wall discontinuity and contrast extravasation from the posterolateral aspect of the aorta (*white arrow*), the most common site of disruption.

length, angulation/configuration of aneurysm neck, and diameter of the iliac arterial system. Additional items to discuss include the presence of mural thrombus, calcifications, and any acute-appearing vascular disease. Iliofemoral vessel patency, tortuosity, and calcification are also particularly important for endovascular repair.

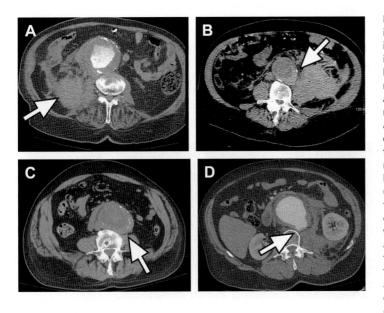

Fig. 17. CT findings of AAA rupture in 4 different patients. (*A*) Axial CTA image shows a large AAA with intraluminal thrombus. There is a large right retroperitoneal hemorrhage (*arrow*). Although no focal aortic wall discontinuity is seen, rupture can be diagnosed based on aneurysm size, the hematoma, and clinical symptoms. (*B*) Axial noncontrast CT image shows a large left retroperitoneal hematoma. The high-attenuation crescent sign (*arrow*) within the AAA is a specific feature of rupture. (*C*) Axial noncontrast CT image shows an AAA with the drape sign (*arrow*), another feature of rupture. Note the obscured fat plane between the posterolateral aorta and the adjacent vertebral body. Intimal calcifications are also displaced posterolaterally to the left. Despite the lack of a large hematoma, rupture or impending rupture can be diagnosed. This patient underwent AAA repair shortly after the CT, when he became hemodynamically unstable. (*D*) Rupture can be easily diagnosed on this axial contrast-enhanced CT image with frank aortic wall disruption (*arrow*), contrast extravasation, and a large adjacent hemorrhage.

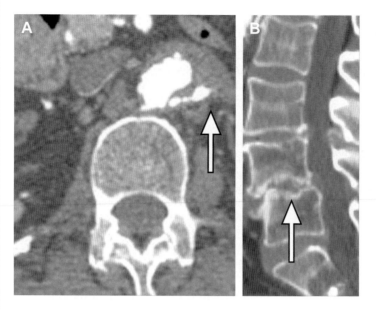

Fig. 18. (*A*) Axial CTA image shows a mycotic aneurysm. Note the eccentric irregular aortic wall thickening (*arrow*). This thickening had rapidly appeared, new from 1 month before (not shown). Additional findings of mycotic aneurysms (which are prone to rupture) include periaortic inflammatory change and gas foci. (*B*) Sagittal CT image in bone window shows irregular destructive changes of diskitis at the L4-L5 disk space (*arrow*), the source of infection in this case. Diskitis osteomyelitis is a frequent source of mycotic aneurysm.

present with severe hypotension, anemia, and hematochezia (**Fig. 23**).

- If renal arteries are sacrificed or accidentally covered by a nonfenestrated graft component, renal infarction can occur (**Fig. 24**).

Pearls and Pitfalls

- Postoperative materials or calcified thrombus in the excluded portion of the aneurysm sac can simulate an endoleak (see **Fig. 9**). Obtaining a noncontrast series if there is a history of previous endograft repair helps to avoid this pitfall.

What the Referring Physician Needs to Know

- Presence of pseudoaneurysm, aortoenteric fistula, aortocaval fistula, infection, or other postoperative complications

- After endograft repair, presence and type of endoleak as well as excluded aneurysm sac size and interval changes from previous imaging sizes

ACUTE AORTIC DISEASE
Clinical Presentation and Pathophysiology

- Acute aortic syndromes involving the abdominal aorta include dissection, IMH, penetrating aortic ulcer (PAU), and traumatic injury.[59]
- Patients generally experience back or abdominal pain, although they occasionally have vague nonspecific symptoms. Traumatic injury may occur in the setting of major closed or penetrating trauma. Hypertension is a common risk factor preceding many acute aortic syndromes.

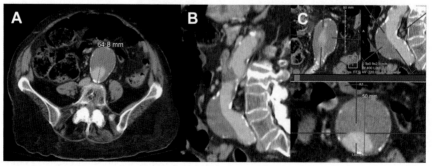

Fig. 19. Multiple axial CT images showing the usefulness of diameter measurement with double oblique technique. (*A*) Axial CT image denotes an AP diameter of 6.5 cm; however, the sagittal CT image (*B*) shows a significant focal bend in the aorta, resulting in an erroneously large measurement of true luminal diameter. (*C*) Double oblique reformatted MPR yields a more accurate diameter of 5.0 cm at this focal bend. Centerline technique can also help accuracy for tortuous vessel measurement.

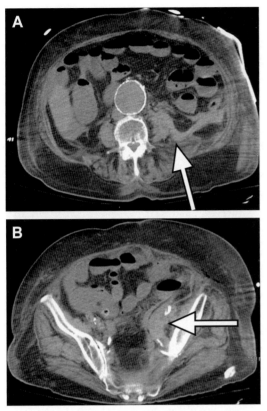

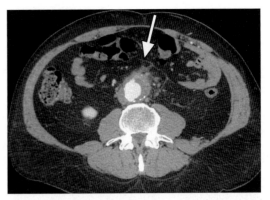

Fig. 21. Axial CTA image shows an AAA with marked wall thickening and adjacent inflammatory change (*arrow*). This finding was in a 42-year-old man with a strong smoking history. Pathology from excision showed this to be an inflammatory AAA, which are more likely to be symptomatic and are frequently seen in younger to middle-aged adults and smokers. Some are steroid responsive, but in adequate candidates, operative treatment is standard of care. Retroperitoneal inflammatory change usually substantially improves or resolves after fixation. The inflammatory change can mimic rupture (no rupture was present in this case).

Fig. 20. (*A*) Axial noncontrast CT image shows a 5.0-cm AAA, with adjacent left retroperitoneal hemorrhage (*arrow*). (*B*) More inferior image in the pelvis shows a left pelvic sidewall hematoma (*arrow*). The initial image mimics findings of AAA rupture, although no drape or crescent signs are present. The source of hemorrhage was a pseudoaneurysm from recent femoral catheterization, which resolved with conservative management.

- Dissection is related to a tear in the intimal layer of the aorta and subsequent blood flow through the tear into the media, whereas IMH is hemorrhage into the media layer, often caused by ruptured vasa vasorum vessels. PAU is usually the result of chronic atherosclerosis and inflammation.

Imaging and Differential Diagnosis

- Dissection presents as a linear filling defect in the aortic lumen. The true lumen is often smaller, and the false lumen is variably

Table 4
What the clinician needs to know: AAA reporting

Essential Information in Report	Use
Maximal AP diameter	Criteria for undergoing repair (typically >5.5 cm)
Relationship of AAA to renal arteries	Infrarenal, juxtarenal, and suprarenal aneurysms require different repair strategies
Distance of AAA neck to lowest renal artery	Determines if endograft repair is feasible and if fenestrated graft components are needed
Total length	Needed for graft repair planning
Angulation of neck/aorta	If severely angulated, an AAA may not be suitable for endograft repair
Iliofemoral artery diameter, tortuosity, and calcification status	Determines if vessels are adequate for endograft delivery

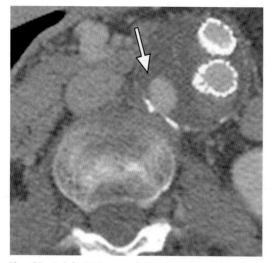

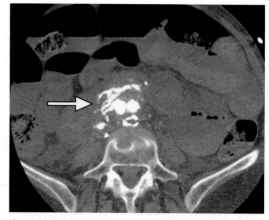

Fig. 22. Axial CT image from the delayed venous acquisition of a 3-phase endograft protocol CT. There is contrast opacification (*arrow*) of the excluded aneurysm sac, consistent with an endoleak. This was a type II endoleak from a lumbar collateral vessel.

Fig. 23. Axial CTA image at the level of the third portion of the duodenum in a patient with a history of complex open AAA repair 10 years previously and current hypotension with hematemesis. The arrow indicates contrast opacification of the duodenal lumen consistent with an aortoenteric fistula. The patient did not survive an open repair attempt.

opacified and can thrombose. The bird's beak sign may aid in differentiation of true and false lumens (**Fig. 25**). This observation is in reference to the acute intraluminal angle in the true lumen formed by the dissection flap and the normal wall of the aorta adjacent to it.

- IMH is seen as a crescentic area of high attenuation in the wall, best seen without contrast (**Fig. 26**).
- PAUs are focal outpouchings of contrast that extend beyond the expected normal aortic wall (**Fig. 27**).
- Traumatic injury is seen as periaortic stranding and hemorrhage, sometimes with contrast extravasation. In catastrophic injury, patients may exsanguinate before hospital arrival.

Pearls and Pitfalls

- Motion artifact and strands of thrombus can simulate an aortic dissection. Key is to recognize motion on other parts of the image.
- Ulcerated intraluminal plaque can mimic a PAU. Key is to recognize the intraluminal location of the ulcerated plaque, within the expected contour of the aortic wall.

What the Referring Physician Needs to Know

- Presence and type of acute aortic disease.
- In IMH and dissection, keys are reporting extent of dissection, description of branch vessel involvement, end organ malperfusion, true and false lumen opacification and extent, and changes from previous imaging (**Fig. 28**).
- PAU: location, size, and changes.

Table 5	
Types of endoleak	
Endoleak Type	**Imaging Findings**
1. Inadequate seal	Typically seen during placement. Contrast arrives via inadequate proximal seal of graft
2. Retrograde leak from collaterals	Most common type, most are inconsequential. Typically fill via IMA or lumbar collaterals
3. Mechanical failure of graft	Leak around inadequately sealed graft components (eg, aortic and iliac limbs). Often requires repair
4. Leak through graft porosity	No specific imaging findings. Rare with currently used endografts
5. Endotension	Aneurysm growth with no identifiable cause/idiopathic

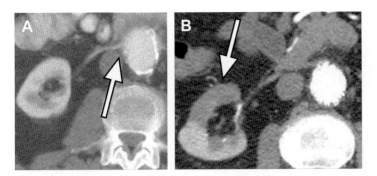

Fig. 24. (*A*) Axial CTA image before endovascular repair of AAA shows a small accessory renal artery supplying part of the right kidney lower pole (*arrow*). (*B*) Postendograft CT shows a renal infarct (*arrow*) in the area supplied by the accessory artery, which was occluded by a nonfenestrated portion of the endograft.

- Trauma: anticipated injury site and presence of any active contrast extravasation.

ATHEROSCLEROTIC OCCLUSIVE DISEASE
Clinical Presentation and Pathophysiology

- Atherosclerotic occlusive disease commonly affects the infrarenal aorta and common iliac vessels, notably at the iliac bifurcation.
- Clinical findings include back, hip, and buttock pain in addition to impotence (Leriche syndrome [**Fig. 29**]).
- Limb claudication symptoms can occur.
- The pathophysiology of atherosclerosis is a complex topic of intense debate and study in the literature. Inflammatory, genetic, and lifestyle (eg, cholesterol, diet, exercise, smoking) factors all play a role in development and progression of vascular disease.[60–62]

Imaging and Differential Diagnosis

- Atherosclerotic occlusive disease generally manifests as narrowing (typically >50% if symptomatic) of the aorta or iliac arteries related to calcified or noncalcified plaque.
- As mentioned previously, assessment of diameter narrowing is greatly aided by postprocessing techniques such as CPR and centerline analysis.

Pearls and Pitfalls

- Blooming artifact shown on CT usually occurs in the setting of severe calcific disease. This result can lead to overestimation of vessel stenosis. Iterative reconstruction and CPR can help to overcome this artifact.[63]

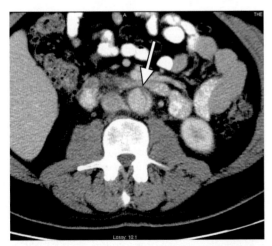

Fig. 25. Axial CT image shows an infrarenal aortic dissection (*arrow*). The smaller true lumen (left aspect of aorta) was separated from the opacified false lumen by a dissection flap. To aid in delineation, the false lumen is often larger and has a bird's beak configuration in relation to the true lumen.

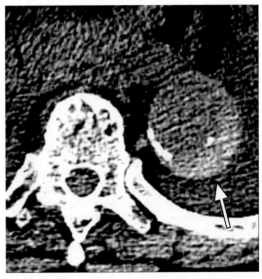

Fig. 26. Axial noncontrast CT image in narrow window setting shows a crescentic high-attenuation IMH at the level of the diaphragmatic hiatus (*arrow*). IMH most commonly occurs in the thoracic aorta, but can occur within or be isolated to the abdomen. Narrow windowing of noncontrast images allows for improved conspicuity.

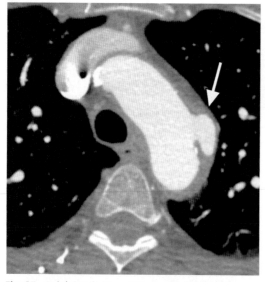

Fig. 27. Axial CTA image at the level of the aortic arch shows a focal contrast outpouching consistent with a PAU (*arrow*). Most commonly seen in the setting of hypertension, these PAUs are more frequently seen in the thoracic aorta but can occur in the abdomen as well.

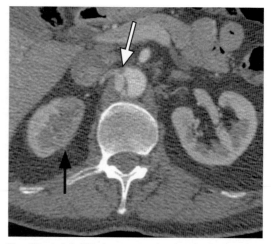

Fig. 28. Axial CTA image at the level of the renal arteries shows a focal dissection flap extending into the right renal artery (*white arrow*). This caused end organ ischemia in the form of an upper pole renal infarct (*black arrow*).

What the Referring Physician Needs to Know

- In addition to the approximate % degree of stenosis/occlusion, the referring physician needs to know the length of involvement, multiplicity of stenoses, unilateral or bilateral iliac involvement, and calcification extent.
- Aortoiliac lesion morphology is typically grouped into the TransAtlantic InterSociety Consensus (TASC) classification grouping (**Table 6**).[64]

VASCULITIS
Clinical Presentation and Pathophysiology

- Giant cell arteritis (GCA) and Takayasu arteritis (TA) are the most common large vessel vasculitides to have imaging findings on CTA. Both are systemic large vessel granulomatous inflammatory processes.
- Both diseases are idiopathic inflammatory disorders with various postulated environmental, autoimmune, and genetic causes.[65]
- GCA typically affects older individuals of northern European heritage, whereas TA is classically associated with younger females of Asian heritage.
- Clinical manifestations of disease include abnormal or absent pulses as well as symptoms related to occlusion or narrowing of large vessels (eg, mesenteric ischemic

symptoms if the splanchnic vasculature is involved or renal failure if the renal arteries are involved).

Imaging and Differential Diagnosis

- Both diseases manifest as areas of nonspecific aortic wall thickening and variable levels of thrombosis and occlusion[66,67] (**Fig. 30**). Rarely, the abdominal aorta or the ascending thoracic aorta may be affected by ectasia or aneurysm formation.
- In the setting of chronic occlusion, arterial collateral pathways may form.

Pearls and Pitfalls

- If discovered in an acute setting, inflammatory vascular wall thickening can be mistaken for an acute aortic disease such as an IMH. IMH is typically higher in attenuation than the nearby normal aortic wall and psoas muscle, whereas the thickened vessel wall in vasculitis is more commonly isoattenuating.
- Advanced noncalcified atherosclerotic disease in individuals (eg, young female type 1 diabetics) can lead to a false-positive suggestion of a vasculitis.

What the Referring Physician Needs to Know

- At initial disease presentation, an index of disease sites and severity is made. Assessment for occlusion or significant narrowing is essential, as is a survey for end organ ischemia in the setting of visceral branch vessel involvement.

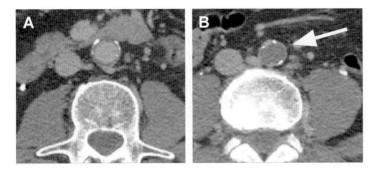

Fig. 29. Axial CTA images from a 70-year-old man with impotence and buttock claudication. (A) The aorta just below the renal arteries is patent, but becomes completely occluded just inferior to that (arrow, B). He had a clinical diagnosis of Leriche syndrome and underwent open aortobifemoral bypass grafting for repair.

Table 6	
TASC classification of aortoiliac occlusive disease	
A	Unilateral or bilateral single stenosis (<3 cm) of CIA or EIA
B	Single 3-cm-long to 10-cm-long stenosis (not into CFA)
	≤2 CIA or EIA stenosis (<5 cm, not into CFA)
	Unilateral CIA occlusion
C	Bilateral stenoses of CIA or EIA (5–10 cm, not into CFA)
	Unilateral EIA occlusion (not into CFA)
	Unilateral EIA stenosis extending into CFA
	Bilateral CIA occlusion
D	Diffuse stenosis of CIA, EIA, and CFA (>10 cm)
	Unilateral occlusion of CIA and EIA
	Bilateral EIA occlusion
	Iliac stenosis + aneurysm of aorta or iliacs

Abbreviation: CFA, common femoral artery.

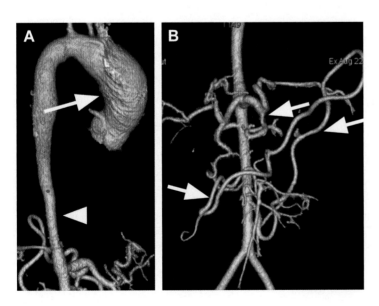

Fig. 30. 3D VR images of the aorta in a 32-year-old female patient with Takayasu arteritis. (A) Thoracic aorta shows aneurysm formation in the aortic root and ascending aorta (arrow). There is diffuse circumferential narrowing (arrowhead) of the descending thoracic and abdominal aorta from wall thickening/arteritis. (B) 3D VR image of the abdominal aorta shows occlusion of the SMA with resultant formation of numerous arterial collateral vessels (arrows) between the CA and IMA.

- Serial examinations while on therapy may be obtained – documenting areas of disease improvement or progression is the main task in this setting.

SUMMARY

State-of-the-art CTA of the abdominal aorta is essential for most aspects of aortic disease evaluation, treatment planning, and postprocedural follow-up. Obtaining quality arterial phase images, performing the correct imaging protocol for the task at hand, and using the lowest contrast dose and limiting radiation dose are goals for optimal patient care. Mastering image acquisition technique and image interpretation/reporting maximizes the radiologist's ability to care for patients with abdominal aortic disease.

REFERENCES

1. Ginat DT, Gupta R. Advances in computed tomography imaging technology. Annu Rev Biomed Eng 2014;16:431–53.
2. Amako M, Yamamoto Y, Nakamura K, et al. Preoperative visualization of the artery of Adamkiewicz by dual-phase CT angiography in patients with aortic aneurysm. Kurume Med J 2011;58(4):117–25.
3. Bilhim T, Pereira JA, Fernandes L, et al. Angiographic anatomy of the male pelvic arteries. AJR Am J Roentgenol 2014;203(4):W373–82.
4. Raman SS, Pojchamarnwiputh S, Muangsomboon K, et al. Utility of 16-MDCT angiography for comprehensive preoperative vascular evaluation of laparoscopic renal donors. AJR Am J Roentgenol 2006; 186(6):1630–8.
5. Koops A, Wojciechowski B, Broering DC, et al. Anatomic variations of the hepatic arteries in 604 selective celiac and superior mesenteric angiographies. Surg Radiol Anat 2004;26(3):239–44.
6. Arjhansiri K, Charoenrat P, Kitsukjit W. Anatomic variations of the hepatic arteries in 200 patients done by angiography. J Med Assoc Thai 2006; 89(Suppl 3):S161–8.
7. Egorov VI, Yashina NI, Fedorov AV, et al. Celiacomesenterial arterial aberrations in patients undergoing extended pancreatic resections: correlation of CT angiography with findings at surgery. JOP 2010;11(4):348–57.
8. Hayashi H, Yoshihara H, Takagi R, et al. Minimally invasive diagnosis of persistent sciatic artery by multidetector-row computed tomographic angiography. Heart Vessels 2006;21(4):267–9.
9. Budovec JJ, Pollema M, Grogan M. Update on multidetector computed tomography angiography of the abdominal aorta. Radiol Clin North Am 2010;48(2): 283–309, viii.
10. Fleischmann D. CT angiography: injection and acquisition technique. Radiol Clin North Am 2010; 48(2):237–47, vii.
11. Rengier F, Geisbusch P, Vosshenrich R, et al. State-of-the-art aortic imaging: part I– fundamentals and perspectives of CT and MRI. Vasa 2013;42(6): 395–412.
12. Rubin GD, Leipsic J, Joseph Schoepf U, et al. CT angiography after 20 years: a transformation in cardiovascular disease characterization continues to advance. Radiology 2014;271(3):633–52.
13. Lell MM, Anders K, Uder M, et al. New techniques in CT angiography. Radiographics 2006;26(Suppl 1): S45–62.
14. von Tengg-Kobligk H, Weber TF, Rengier F, et al. Image postprocessing of aortic CTA and MRA. Radiologe Nov 2007;47(11):1003–11 [in German].
15. Apfaltrer P, Hanna EL, Schoepf UJ, et al. Radiation dose and image quality at high-pitch CT angiography of the aorta: intraindividual and interindividual comparisons with conventional CT angiography. AJR Am J Roentgenol 2012;199(6):1402–9.
16. Puippe GD, Winklehner A, Hasenclever P, et al. Thoraco-abdominal high-pitch dual-source CT angiography: experimental evaluation of injection protocols with an anatomical human vascular phantom. Eur J Radiol 2012;81(10):2592–6.
17. Shen Y, Sun Z, Xu L, et al. High-pitch, low-voltage and low-iodine-concentration CT angiography of aorta: assessment of image quality and radiation dose with iterative reconstruction. PLoS One 2015; 10(2). e0117469.
18. Fleischmann D. How to design injection protocols for multiple detector-row CT angiography (MDCTA). Eur Radiol 2005;15(Suppl 5):E60–5.
19. Fleischmann D. Use of high concentration contrast media: principles and rationale-vascular district. Eur J Radiol 2003;45(Suppl 1):S88–93.
20. Hallett RL, Fleischmann D. Tools of the trade for CTA: MDCT scanners and contrast medium injection protocols. Tech Vasc Interv Radiol 2006;9(4): 134–42.
21. Orlandini F, Boini S, Iochum-Duchamps S, et al. Assessment of the use of a saline chaser to reduce the volume of contrast medium in abdominal CT. AJR Am J Roentgenol 2006;187(2):511–5.
22. Cademartiri F, van der Lugt A, Luccichenti G, et al. Parameters affecting bolus geometry in CTA: a review. J Comput Assist Tomogr 2002;26(4):598–607.
23. Bae KT. Test-bolus versus bolus-tracking techniques for CT angiographic timing. Radiology 2005;236(1): 369–70 [author reply: 370].
24. Cademartiri F, Nieman K, van der Lugt A, et al. Intravenous contrast material administration at 16-detector row helical CT coronary angiography: test bolus versus bolus-tracking technique. Radiology 2004; 233(3):817–23.

25. Ippolito D, Talei Franzesi C, Fior D, et al. Low kV settings CT angiography (CTA) with low dose contrast medium volume protocol in the assessment of thoracic and abdominal aorta disease: a feasibility study. Br J Radiol 2015;88(1049):20140140.
26. Lell MM, Jost G, Korporaal JG, et al. Optimizing contrast media injection protocols in state-of-the art computed tomographic angiography. Invest Radiol 2015;50(3):161–7.
27. Ichikawa S, Ichikawa T, Motosugi U, et al. Computed tomography (CT) venography with dual-energy CT: low tube voltage and dose reduction of contrast medium for detection of deep vein thrombosis. J Comput Assist Tomogr 2014;38(5):797–801.
28. Zheng M, Liu Y, Wei M, et al. Low concentration contrast medium for dual-source computed tomography coronary angiography by a combination of iterative reconstruction and low-tube-voltage technique: feasibility study. Eur J Radiol 2014;83(2):e92–9.
29. Yin WH, Lu B, Gao JB, et al. Effect of reduced x-ray tube voltage, low iodine concentration contrast medium, and sinogram-affirmed iterative reconstruction on image quality and radiation dose at coronary CT angiography: results of the prospective multicenter REALISE trial. J Cardiovasc Comput Tomogr 2015;9(3):215–24.
30. Nakaura T, Nakamura S, Maruyama N, et al. Low contrast agent and radiation dose protocol for hepatic dynamic CT of thin adults at 256-detector row CT: effect of low tube voltage and hybrid iterative reconstruction algorithm on image quality. Radiology 2012;264(2):445–54.
31. Liu J, Lv PJ, Wu R, et al. Aortic dual-energy CT angiography with low contrast medium injection rate. J Xray Sci Technol 2014;22(5):689–96.
32. Clark ZE, Bolus DN, Little MD, et al. Abdominal rapid-kVp-switching dual-energy MDCT with reduced IV contrast compared to conventional MDCT with standard weight-based IV contrast: an intra-patient comparison. Abdom Imaging 2015;40(4):852–8.
33. Strobl FF, Sommer WH, Haack M, et al. Computed tomography angiography as the basis for optimized therapy planning before endovascular aneurysm repair (EVAR). Radiologe 2013;53(6):495–502 [in German].
34. Ahmed S, Zimmerman SL, Johnson PT, et al. MDCT interpretation of the ascending aorta with semiautomated measurement software: improved reproducibility compared with manual techniques. J Cardiovasc Comput Tomogr 2014;8(2):108–14.
35. Entezari P, Kino A, Honarmand AR, et al. Analysis of the thoracic aorta using a semi-automated post processing tool. Eur J Radiol 2013;82(9):1558–64.
36. Kanematsu M, Goshima S, Miyoshi T, et al. Whole-body CT angiography with low tube voltage and low-concentration contrast material to reduce radiation dose and iodine load. AJR Am J Roentgenol 2014;202(1):W106–16.
37. Qi L, Zhao Y, Zhou CS, et al. Image quality and radiation dose of lower extremity CT angiography at 70 kVp on an integrated circuit detector dual-source computed tomography. Acta Radiol 2015;56(6):659–65.
38. Buffa V, Solazzo A, D'Auria V, et al. Dual-source dual-energy CT: dose reduction after endovascular abdominal aortic aneurysm repair. Radiol Med 2014;119(12):934–41.
39. Stolzmann P, Frauenfelder T, Pfammatter T, et al. Endoleaks after endovascular abdominal aortic aneurysm repair: detection with dual-energy dual-source CT. Radiology 2008;249(2):682–91.
40. Marin D, Boll DT, Mileto A, et al. State of the art: dual-energy CT of the abdomen. Radiology 2014;271(2):327–42.
41. Kaza RK, Platt JF, Goodsitt MM, et al. Emerging techniques for dose optimization in abdominal CT. Radiographics 2014;34(1):4–17.
42. Maturen KE, Kleaveland PA, Kaza RK, et al. Aortic endograft surveillance: use of fast-switch kVp dual-energy computed tomography with virtual noncontrast imaging. J Comput Assist Tomogr 2011;35(6):742–6.
43. Hansen NJ, Kaza RK, Maturen KE, et al. Evaluation of low-dose CT angiography with model-based iterative reconstruction after endovascular aneurysm repair of a thoracic or abdominal aortic aneurysm. AJR Am J Roentgenol 2014;202(3):648–55.
44. Caywood D, Paxton B, Boll D, et al. Effects of model-based iterative reconstruction on image quality for low-dose computed tomographic angiography of the thoracic aorta in a swine model. J Comput Assist Tomogr 2015;39(2):196–201.
45. Pontana F, Pagniez J, Duhamel A, et al. Reduced-dose low-voltage chest CT angiography with Sinogram-affirmed iterative reconstruction versus standard-dose filtered back projection. Radiology 2013;267(2):609–18.
46. Lederle FA, Johnson GR, Wilson SE, et al. The aneurysm detection and management study screening program: validation cohort and final results. Aneurysm Detection and Management Veterans Affairs Cooperative Study Investigators. Arch Intern Med 2000;160(10):1425–30.
47. Kent KC. Clinical practice. Abdominal aortic aneurysms. N Engl J Med 2014;371(22):2101–8.
48. Brown LC, Powell JT. Risk factors for aneurysm rupture in patients kept under ultrasound surveillance. UK Small Aneurysm Trial Participants. Ann Surg 1999;230(3):289–96 [discussion: 296–7].
49. Davis FM, Rateri DL, Daugherty A. Mechanisms of aortic aneurysm formation: translating preclinical studies into clinical therapies. Heart 2014;100(19):1498–505.

50. Crawford ES, Beckett WC, Greer MS. Juxtarenal infrarenal abdominal aortic aneurysm. Special diagnostic and therapeutic considerations. Ann Surg 1986;203(6):661–70.

51. Ayari R, Paraskevas N, Rosset E, et al. Juxtarenal aneurysm. Comparative study with infrarenal abdominal aortic aneurysm and proposition of a new classification. Eur J Vasc Endovasc Surg 2001;22(2):169–74.

52. Rakita D, Newatia A, Hines JJ, et al. Spectrum of CT findings in rupture and impending rupture of abdominal aortic aneurysms. Radiographics 2007; 27(2):497–507.

53. Schwartz SA, Taljanovic MS, Smyth S, et al. CT findings of rupture, impending rupture, and contained rupture of abdominal aortic aneurysms. AJR Am J Roentgenol 2007;188(1):W57–62.

54. Arita T, Matsunaga N, Takano K, et al. Abdominal aortic aneurysm: rupture associated with the high-attenuating crescent sign. Radiology 1997;204(3): 765–8.

55. Siegel CL, Cohan RH, Korobkin M, et al. Abdominal aortic aneurysm morphology: CT features in patients with ruptured and nonruptured aneurysms. AJR Am J Roentgenol 1994;163(5):1123–9.

56. Halliday KE, al-Kutoubi A. Draped aorta: CT sign of contained leak of aortic aneurysms. Radiology 1996;199(1):41–3.

57. Khan S, Verma V, Verma S, et al. Assessing the potential risk of rupture of abdominal aortic aneurysms. Clin Radiol 2015;70(1):11–20.

58. Qin C, Chen L, Xiao YB. Emergent endovascular vs. open surgery repair for ruptured abdominal aortic aneurysms: a meta-analysis. PLoS One 2014;9(1): e87465.

59. Bonaca MP, O'Gara PT. Diagnosis and management of acute aortic syndromes: dissection, intramural hematoma, and penetrating aortic ulcer. Curr Cardiol Rep 2014;16(10):536.

60. Borissoff JI, Spronk HM, ten Cate H. The hemostatic system as a modulator of atherosclerosis. N Engl J Med 2011;364(18):1746–60.

61. Hansson GK. Inflammation, atherosclerosis, and coronary artery disease. N Engl J Med 2005;352(16): 1685–95.

62. Nahrendorf M, Swirski FK. Lifestyle effects on hematopoiesis and atherosclerosis. Circ Res 2015;116(5): 884–94.

63. Renker M, Nance JW Jr, Schoepf UJ, et al. Evaluation of heavily calcified vessels with coronary CT angiography: comparison of iterative and filtered back projection image reconstruction. Radiology 2011;260(2):390–9.

64. Norgren L, Hiatt WR, Dormandy JA, et al. Inter-society consensus for the management of peripheral arterial disease (TASC II). J Vasc Surg 2007;45(Suppl S): S5–67.

65. Chaigne-Delalande S, de Menthon M, Lazaro E, et al. Giant-cell arteritis and Takayasu arteritis: epidemiological, diagnostic and treatment aspects. Presse Med 2012;41(10):955–65 [in French].

66. Zhu FP, Luo S, Wang ZJ, et al. Takayasu arteritis: imaging spectrum at multidetector CT angiography. Br J Radiol 2012;85(1020):e1282–92.

67. Khandelwal N, Kalra N, Garg MK, et al. Multidetector CT angiography in Takayasu arteritis. Eur J Radiol 2011;77(2):369–74.

Computed Tomography Angiography of the Hepatic, Pancreatic, and Splenic Circulation

 CrossMark

Melissa Price, MD[a], Manuel Patino, MD[a],
Dushyant Sahani, MD[b],*

KEYWORDS

• Liver • Pancreas • Spleen • CT angiography • Dual-energy CT

KEY POINTS

• MDCTA allows acquisition of data with enhanced spatial and temporal resolution that can be reconstructed for robust preoperative road mapping.
• MDCTA can detect normal and variant vascular anatomy as well as allow accurate lesion characterization within the liver and pancreas.
• Using dual-energy CT, virtual unenhanced images can be generated, thereby reducing overall radiation dose. In addition, material composition allows for robust delineation of enhancement.

MULTIDETECTOR COMPUTED TOMOGRAPHY ANGIOGRAPHY TECHNIQUES

Multidetector computed tomography angiography (MDCTA) of the hepatic, pancreatic, and splenic circulations delineates both vascular anatomy and parenchymal pathology. This has important implications for preoperative planning and tumor staging. With the advent of modern multidetector CT scanners, it is now possible to temporally acquire fast multiphasic acquisitions of abdominal organs in the optimal phase of enhancement with enhanced 2-dimensional (2D) and 3D image display. In general, rapid acquisition with thin slices and scanning delays are critical components of an optimal MDCTA protocol.[1]

Technical Factors

Adequate distention of the stomach and duodenum is obtained by having patients drink 500 to 1000 mL of water 20 to 30 minutes before the scan and an additional 300 to 500 mL immediately before the scan. Water is preferred to radiopaque contrast, as the latter may make identification of high-attenuation structures, such as hyperenhancing tumors and vessels in the vicinity of stomach and duodenum, on the 2D and 3D image display difficult. Moreover, the natural density of water on CT also clearly delineates the periampullary anatomy and adjacent lesions.[1]

Hepatic Phases

The liver has a dual blood supply from the hepatic artery and portal vein, with the portal vein supplying most blood to the liver (75%–80%). Biphasic hepatic CT protocols include an arterial phase as well as a portal venous phase to detect tumors that have arterial neovascularization and relatively diminished portal supply, such as hepatocellular

a Division of Abdominal Imaging, Massachusetts General Hospital, 55 Fruit Street, White 270, Boston, MA 02114, USA; b Division of Abdominal Imaging, Massachusetts General Hospital, Harvard Medical School, 55 Fruit Street, White 270, Boston, MA 02114, USA
* Corresponding author.
E-mail address: dsahani@mgh.harvard.edu

Radiol Clin N Am 54 (2016) 55–70
http://dx.doi.org/10.1016/j.rcl.2015.08.009
0033-8389/16/$ – see front matter

radiologic.theclinics.com

carcinoma (HCC).[2] Biphasic hepatic CT improves sensitivity in detecting hypervascular primary and metastatic hepatic tumors compared with a single portal venous phase, although the greatest tumor-to-liver contrast typically occurs in the portal venous phase, in both patients with and without cirrhosis.[3]

At our institution, the timing of the arterial phase in MDCTA of the liver is determined with automatic bolus tracking: contrast is injected and 15 seconds after the attenuation of the abdominal aorta reaches 150 Hounsfield units (HU), image acquisition starts. The portal venous phase images are acquired 55 to 70 seconds after the contrast material (CM) injection. A delayed phase also can be added for a triple-phase hepatic CT, which has been shown to have improved sensitivity for detection of HCC over biphasic CT. When automated bolus tracking is used, scanning for the delayed phase occurs 180 seconds after injection of the CM[2] (Table 1).

Pancreatic Protocol

For accurate detection and staging of pancreatic adenocarcinoma, it is important to perform a biphasic pancreatic protocol CTA that includes a pancreatic parenchymal phase at 40 to 50 seconds (if using a fixed delay) and a portal venous phase. The pancreatic parenchymal phase allows for optimal pancreatic parenchymal enhancement and provides maximal contrast difference between normal pancreatic parenchyma and tumor; for pancreatic ductal adenocarcinoma, the tumor is hypoattenuating versus background parenchyma. The pancreatic phase also allows depiction of the arterial anatomy. The portal venous phase delineates the portal and mesenteric venous anatomy and hepatic parenchymal pathology[4] (Tables 2 and 3).

Recently, utilization of split-bolus injection in conjunction with spectral CT has been shown to improve pancreatic tumor conspicuity and reduce radiation dose by combing the pancreatic and portal venous phases into one scan. This is done by initially administering 100 mL iodinated intravenous contrast before the CT for the portal venous phase and then injecting an additional 40 mL of contrast 35 seconds later to enhance the pancreatic phase. Bolus tracking initiates scanning 15 seconds after the abdominal aorta reaches an attenuation of 280 HU. Images are then reconstructed at 60 and 77 keV. This scanning protocol offers marked reduction in radiation dose and higher tumor conspicuity with the 60 keV compared with a standard pancreatic protocol CT.[5]

Dual-Energy Computed Tomography and Low Peak Kilovoltage Imaging

Dual-energy CT (DECT) can now be used in conjunction with MDCTA to provide additional information about tissue composition and enhance

---

Table 1
Sample liver computed tomography angiography

	Noncontrast (Only 4 Slices Through Mid Liver)	Arterial Phase	Portal Venous
Scan delay	—	Bolus tracking	70 s after contrast injection
Ref kV	120	120	120
Quality ref mAs	180	220	200
Slice thickness	5 mm	1 mm	5 mm
Slice increment	5 mm	0.6 mm	5 mm
Pitch	0.95	0.95	0.95
Rotation time	0.5	0.5	0.5
ACQ	128 × 0.6	128 × 0.6	128 × 0.6
Kernel	I30F medium smooth	I30F medium smooth	I30F medium smooth

Liver multidetector computed tomography angiography: Siemens Definition Edge 128 CT scanner (Siemens Medical Solutions, Malvern, PA, USA).
  Intravenous (IV) contrast: 370 mg/mL.
  Weight-based dose: <135 lb: 80 mL, 135–200 lb: 90 mL, >200 lb: 120 mL.
  IV gauge: 18 gauge.
  IV contrast rate: 4 mL/s.
  Oral contrast: water.
  Bolus tracking: 150 HU of abdominal aorta measured at the level of the mid liver, monitored delay of 10 seconds and scan delay of 15 seconds for arterial phase.

Table 2
Sample pancreatic computed tomography angiography (CTA) protocol

	Pancreatic CTA	Portal Venous Phase
Delay (fixed)	50 s	70 s
Care kV	Ref 120	Ref 120
Quality ref mAs	220	200
Slice thickness	2 mm	5 mm
Slice increment	2 mm	5 mm
Pitch	0.95	0.95
Rotation time	0.5	0.5
Collimation	128 × 0.6 mm	128 × 0.6 mm
Kernel	I30F medium smooth	I30F medium smooth

Pancreatic multidetector computed tomography angiography: Siemens Definition Edge 128 CT scanner.
Intravenous (IV) contrast: 370 mg/mL.
Weight-based dose: <135 lb: 80 mL, 135–200 lb: 90 mL, >200 lb: 120 mL.
IV gauge: 18–20 gauge.
IV contrast rate: 4 mL/s.
Oral contrast: water.

contrast resolution by imaging at 2 different energies: 80 and 140 kVp. Iodinated contrast demonstrates increased attenuation at lower energy levels because the K-edge of iodine (33.2 KeV) is closer to the lower energy of 80 kVp than the higher energy level. Imaging at a lower energy of 80 kVp can improve hypervascular lesion conspicuity as well as reduce the effective radiation dose, and the amount of iodinated contrast required for an examination. The disadvantage of using a lower kVp is that image noise increases

Table 3
Protocol for pancreatic CTA reconstruction and reformatted images

	CTA Thin Reconstructions	3D MPR: CTA Sagittal and Coronal Reformats
Kernel	I31F S3	I31F S3
Thickness	1 mm	3 mm
Interval	0.6 mm	3 mm

Pancreatic multidetector computed tomography angiography: Reconstruction and Reformats.
Siemens Definition Edge 128 CT scanner.
Abbreviations: 3D, three dimensional; CTA, computed tomography angiography; MPR, multiplanar reconstruction.

due to attenuation of the x-ray beam by the patient, which is exacerbated in larger patients. Certain structures, such as gallstones and urinary stones, also demonstrate greater conspicuity when imaged at a higher kVp. By imaging at the 2 energy levels, the benefits of both low and higher energy levels can be achieved in a single examination.[6,7]

With DECT, 80 kVp and 140 kVp datasets are acquired with a single acquisition, and virtual unenhanced and weighted average images (WAIs) are then created from these raw datasets. WAIs combine the HU data acquired by the 80 kVp and 140 kVp datasets to simulate a 120 kVp acquisition. This results in optimal lesion conspicuity, high contrast, low noise, and artifact reduction. The quality of vascular imaging can be improved with the lower kVp dataset.[8,9]

Dual-Energy Computed Tomography Image Reconstruction and Postprocessing Techniques

Material-specific applications in DECT allow for the generation of images based on differences in attenuation and changes in attenuation at different energy levels, which help to differentiate the composition of materials. With dual-source dual-energy CT, a 3-material decomposition algorithm of iodine, soft tissue, and fat is used, and separate material-specific images can be generated based on them. Single-source dual-energy CT uses a 2-material decomposition algorithm composed of iodine and water.[10]

Dual-energy techniques can reduce effective radiation dose by reconstructing virtual unenhanced images, which obviate the need for an unenhanced scan in multiphase MDCTA. The virtual unenhanced images are obtained by digitally subtracting iodine from the data set of contrast-enhanced images.[6] The iodine-specific images in dual-energy CT are derived from material decomposition and demonstrate true iodine content of tissues. These images are not dependent on inherent tissue attenuation and therefore can more reliably demonstrate true tissue enhancement. The iodine content of each voxel is quantified in iodine-specific maps, allowing for detection of very small amounts of enhancement.[10]

Virtual monochromatic (VMC) images are created from material-specific algorithms and postprocessed from the dual-energy data set. The selected VMC energy level depicts structures as though they were acquired from a monochromatic beam. Low-energy VMC images show greater attenuation of iodine leading to better contrast between structures, although at the expense of higher noise.[10]

Volumetric material-specific datasets acquired with DECT can be reconstructed as axial images or even processed by conventional 3D applications like maximum intensity projection (MIP), multiplanar reconstruction (MPR), and volume-rendered reformation. MPR, MIP, and volume-rendered reconstructions of the iodine-specific maps make virtual bone subtraction possible, which in turn helps visualization of the vessels with removal of bones and calcified plaques. Virtual nonenhanced images aid in the detection of vascular calcification by removing contrast from images, although they contain higher noise and lower resolution.[9]

ARTERIAL ANATOMY

The vascular anatomy of the liver and pancreas influences surgical decisions for tumor resection so as to minimize surgical morbidity. Moreover, because primary and metastatic hepatic malignancies are increasingly being treated with minimally invasive interventional and surgical techniques, MDCTA has become an essential modality to accurately define hepatic arterial anatomy. It is crucial for interventional radiologists and surgeons to be familiar with variant arterial anatomy to avoid procedural and surgical complications.[11]

CELIAC AXIS

The celiac artery is the first major anterior infradiaphragmatic branch of the abdominal aorta, followed by the superior mesenteric artery (SMA) and inferior mesenteric artery. With the most common branching pattern of the celiac axis, the left gastric artery branches first and the celiac trunk then divides into the common hepatic and splenic arteries. This pattern is seen in approximately 70% of individuals. Several other variants have been described, such as a true trifurcation of all 3 vessels from the terminal portion of the celiac axis, and combined trunks when one vessel is replaced from a different arterial bed.[12]

HEPATIC ARTERY

The common hepatic artery (CHA) originates from the celiac trunk, giving off the gastroduodenal artery as the first branch, and continues to the porta hepatis as the proper hepatic artery. The right gastric artery originates from the proper hepatic artery at the portal hilum. The proper hepatic artery then finally divides into its 3 terminal branches: the right, middle, and left hepatic arteries.[12]

The proper hepatic artery is located anterior to the portal vein within the porta hepatis and to the left of the common bile duct. Following its take-off from the proper hepatic artery, the right hepatic artery courses between the common bile duct and the portal vein.[13]

Classic branching of the hepatic artery is observed in approximately 60% of people.[12] Variant origins of the CHA are rare and seen in only approximately 4% of individuals. In people with a replaced CHA, 50% have an origin from the SMA and the remainder are usually replaced to the abdominal aorta.[11] In patients who have a CHA that arises from the SMA, the artery typically maintains a suprapancreatic position but courses posterior to the main portal vein and superior mesenteric vein (SMV), unlike in the normal CHA anatomy. The CHA maintains a suprapancreatic, preportal pathway when it arises from the abdominal aorta[14] (Fig. 1).

The most frequent anatomic variation of the hepatic arterial system is a replaced right hepatic artery arising from the SMA, present in up to 18% of patients (Fig. 2). The next most common variation is a replaced left hepatic artery arising from the left gastric artery.[14]

Pancreatic Arterial Anatomy

The pancreatic blood supply is derived from branches of the celiac trunk and the SMA. The dorsal pancreatic artery and pancreatica magna artery arise from the splenic artery, which also gives off distal arterial branches to supply the pancreatic tail. The SMA branches off the abdominal aorta just inferior to the celiac trunk and posterior to the neck of the pancreas. The SMA courses anterior to the pancreatic uncinate and to the left of the SMV.[1,15]

The gastroduodenal artery originates from the CHA and gives off the anterior and superior pancreatoduodenal arteries, which form an anastomosis with the inferior pancreaticoduodenal artery. This anastomosis creates an arterial arcade that surrounds the head and uncinate process of the pancreas. The transverse pancreatic artery forms a connection between pancreaticoduodenal arcade and the dorsal pancreatic and pancreatica magna arteries.[1]

Splenic Artery

The splenic artery has the most torturous course of all the branches of the celiac axis and is usually the largest branch, with a diameter of approximately 6 to 10 mm and an average length of 13 cm. Aberrant origins of the splenic artery are uncommon and seen in fewer than 1% of individuals. When

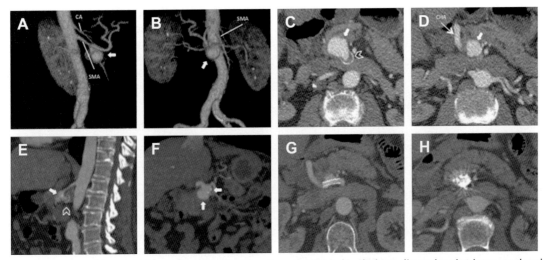

Fig. 1. A 62-year-old man with a replaced CHA arising from the SMA. (*A, B*) Three-dimensional volume-rendered images. (*C, D*) Axial contrast-enhanced CTA images. (*E, F*) Sagittal and coronal reformatted images. A bilobed aneurysm (*arrows*) with calcification and mural thrombus (*arrowhead*) arises from the CHA. (*G, H*) CTA images following coil embolization of the aneurysm.

present, the most common variant origins of the splenic artery are the abdominal aorta, SMA, and right hepatic artery.[12]

The splenic artery courses along the superior margin of the pancreas, anterior and superior to the splenic vein. At the hilum, the splenic artery divides into superior and inferior terminal branches, which then subsequently divide into segmental intrasplenic branches. The superior terminal branches are the dominant arterial supply to the spleen and tend to be longer than the inferior terminal branches. As previously mentioned, the splenic artery supplies multiple arterial branches to the pancreas. The dorsal pancreatic artery is the first branch and is followed by the pancreatica magna, which typically arises from the middle portion of the splenic artery.[16]

VENOUS ANATOMY
Portal Venous Anatomy

The portal vein forms posterior to the pancreatic neck when the superior mesenteric and splenic veins converge. Within the porta hepatis, the portal vein is located posterior to the proper hepatic artery and common bile duct and normally has a diameter of 11 to 13 mm.[13]

Conventional Anatomy

- Main portal vein branches into the right and left portal veins
- Right portal vein divides into the anterior and posterior branches
- Right anterior branch supplies hepatic segments V and VIII

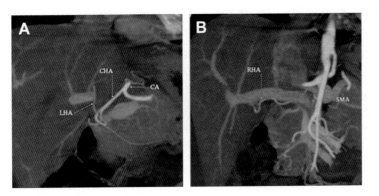

Fig. 2. A 35-year-old woman before liver donor evaluation. Multiplanar MIP images. (*A*) Celiac artery (CA), CHA, and left hepatic artery (LHA). (*B*) Replaced right hepatic artery (RHA) arising from the SMA.

- Right posterior branch supplies segments VI and VII

Variant Anatomy

- "Z type" variant: right posterior portal vein is the first branch to arise from the main portal vein and is subsequently followed by the right anterior and finally the left portal veins
- Trifurcation: right anterior, right posterior, and left portal veins share a common origin from the main portal vein[17]

Hepatic Venous Anatomy

- The liver is conventionally drained via 3 hepatic veins that converge into the inferior vena cava
- Right hepatic vein drains segments V to VIII
- Middle hepatic vein drains segments IV, V, and VIII
- Left hepatic vein drains segments II and III[18]

LIVER MULTIDETECTOR COMPUTED TOMOGRAPHY ANGIOGRAPHY
Preoperative Assessment for Hepatic Transplantation

MDCTA is an excellent modality for demonstrating a patient's hepatic vascular anatomy before liver transplantation and has become the first-line imaging modality for surgical planning of living donor liver transplantation.

Hepatic vascular variants are important to identify with preoperative imaging, as they can dramatically impact surgical technique and rarely result in donor exclusion. In adult-to-adult living donor preoperative imaging, it is essential to identify the location of and course of the middle hepatic vein because the hepatectomy plane is typically along the gallbladder fossa, approximately 1 cm to the right of the middle hepatic vein.[19]

The middle hepatic artery, supplying segment IV, is also included in the hepatectomy plane of adult-to-adult live donor liver transplantation, and its origin and course are important to delineative preoperatively. One variant that has important surgical implications is a middle hepatic artery arising from the right hepatic artery, as this crosses the planned hepatectomy line.[18]

Postoperative Evaluation for Liver Transplantation

MDCTA has a critical role in detecting arterial complications after liver transplantation, and is commonly used as the next imaging modality when abnormalities are detected on liver Doppler ultrasound. Hepatic arterial complications following transplantation that can be diagnosed with MDCTA include the following:

- Thrombosis
- Dissection
- Stenosis
- Pseudoaneurysm formation

Hepatic Artery Thrombosis

Hepatic arterial thrombosis (HAT) is a potentially devastating arterial complication following transplantation and also the most common vascular complication. Undetected HAT can result in biliary ischemia, necrosis, bilomas, sepsis, fulminant hepatic necrosis, and graft failure. Although early diagnosis of HAT may enhance the success of attempts at revascularization with surgical thrombectomy or thrombolysis, most patients with HAT will require retransplantation.[20] Absence of hepatic arterial flow on Doppler ultrasonography should raise concern for hepatic arterial thrombosis and prompt further evaluation with CTA, magnetic resonance angiography, or catheter angiography (**Fig. 3**).

- "Early" HAT is defined as occurring within the first month following transplantation

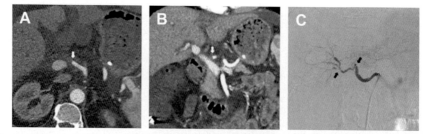

Fig. 3. A 64-year-old man 10 days status post orthotopic liver transplant with hepatic artery thrombosis. (*A*) Axial arterial-phase CTA image and (*B*) coronal arterial-phase image demonstrating abrupt cutoff of the hepatic artery (*white arrows*). (*C*) Angiographic image after surgical thrombectomy showing multifocal stenosis of the proper hepatic artery (*black arrows*).

- "Late" HAT occurs 1 month or more after transplantation
- HAT is more common in the early posttransplant period and may present with fulminant hepatic failure[21]

Hepatic Artery Stenosis

The incidence of hepatic artery stenosis in liver transplant recipients is 5% to 11%.[20,22,23] Hepatic artery stenosis most commonly occurs at the site of anastomosis within the first 3 months after transplantation. It is critical to detect hepatic arterial stenosis, as it can lead to graft dysfunction, hepatic artery thrombosis, and biliary structuring if untreated. When detected early with imaging modalities such as MDCTA, there is a greater likelihood that hepatic artery stenosis can be successfully treated with catheter angioplasty or surgical reconstruction so that retransplantation is not required.[22,23]

Hepatic Artery Aneurysms

MDCT serves as an excellent noninvasive imaging modality for diagnosis and surveillance of hepatic artery aneurysms (HAAs). HAAs are the second most common type of visceral artery aneurysm, after splenic artery aneurysms.[24] Most HAAs are incidentally detected with cross-sectional imaging and patients will be asymptomatic unless the aneurysm ruptures. Unlike splenic artery aneurysms, HAAs most frequently occur in men.[25] When imaging HAAs, it is critical to assess for the presence of any anatomic vascular variants, particularly in the presence of planned endovascular or surgical intervention (see **Fig. 1**).

Hepatocellular Carcinoma

HCC most frequently occurs in individuals with hepatitis or cirrhosis. HCC classically demonstrates arterial enhancement with washout on the portal venous phase and may show delayed capsule appearance. Although HCC can present as a well-defined lesion at imaging, it can also diffusely infiltrate the liver and invade hepatic and portal veins. The sensitivity of MDCT for detection of HCC varies by tumor size. In larger lesions, it can exceed 70%; however, when tumors are smaller than 20 mm, the sensitivity of MDCT decreases to approximately 50% in patients with cirrhosis undergoing multiphase CT examinations with unenhanced, arterial, and portal venous phases.[26] (**Fig. 4**)

Although HCC most frequently develops in the setting of cirrhosis, in the United States approximately 22% of HCC will occur in noncirrhotic livers. Individuals who develop HCC without cirrhosis are more likely to present with a symptomatic solitary or dominant hepatic mass, and the tumor is typically moderately or well differentiated at pathology. Most of these lesions in patients without cirrhosis show necrosis, and approximately one-quarter will have hemorrhagic components.[27]

The United Network for Organ Sharing (UNOS), which administers the Organ Procurement and Transplant Network (OPTN), gives increased priority on the transplant waitlist to individuals who have HCC and remain within the Milan Criteria; namely, 1 HCC that is 5 cm or smaller, or as many as 3 HCCs that are all 3 cm or smaller. UNOS allows for the diagnosis of HCC to be made with imaging alone, either with dynamic contrast-enhanced MDCT or MR. In 2011, the UNOS/OPTN board of directors issued an amended policy delineating the technical parameters that should be followed for dynamic liver protocols and the criteria required to diagnose HCC with imaging, with an emphasis on specificity over sensitivity. OPTN Class 5 lesions in cirrhotic livers meet radiologic criteria for HCC, which are outlined in **Table 4**.[28]

There are several advantages of using dual-energy CT in conjunction with MDCTA for imaging evaluation of HCC. Hypervascular hepatic tumors such as HCC have enhanced conspicuity when imaged at 80 kVp rather than 140 kVp, and the effective radiation dose is also lower at 80 kVp.[6] The low-energy VMC images, which are available with both single-source and dual-source DECT,

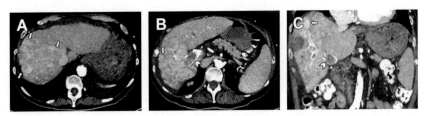

Fig. 4. An 80-year-old man with HCC. (*A, B*) Arterial-phase axial images. (*C*) Coronal arterial-phase image. There is an arterially enhancing tumor infiltrating most of the right hepatic lobe (*arrows*). Tumor thrombus extends into the right portal vein (*arrowhead*).

Table 4
OPTN imaging guidelines for class 5 nodules in cirrhotic livers

OPTN class 5A	• Nodule <2 cm and ≥1 cm in size • Late arterial hyperenhancement relative to hepatic parenchyma • Washout on the later contrast phases and pseudocapsule formation (peripheral rim enhancement)
OPTN class 5A-g (growth)	• Nodule <2 cm and ≥1 cm in size • Late arterial hyperenhancement relative to hepatic parenchyma • Lesion growth by 50% or greater on serial CT or MRI examinations performed ≤6 mo apart (not applicable to ablated lesions)

OPTN class 5B	• Nodule ≥2 cm and ≤5 cm in size
	• Late arterial hyperenhancement relative to hepatic parenchyma
	• One of the following criteria:
	  ○ Portal venous or delayed phase washout
	  ○ Late capsule or pseudocapsule formation
	  ○ Lesion growth by 50% or greater on serial CT or MRI examinations performed ≤6 mo apart
	  ○ Biopsy proven

OPTN 5T (treated)	• OPTN class 5 lesion or biopsy-proven HCC that has been treated with locoregional therapy • Findings suggestive of residual or recurrent tumor, such as nodular enhancement along the ablation zone can be present

Abbreviations: CT, computed tomography; HCC, hepatocellular carcinoma; OPTN, Organ Procurement and Transplant Network.

From HRSA/OPTN. OPTN policy 9: allocation of livers and liver-intestines. 2015. Available at: http://optn.transplant.hrsa.gov/resources/by-organ/liver-intestine. Accessed June 27, 2015.

increase the contrast-to-noise ratio (CNR) between hypervascular hepatic tumors and the adjacent liver.[10] Iodine-specific image maps increase the conspicuity of the ablation zone margin compared with the blended VMC images in patients who have undergone radiofrequency ablation and can be particularly useful when assessing for local tumor recurrence[29,30] (**Fig. 5**).

SPLENIC MULTIDETECTOR COMPUTED TOMOGRAPHY ANGIOGRAPHY
Splenic Artery Aneurysms

Splenic artery aneurysms (SAAs) are the most common type of visceral artery aneurysm, making up 60% of cases, and have a prevalence of 0.04% to 0.10% at autopsy.[16,25,31] They are typically asymptomatic and incidentally diagnosed at imaging. By definition, SAAs occur when the artery size exceeds 1 cm and involves dilatation of all layers of the artery wall. Women are more commonly affected than men. When SAAs exceed 2 cm in size, intervention is usually favored, either with endovascular or open surgical repair due to the risk of rupture; however, there are no definitive management guidelines.[32] In addition, enlargement of the aneurysm, pregnancy or planned pregnancy, or the presence of symptoms also may prompt intervention.[25]

SAAs are usually saccular and tend to occur either at the distal aspect of the artery or at a bifurcation in the middle or distal segment of the

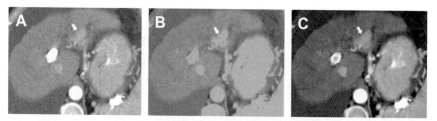

Fig. 5. Contrast-enhanced dual-energy CT images of a 62-year-old showing HCC in hepatic segment II (*arrow*). (*A*) Single-energy CT image 140 kVp. (*B*) Virtual monochromatic image 50 keV. (*C*) Material-density iodine image. Note the increase in iodine attenuation and high image contrast observed on the low-keV and iodine images, compared with the conventional single-energy image.

artery.[16,33] Multiparous women and individuals with portal hypertension have the most frequent incidence of SAAs. The association with multiparity has been postulated to be due to hormonal alterations that result in intimal hyperplasia and subsequent aneurysm formation.[16,34] (**Fig. 6**)

PANCREATIC MULTIDETECTOR COMPUTED TOMOGRAPHY ANGIOGRAPHY
Pancreatic Cancer

Pancreatic ductal adenocarcinoma (PDA) is an aggressive cancer with high mortality. Accurate staging of PDA at the time of diagnosis is important to triage patients to surgical resection or chemotherapy, as well as help determine overall prognosis. Evaluation with imaging plays a primary role in the initial decision-making process of patients with PDA by providing staging information.[4] MDCTA has been shown to have positive predictive value of 89% for preoperative prediction of resectability of PDA across multiple generations of CT scanners.[35]

Achieving high CNR and lesion conspicuity are particularly critical in pancreatic imaging, as PDAs can appear relatively inconspicuous and in some cases isoattenuating to pancreatic parenchyma on CT.[6] It has been shown that imaging with a lower voltage (80 kVp) and higher tube current results in greater pancreas-to-tumor CNR.[36] The iodine-specific maps in dual-energy CT can improve conspicuity of hypoattenuating PDAs and the low-voltage dataset can better delineate tumor margins due to the increased tumor-to-pancreas CNR.[37] (**Fig. 7**)

Based on imaging features of PDA demonstrated at MDCTA, these tumors are classified as resectable, borderline resectable, or unresectable. The National Comprehensive Cancer Network criteria for placing patients in 1 of these 3 categories is outlined in **Table 5**. The pertinent findings recommended in the Consensus Statement of the Society of Abdominal Radiology and American Pancreatic Association on the pancreatic radiology reporting template should be included in the imaging report for patients with known or suspected PDA, as summarized in **Table 6**[4] (**Figs. 8 and 9**).

Hypervascular Pancreatic Tumors

The differential diagnosis of focal hypervascular pancreatic lesions includes primary neuroendocrine tumors, metastases, intrapancreatic accessory spleen, and vascular lesions, such as arteriovenous fistulas or aneurysms of the splenic artery.

Although pancreatic neuroendocrine tumors comprise fewer than 5% of all primary pancreatic malignancies,[38] they are the most common hypervascular tumors of the pancreas. These lesions are usually well demarcated and usually show avid enhancement on the early arterial-phase images, owing to the rich capillary network present within the lesions (**Fig. 10**).[39] Smaller functioning tumors show homogeneous enhancement, whereas

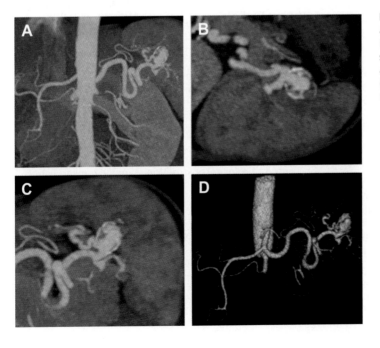

Fig. 6. A 54-year-old woman with an SAA. (*A–C*). Multiplanar MIP images show the aneurysm at the splenic hilum with mural thrombus and peripheral rim calcification. (*D*) Three-dimensional volume-rendered image.

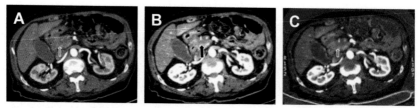

Fig. 7. A 79-year-old man with PDA involving the head and invading the duodenum. Dual-energy axial CTA images show a hypoattenuating tumor within the pancreatic head (*arrows*) that appears more conspicuous on the monochromatic 50-keV and iodine-specific images. (*A*) Single-energy CT (SECT) 140 kVp arterial-phase image. (*B*) Monochromatic 50 keV image. (*C*) Material-density iodine image.

larger nonfunctioning lesions may show heterogeneity and necrosis. It is crucial to perform pancreatic protocol MDCTA in patients with a known neuroendocrine lesion so as to assess the primary lesion within the pancreas as well as evaluate the liver for hypervascular metastases (**Fig. 11**).

Pancreatic Metastases

Metastatic lesions to the pancreas are uncommon and account for fewer than 5% of all pancreatic malignancies.[40] Primary tumors of the kidney, thyroid, lung, and breast, as well as melanoma have been reported to metastasize to the pancreatic parenchyma. It is important to note that because these metastatic lesions can invade the ductal epithelium, they may produce ductal dilatation and mimic pancreatic adenocarcinoma.[41] Metastases from renal cell carcinoma (RCC) may be found at the time of primary tumor diagnosis or, more frequently, during follow-up after surgery,[42] and though these lesions can be solitary, they have been reported to be multiple in 20% to 45% of patients.[43] RCC is the most common primary tumor leading to solitary pancreatic metastases.[44] These lesions are usually round or ovoid masses, well-delineated, and show brisk enhancement in the pancreatic late arterial phase and washout on delayed phase images.[45] Based on enhancement alone, it can be difficult to differentiate these metastatic lesions from hypervascular neuroendocrine tumors of the pancreas (**Fig. 12**).

Table 5
National Comprehensive Cancer Network Guidelines for PDA Staging

Stage	Arterial Findings	Venous Findings	Nodal and Distant Metastases
Resectable	Preserved fat planes around celiac axis, SMA, and hepatic artery	No SMV or portal vein involvement	—
Borderline resectable	• Gastroduodenal artery encasement up to the hepatic artery or direct abutment of hepatic artery • Tumor abutment of SMA should be <180°	SMV involvement or portal vein distortion or narrowing with sufficient vessel length proximal and distal for safe resection and reconstruction	
Unresectable	• Aortic invasion or encasement • Pancreatic head tumors: SMA encasement of more than 180°, celiac axis abutment, or inferior vena cava invasion • Pancreatic body/tail tumors: SMA or celiac axis encasement of more than 180°	SMV and portal vein occlusion unsuitable for reconstruction	Distant metastases; metastases to lymph nodes beyond field of resection

Abbreviations: PDA, pancreatic ductal adenocarcinoma; SMA, superior mesenteric artery; SMV, superior mesenteric vein.
From Al-Hawary MM, Francis IR, Chari ST, et al. Pancreatic ductal adenocarcinoma radiology reporting template: consensus statement of the Society of Abdominal Radiology and the American Pancreatic Association. Radiology 2014;270(1):248–60.

Table 6 Pancreatic ductal adenocarcinoma reporting template: Society of Abdominal Radiology and American Pancreatic Association	
Tumor location	• Right of superior mesenteric vein (SMV): pancreatic head or uncinate process • Left of SMV: pancreatic body or tail
Tumor size	—
Presence and extent of vascular involvement: arterial	Celiac axis, superior mesenteric artery and common hepatic artery: • ≤180° vessel contact • >180° vessel contact
Presence and extent of vascular involvement: venous	Portal vein and SMV: • Circumferential degree of tumor vessel contact • Focal caliber narrowing • Contour abnormality • Presence of bland thrombus
Presence of arterial anatomic variants	—
Extrapancreatic tumor extension	• Local (to adjacent organs): stomach, small bowel, spleen, colon/mesocolon • Distant: liver, peritoneum, abnormal-appearing lymph nodes outside local drainage pathway

Data from Al-Hawary MM, Francis IR, Chari ST, et al. Pancreatic ductal adenocarcinoma radiology reporting template: consensus statement of the Society of Abdominal Radiology and the American Pancreatic Association. Radiology 2014;270(1):248–60.

Vascular Complications of Pancreatitis

Acute pancreatitis is associated with trypsin activation within pancreatic acinar cells with resulting autodigestion of the pancreas. When severe, the enzymatic autodigestion can extend beyond the pancreatic parenchyma and result in vascular and hemorrhagic complications. Reports in the literature state that major vascular complications following pancreatitis occur with a greater incidence in individuals with chronic pancreatitis compared with acute pancreatitis.[46]

As the pancreas is anatomically associated with the splenic, superior mesenteric, and portal veins, these can be involved in pancreatitis. Thrombosis

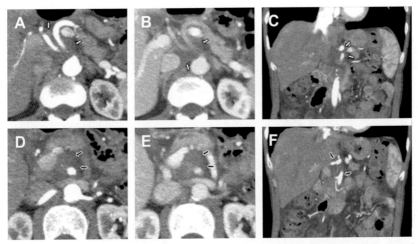

Fig. 8. CTA images for staging of a 65-year-old man with locally advanced adenocarcinoma arising from the head and uncinate process of the pancreas. (*A–C*) Arterial and portal venous phase axial and coronal images showing encasement of celiac artery and common hepatic artery by tumor (*white arrows*). (*D–F*) Arterial and portal venous phase axial and coronal images showing encasement of the superior mesenteric and common hepatic arteries (*black arrows*).

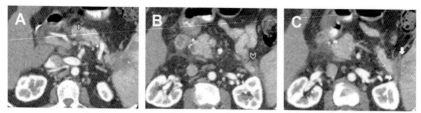

Fig. 9. A 68-year-old man with adenocarcinoma of the pancreatic tail. (*A*) Hypodense lesion in the body of the pancreas (*arrow*) without associated pancreatic duct dilatation or enhancing mural nodules, consistent with an intraductal papillary mucinous neoplasm (IPMN). (*B, C*) Ill-defined soft tissue mass in the tail of the pancreas (*arrowhead*), invading the splenic hilum and left anterior pararenal space (*white arrows*). The patient underwent distal pancreatectomy and splenectomy; pathology confirmed pancreatic ductal adenocarcinoma with splenic involvement.

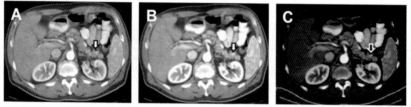

Fig. 10. Dual-energy CTA images from a 68-year-old man with an 8-mm enhancing lesion in the pancreatic tail. (*A*) A 140-kVp image. (*B*) Virtual monochromatic 65-keV image. (*C*) Material-density iodine image. The pancreatic tail lesion (*arrow*) is most conspicuous on the low-keV and iodine-specific images. The patient underwent endoscopic ultrasound and transgastric biopsy. Histopathology confirmed a well-differentiated endocrine neoplasm, strongly positive for chromogranin and synaptophysin.

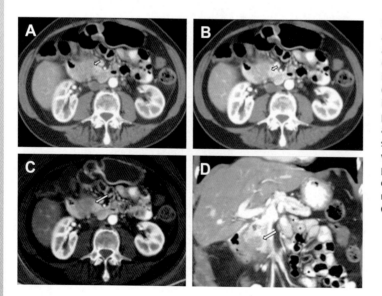

Fig. 11. Dual-energy CTA images of a 64-year-old woman with a hypo-attenuating pancreatic head mass (*arrows*). (*A*) Axial, SECT 140-kVp image. (*B*) Axial, monochromatic 65-keV image. (*C*) Material-density iodine image. (*D*) Coronal arterial-phase image. The lesion borders are delineated best on the iodine-specific images. The patient underwent a Whipple resection and pathology confirmed a well-differentiated neuroendocrine tumor, World Health Organization Grade 2 of 3.

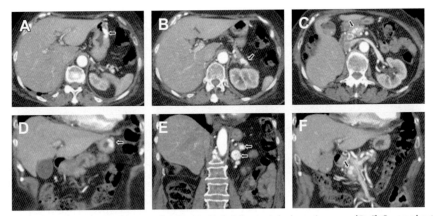

Fig. 12. A 74-year-old woman with history of RCC. (*A–C*) Axial arterial-phase images. (*D–F*) Coronal arterial-phase images. The images show arterially enhancing metastases involving the greater curvature of the stomach, left adrenal gland, and pancreas (*arrows*).

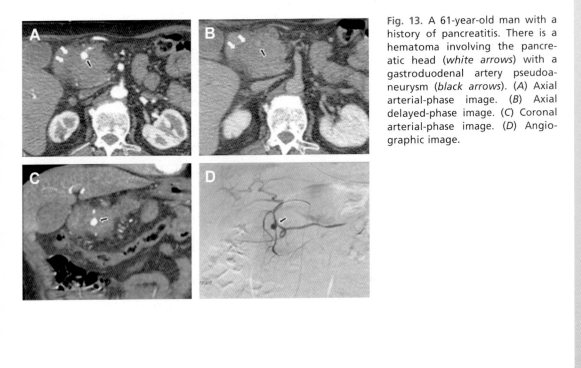

Fig. 13. A 61-year-old man with a history of pancreatitis. There is a hematoma involving the pancreatic head (*white arrows*) with a gastroduodenal artery pseudoaneurysm (*black arrows*). (*A*) Axial arterial-phase image. (*B*) Axial delayed-phase image. (*C*) Coronal arterial-phase image. (*D*) Angiographic image.

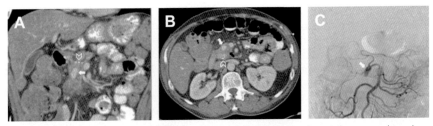

Fig. 14. A 55-year-old man with history of chronic pancreatitis. (*A*) Coronal portal venous phase image. (*B*) Axial portal venous phase image. Note the presence of punctate calcifications in the pancreas (*arrowheads*). There is a hematoma involving the head and uncinate process of the pancreas (*black arrow*), and a pseudoaneurysm (*white arrows*) arising from the middle colic artery. (*C*) Angiographic image.

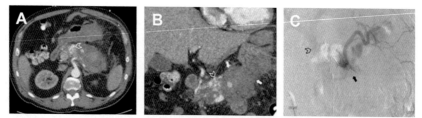

Fig. 15. A 54-year-old man with hemorrhagic, necrotizing pancreatitis. (*A*) Axial arterial-phase CTA image. (*B*) Coronal arterial-phase CTA image. (*C*) Angiographic image. The CTA images show extensive pancreatic necrosis and a heterogeneous collection (*white arrows*). There is a complex arteriovenous fistula (*arrowhead*) in the neck of the pancreas with branches from the celiac artery, left gastric artery, and SMV. Angiographic image (*C*) shows the arteriovenous fistula (*black arrow*) draining into the splenoportal junction (*black arrowhead*).

of the splanchnic veins, defined as the portal, splenic, or SMVs, either in combination or isolation, occurs in approximately 1.8% of individuals with acute pancreatitis. Isolated splenic vein thrombosis (SPV) is the most common form of splanchnic vein thrombosis.[47] SPV is more likely to occur in the presence of pancreatic fluid collections with severe necrotizing pancreatitis and can be caused by inflammation or compression from an adjacent fluid-collection.[48] When present, these complications are important to accurately diagnosis, because in some cases untreated splenic vein thrombosis can result in gastric varices, and SMV occlusion may lead to small bowel ischemia.[47]

Direct vascular injuries, although rare, can lead to pseudoaneurysm formation and, rarely, arterial rupture into the gastrointestinal tract.[49] Pseudoaneurysm formation is a severe complication of pancreatitis and can be identified at MDCTA as a focal outpouching arising from the involved artery, typically in a region of pancreatic necrosis.[50] The most common sites of pseudoaneurysm formation secondary to pancreatitis in order of decreasing frequency are the splenic, gastroduodenal, pancreaticoduodenal, hepatic, and left gastric arteries[50,51] (**Fig. 13**). Rarely, superior mesenteric, jejunal, or colic arterial branches are affected[52] (**Fig. 14**).

In rare cases of severe hemorrhagic pancreatitis, more complex vascular injuries may occur (**Fig. 15**).

CTA allows accurate diagnosis of arterial injures and can demonstrate the extent of a pseudoaneurysm along with the degree of thrombosis within the pseudoaneurysm. The 3D postprocessing of images, with MIPs and volume rendering, assist with surgical planning and interventional procedures.

SUMMARY

MDCTA of the hepatic, pancreatic, and splenic circulations is a highly effective noninvasive imaging modality that delineates complex vascular anatomy and anatomic variants as well as parenchymal organ pathology with high spatial resolution. Newer imaging techniques, such as DECT, can increase contrast resolution and enhance diagnostic capabilities while limiting radiation dose.

REFERENCES

1. Perez-Johnston R, Lenhart DK, Sahani DV. CT angiography of the hepatic and pancreatic circulation. Radiol Clin North Am 2010;48(2):311–30, viii.
2. Iannaccone R, Laghi A, Catalano C, et al. Hepatocellular carcinoma: role of unenhanced and delayed phase multi-detector row helical CT in patients with cirrhosis. Radiology 2005;234(2):460–7.
3. Foley WD, Mallisee TA, Hohenwalter MD, et al. Multiphase hepatic CT with a multirow detector CT scanner. AJR Am J Roentgenol 2000;175(3):679–85.
4. Al-Hawary MM, Francis IR, Chari ST, et al. Pancreatic ductal adenocarcinoma radiology reporting template: consensus statement of the Society of Abdominal Radiology and the American Pancreatic Association. Radiology 2014;270(1):248–60.
5. Brook OR, Gourtsoyianni S, Brook A, et al. Split-bolus spectral multidetector CT of the pancreas: assessment of radiation dose and tumor conspicuity. Radiology 2013;269(1):139–48.
6. Heye T, Nelson RC, Ho LM, et al. Dual-energy CT applications in the abdomen. AJR Am J Roentgenol 2012;199(5 Suppl):S64–70.
7. Yeh BM, Shepherd JA, Wang ZJ, et al. Dual-energy and low-kVp CT in the abdomen. AJR Am J Roentgenol 2009;193(1):47–54.
8. Macari M, Spieler B, Kim D, et al. Dual-source dual-energy MDCT of pancreatic adenocarcinoma: initial observations with data generated at 80 kVp and at simulated weighted-average 120 kVp. AJR Am J Roentgenol 2010;194(1):W27–32.
9. Vlahos I, Chung R, Nair A, et al. Dual-energy CT: vascular applications. AJR Am J Roentgenol 2012; 199(5 Suppl):S87–97.

10. Agrawal MD, Pinho DF, Kulkarni NM, et al. Onco-logic applications of dual-energy CT in the abdomen. Radiographics 2014;34(3):589–612.

11. Covey AM, Brody LA, Maluccio MA, et al. Variant hepatic arterial anatomy revisited: digital subtraction angiography performed in 600 patients. Radiology 2002;224(2):542–7.

12. Hazirolan T, Metin Y, Karaosmanoglu AD, et al. Mesenteric arterial variations detected at MDCT angiography of abdominal aorta. AJR Am J Roentgenol 2009;192(4):1097–102.

13. Tirumani SH, Shanbhogue AK, Vikram R, et al. Imaging of the porta hepatis: spectrum of disease. Radiographics 2014;34(1):73–92.

14. Song SY, Chung JW, Yin YH, et al. Celiac axis and common hepatic artery variations in 5002 patients: systematic analysis with spiral CT and DSA. Radiology 2010;255(1):278–88.

15. Johnson PT, Heath DG, Kuszyk BS, et al. CT angiography with volume rendering: advantages and applications in splanchnic vascular imaging. Radiology 1996;200(2):564–8.

16. Madoff DC, Denys A, Wallace MJ, et al. Splenic arterial interventions: anatomy, indications, technical considerations, and potential complications. Radiographics 2005;25(Suppl 1):S191–211.

17. Covey AM, Brody LA, Getrajdman GI, et al. Incidence, patterns, and clinical relevance of variant portal vein anatomy. AJR Am J Roentgenol 2004;183(4):1055–64.

18. Sahani D, Mehta A, Blake M, et al. Preoperative hepatic vascular evaluation with CT and MR angiography: implications for surgery. Radiographics 2004;24(5):1367–80.

19. Singh AK, Cronin CG, Verma HA, et al. Imaging of preoperative liver transplantation in adults: what radiologists should know. Radiographics 2011;31(4):1017–30.

20. Itri JN, Heller MT, Tublin ME. Hepatic transplantation: postoperative complications. Abdom Imaging 2013;38(6):1300–33.

21. Pareja E, Cortes M, Navarro R, et al. Vascular complications after orthotopic liver transplantation: hepatic artery thrombosis. Transplant Proc 2010;42(8):2970–2.

22. Caiado AH, Blasbalg R, Marcelino AS, et al. Complications of liver transplantation: multimodality imaging approach. Radiographics 2007;27(5):1401–17.

23. Quiroga S, Sebastia MC, Margarit C, et al. Complications of orthotopic liver transplantation: spectrum of findings with helical CT. Radiographics 2001;21(5):1085–102.

24. Horton KM, Fishman EK. CT angiography of the mesenteric circulation. Radiol Clin North Am 2010;48(2):331–45, viii.

25. Horton KM, Smith C, Fishman EK. MDCT and 3D CT angiography of splanchnic artery aneurysms. AJR Am J Roentgenol 2007;189(3):641–7.

26. Addley HC, Griffin N, Shaw AS, et al. Accuracy of hepatocellular carcinoma detection on multidetector CT in a transplant liver population with explant liver correlation. Clin Radiol 2011;66(4):349–56.

27. Brancatelli G, Federle MP, Grazioli L, et al. Hepatocellular carcinoma in noncirrhotic liver: CT, clinical, and pathologic findings in 39 U.S. residents. Radiology 2002;222(1):89–94.

28. Wald C, Russo MW, Heimbach JK, et al. New OPTN/UNOS policy for liver transplant allocation: standardization of liver imaging, diagnosis, classification, and reporting of hepatocellular carcinoma. Radiology 2013;266(2):376–82.

29. Lee SH, Lee JM, Kim KW, et al. Dual-energy computed tomography to assess tumor response to hepatic radiofrequency ablation: potential diagnostic value of virtual noncontrast images and iodine maps. Invest Radiol 2011;46(2):77–84.

30. Morgan DE. Dual-energy CT of the abdomen. Abdom Imaging 2014;39(1):108–34.

31. Abbas MA, Stone WM, Fowl RJ, et al. Splenic artery aneurysms: two decades experience at Mayo clinic. Ann Vasc Surg 2002;16(4):442–9.

32. Hogendoorn W, Lavida A, Hunink MG, et al. Open repair, endovascular repair, and conservative management of true splenic artery aneurysms. J Vasc Surg 2014;60(6):1667–76.e1.

33. Liu Q, Lu JP, Wang F, et al. Visceral artery aneurysms: evaluation using 3D contrast-enhanced MR angiography. AJR Am J Roentgenol 2008;191(3):826–33.

34. Mattar SG, Lumsden AB. The management of splenic artery aneurysms: experience with 23 cases. Am J Surg 1995;169(6):580–4.

35. Zamboni GA, Kruskal JB, Vollmer CM, et al. Pancreatic adenocarcinoma: value of multidetector CT angiography in preoperative evaluation. Radiology 2007;245(3):770–8.

36. Marin D, Nelson RC, Barnhart H, et al. Detection of pancreatic tumors, image quality, and radiation dose during the pancreatic parenchymal phase: effect of a low-tube-voltage, high-tube-current CT technique–preliminary results. Radiology 2010;256(2):450–9.

37. De Cecco CN, Darnell A, Rengo M, et al. Dual-energy CT: oncologic applications. AJR Am J Roentgenol 2012;199(5 Suppl):S98–105.

38. Bhosale PR, Menias CO, Balachandran A, et al. Vascular pancreatic lesions: spectrum of imaging findings of malignant masses and mimics with pathologic correlation. Abdom Imaging 2013;38(4):802–17.

39. Lewis RB, Lattin GE Jr, Paal E. Pancreatic endocrine tumors: radiologic-clinicopathologic correlation. Radiographics 2010;30(6):1445–64.

40. Crippa S, Angelini C, Mussi C, et al. Surgical treatment of metastatic tumors to the pancreas: a single

center experience and review of the literature. World J Surg 2006;30(8):1536–42.

41. Scatarige JC, Horton KM, Sheth S, et al. Pancreatic parenchymal metastases: observations on helical CT. AJR Am J Roentgenol 2001;176(3):695–9.

42. Koide N, Yokoyama Y, Oda K, et al. Pancreatic metastasis from renal cell carcinoma: results of the surgical management and pathologic findings. Pancreas 2008;37(1):104–7.

43. Law CH, Wei AC, Hanna SS, et al. Pancreatic resection for metastatic renal cell carcinoma: presentation, treatment, and outcome. Ann Surg Oncol 2003;10(8):922–6.

44. Tsitouridis I, Diamantopoulou A, Michaelides M, et al. Pancreatic metastases: CT and MRI findings. Diagn Interv Radiol 2010;16(1):45–51.

45. Vincenzi M, Pasquotti G, Polverosi R, et al. Imaging of pancreatic metastases from renal cell carcinoma. Cancer Imaging 2014;14:5.

46. Sharma PK, Madan K, Garg PK. Hemorrhage in acute pancreatitis: should gastrointestinal bleeding be considered an organ failure? Pancreas 2008; 36(2):141–5.

47. Harris S, Nadkarni NA, Naina HV, et al. Splanchnic vein thrombosis in acute pancreatitis: a single-center experience. Pancreas 2013;42(8):1251–4.

48. Flati G, Andren-Sandberg A, La Pinta M, et al. Potentially fatal bleeding in acute pancreatitis: pathophysiology, prevention, and treatment. Pancreas 2003;26(1):8–14.

49. Barge JU, Lopera JE. Vascular complications of pancreatitis: role of interventional therapy. Korean J Radiol 2012;13(Suppl 1):S45–55.

50. Shyu JY, Sainani NI, Sahni VA, et al. Necrotizing pancreatitis: diagnosis, imaging, and intervention. Radiographics 2014;34(5):1218–39.

51. Kirby JM, Vora P, Midia M, et al. Vascular complications of pancreatitis: imaging and intervention. Cardiovasc Intervent Radiol 2008;31(5):957–70.

52. Verde F, Fishman EK, Johnson PT. Arterial pseudoaneurysms complicating pancreatitis: literature review. J Comput Assist Tomogr 2015;39(1):7–12.

Computed Tomograpy Angiography of the Renal Circulation

 CrossMark

Luke A. Falesch, MD*, William Dennis Foley, MD

KEYWORDS

- Computed tomography angiography • Renal artery stenosis • Atherosclerotic stenosis
- Fibromuscular dysplasia • Curved planar reformat • Three-dimensional volume-rendered display
- Dual energy computed tomography • Renal cell carcinoma

KEY POINTS

- There are 4 distinct phases of enhancement of the kidneys: arterial, cortical, medullary, and excretory/pyelographic phases.
- Using various reformatted displays of the renal circulation aids in accurate depiction of the vessels and degree of arterial stenosis.
- It is not always possible to distinguish acute renal arterial occlusion because of dissection versus thromboembolic disease; therefore, adequate angiographic phase acquisition of the aorta and mesenteric vasculature may provide a full picture of the pathology.
- Acute occlusion of the renal artery can be a diagnostic challenge given significant overlap of disease clinical presentation, and complete imaging of the kidneys may aid timely diagnosis (ie, noncontrast, complete angionephrogram, and excretory phases).
- Dual energy computed tomography can eliminate additional radiation by providing virtual noncontrast imaging and may possibly be able to differentiate various subtypes of renal cell carcinoma.

INTRODUCTION

The kidneys are critical organs maintaining fluid and electrolyte balance and hormonal homeostasis. The arterial blood supply is critical to maintaining these homeostatic functions. Renal arterial blood flow may be compromised by a variety of pathologic conditions that affect the pediatric and adult population. These conditions may be clinically suspect or relatively occult.

Modern medicine has produced substantial literature on the indications for and clinical value of varying approaches to imaging the renal arterial circulation. Within the last 20 years, computed tomography (CT) angiography has evolved as the dominant imaging modality that provides high-resolution 2- and 3-dimensional imaging of the renal arterial circulation together with 3-dimensional display of the renal parenchyma and imaging of the renal veins.[1] Doppler renal sonography, more particularly in pediatric and young adult populations, serves a role as an initial screening modality.[2] Magnetic resonance (MR) angiography has also developed into a high-resolution 2- and 3-dimensional imaging process, but spatial resolution is still inferior to that of CT angiography. MR angiography is of most benefit when used in the pediatric population as a nonionizing imaging modality or in adults with renal dysfunction in whom intravenous iodinated contrast material is relatively contraindicated.[3] However, MR in the adult population with renal dysfunction less than an estimated

Department of Radiology, Medical College of Wisconsin, 9200 West Wisconsin Avenue, Milwaukee, WI 53226, USA
* Corresponding author.
E-mail address: falesch@gmail.com

Radiol Clin N Am 54 (2016) 71–86
http://dx.doi.org/10.1016/j.rcl.2015.08.003

glomerular filtration rate value of 30 also runs the potential risk of nephrogenic systemic fibrosis.

In this article, the clinical indications, techniques, and findings associated with the appropriate use of CT angiography are described.

COMPUTED TOMOGRAPHY ANGIOGRAPHY: TECHNIQUE

In the resting state, renal arterial flow constitutes 25% of cardiac output. This flow is distributed most prominently to the renal cortex, which receives 90% of the renal arterial flow input and also constitutes the most rapid flow component with a renal arteriovenous circulation time of 6 seconds. Flow to the renal medulla and renal sinus tissues occurs at a considerably lower rate and smaller volume flow rate component.

After contrast material delivery into the renal circulation, an initial cortical angionephrogram effect is observed reflecting the fast flow rate and volume flow component to the renal cortex. In a healthy young adult, the cortical angionephrogram effect is observed with diminishing cortical to medullary contrast observed up to 80 seconds after injection. In the timeframe of 80 to 120 seconds, renal medullary enhancement increases secondary to glomerular filtration of contrast material resulting in a uniform nephrogram, which is usually observed up to 180 seconds after injection. At that stage, the excretory phase begins with calyceal excretion of contrast material.[4]

On imaging studies, the renal flow physiology results in the sequential appearance of an arterial and venous flow imaging phase with a cortical angionephrogram, a uniform nephrogram phase, and an excretory phase. CT angiography for depiction of the renal arteries preferably uses first circulation contrast bolus with an accompanying well-defined cortical angionephrogram. Concurrent imaging of the main renal vein is caused by the rapid parenchymal contrast circulation from the renal arteries to renal veins.[4]

Appropriate acquisition timing depends on either preliminary mini bolus or bolus tracking software.

High-resolution CT angiographic images are provided by 64-channel and above detector arrays with submillimeter isotropic volume acquisition.

The more modern CT platforms use either a wide detector approach with 256-channel or greater acquisition or a dual source system in a high-pitch mode resulting in rapid acquisition and high temporal resolution.

Contrast material injection and acquisition parameters are critical elements in the production of high-resolution CT angiographic, cortical angiographic, and uniform nephrographic phase display.

Contrast material concentration of 300 mg of iodine per milliliter or greater with an injection rate of 4 to 6 mL/s and contrast volume appropriate for increasing the attenuation of the abdominal aorta and renal arteries by 300 to 400 Hounsfield units is a relatively standard acquisition approach. The volume of contrast material depends on both the duration of acquisition and the patient weight (**Table 1**). In our practice, the standard interval for contrast medium injection is equal to a delay time between the arrival of contrast material in the abdominal aorta and the beginning of acquisition plus the acquisition interval is used (**Fig. 1**). Using preliminary mini bolus technique, the arrival time of contrast material is determined by the time to peak in the abdominal aorta at the level of renal arteries. Only 12 to 15 mL of contrast is needed for this determination. A 4- to 6-second delay between arrival and the beginning of acquisition is used so that imaging is performed during peak aortic enhancement. With an acquisition interval equal to 4 seconds (determined by beam width, pitch, and rotation speed) and a delay time between bolus arrival in the aorta and beginning of scan acquisition equal to 6 seconds, a total contrast material injection interval of 10 seconds is chosen. With an injection rate of 6 mL/s, this results in a total contrast volume of 60 mL.

A sliding scale of total contrast material volume versus patient weight is also used, as larger body weight correlates with higher circulating arterial blood volume, resulting in relative dilution of contrast material bolus. Thus, in patients with larger body weights, a longer contrast medium injection duration and a longer delay between bolus arrival in the aorta and the beginning of scan acquisition are used (**Fig. 2**).

In patients with suspected renal artery stenosis or aneurysm or in patients studied after intravascular

Table 1					
Weight/velocity compensated CT Angiography					
Patient weight (lbs)	<150	151–200	201–250	251–300	>300
Peak plus delay (s)	4–7	7	11	14	14
Contrast volume (mL)	60–80	80–100	100–125	125–140	140–160

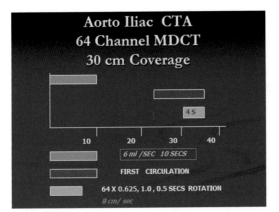

Fig. 1. Schematic illustration of injection/acquisition for renal multidetector CT angiography. Timeline on the X axis. Contrast injection interval of 10 seconds equals the time between the aortic arrival of contrast material (*red arrow*) and the beginning of acquisition (6 seconds) plus the acquisition interval (4 seconds). Table speed is determined by beam width, pitch, and rotation speed. In this illustration, beam width of 4 cm, pitch value of 1, and rotation time of 0.5 seconds results in a table speed of 8 cm/s.

stent placement, a single arterial phase acquisition is usually appropriate. Because of rapid intrarenal circulation and delay between bolus arrival in the aorta and the beginning of scan acquisition, early venous opacification is achieved in this phase.

In patients with known or suspected renal tumor, a dual-phase acquisition of arterial phase plus nephrographic phase is used. Nephrographic phase provides the best definition of renal tumor margins, adjacent renal parenchyma, and renal sinus tissue.

A double pass acquisition is also used in potential renal donors because the arterial phase

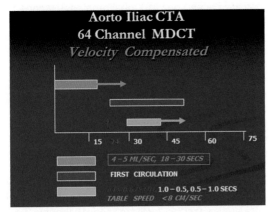

Fig. 2. Adaption to slower flow velocity with lengthening of the injection interval (accompanied by decrease in injection rate) to accommodate a decrease in table speed. The injection acquisition parameters are adjusted flexibly for each patient.

provides optimal delineation of accessory renal arteries, and the nephrographic phase provides a clear display of the renal venous anatomy and identifies the presence or absence of a duplicated collecting system.

RENAL ARTERY STENOSIS

Renal artery stenosis (RAS) is most commonly secondary to atherosclerotic disease. Less often, fibromuscular dysplasia (FMD), radiation, phakomatoses, or radiation therapy can lead to RAS. In the elderly, RAS is a major cause of end-stage renal disease.[5]

RAS may result in renovascular hypertension.[6] RAS is usually unilateral but may be bilateral. Bilateral RAS can result in both renovascular hypertension and renal insufficiency. In patients with solitary or dysplastic kidneys, RAS to the normal kidney may result in hypertension and renal insufficiency. RAS results in a decrease in pulse pressure distal to the stenosis, which is sensed as inadequate flow to the glomeruli by the juxtaglomerular apparatus, resulting in release of renin and activation of the renin-angiotensin-aldosterone system. Although the hormone response is appropriate in maintaining glomerular perfusion, it can result in systemic hypertension.[7] Renovascular hypertension is suspected in young adult patients with otherwise undiagnosed systemic hypertension, in middle age or older adults in whom hypertension is resistant to standard 3-drug medical regimens, patients with hypertension with rapid progression, or patients in whom the initial onset of severe hypertension is rapid.[6]

The most common cause of RAS in the young adult population is fibrodysplastic disease, and atherosclerosis in the middle age to elderly population. Fibrodysplastic renal artery disease is most common in young adult women and typically involves the mid and distal main renal artery or primary division branches. It is not uncommonly bilateral and may involve accessory renal arteries. The imaging appearance is most commonly a "string of beads" appearance of medial fibrodysplasia caused by ridges of fibrodysplastic tissue separated by small segments of mildly dilated renal artery (**Fig. 3**).[8]

CT angiography is accurate in displaying almost all but the more limited areas of fibrodysplasia and is superior to MR angiography in this regard. The hemodynamic significance of the stenosis is inferred by the luminal diameter reduction, which, if hemodynamically significant, should be at least 60% to 70% of expected luminal diameter. This is best seen in a combination of subvolume maximal intensity projection (MIP) images and curved plantar reformations.

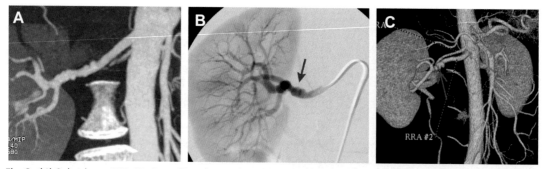

Fig. 3. (A) Subvolume MIP. "String of beads" appearance (arrows) of FMD in the typical distribution of the distal two-thirds of the main renal artery. (B) Digital subtraction angiography correlation of the same artery with FMD (arrow) in (A). (C) Three-dimensional volume-rendered display of FMD (arrow). RRA, right renal artery.

Atherosclerotic renal artery stenosis is common, affecting 6.8% of the adult Medicare population.[9] Unlike fibrodysplastic disease, renal artery atherosclerosis usually involves the ostium or the proximal segment of the main renal arteries and may also involve accessory renal arteries. The disease is often a combination of fibrofatty and fibrocalcific plaque. Both concentric luminal stenosis and eccentric stenosis can occur.[10] As with fibrodysplastic disease, a combination of subvolume MIP and curved plantar reformations best displays the renal artery stenosis (Fig. 4).

Although the Renal Artery Diagnostic Imaging Study in Hypertension (RADISH) trial has questioned the usefulness of CT angiography for the evaluation of RAS, subsequent studies using newer, more advanced CT technology with thinner sections have shown more accurate and reliable results when using reformatted images and automated analysis software for the diagnoses of significant atherosclerotic stenosis and FMD.[7,11–13] One study found sensitivity/specificity of 96%/90% and positive predictive value/negative predictive value of 85%/95% for atheromatous stenosis of greater than 50% when using automated vessel analysis software that is edited by a radiologist.[11] Another study found 100% sensitivity for detection of FMD with CT angiography when interpreted with image reconstructions (multiplanar reformat [MPR], MIP, and shaded-surface display) and subsequently confirmed by conventional angiography.[8]

MR angiography and CT angiography also have comparable negative predictive values for significant renal artery stenosis.[7]

Although hemodynamically significant fibrodysplastic disease in a young adult patient may be treated by transluminal angioplasty with or without stent, atherosclerotic renal artery stenosis is usually treated medically. Most cases of atherosclerotic renal artery stenosis are detected on CT imaging performed for reasons other than suspected renovascular hypertension. Only in patients with severe hypertension resistant to 3-drug regimens or patients with sudden acceleration of hypertension would interventional angiography be considered appropriate.[14]

Another potential outcome of atherosclerotic renal artery disease is progressive renal insufficiency in patients with a solitary kidney, an atrophic dysplastic or hydronephrotic kidney with relatively normal opposite kidney, or bilateral renal artery stenoses. In these circumstances, angioplasty treatment may be used to preserve renal function.[15,16]

RENAL ARTERY ANEURYSMS

Aneurysms of the renal arteries are rare, seen in 0.01% to 0.1% of the population.[17] Although they are uncommon, they account for 22% of aneurysms of arteries supplying the viscera, second only to splenic artery aneurysms. Most aneurysms are related to atherosclerosis. Less commonly they are caused by FMD, phakomatoses, connective tissue disease, or pregnancy. Pseudoaneurysms usually occur after trauma, infections, or vasculitides. Aneurysms are typically asymptomatic but can cause back pain or secondary hypertension related to embolic phenomenon or compression of the artery itself. Aneurysms less than 2 cm are typically followed up with and managed conservatively. Interventions are typically reserved for aneurysms larger than 2 cm, symptomatic patients, or pregnant (or anticipated pregnancy) women, as the risk for death from rupture is significantly higher in this population.[18]

Four types of aneurysms have been described: intrarenal, saccular, fusiform, and dissecting. The saccular type is usually found with FMD and atherosclerotic disease and usually distally located within the main renal artery (Fig. 5). The fusiform types usually occur with FMD and usually

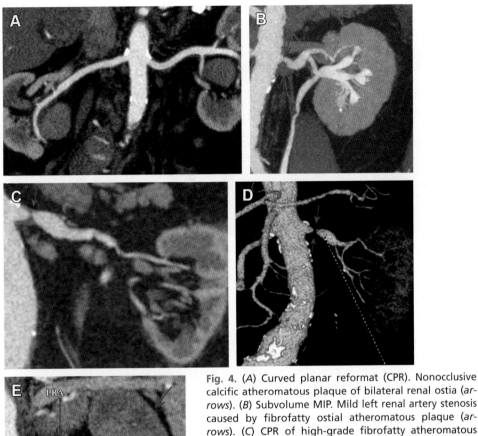

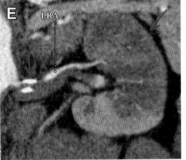

Fig. 4. (*A*) Curved planar reformat (CPR). Nonocclusive calcific atheromatous plaque of bilateral renal ostia (*arrows*). (*B*) Subvolume MIP. Mild left renal artery stenosis caused by fibrofatty ostial atheromatous plaque (*arrows*). (*C*) CPR of high-grade fibrofatty atheromatous proximal left renal artery stenosis (*arrows*). (*D*) Three-dimensional volume-rendered display of the stenosis (*arrows*) demonstrated in (*C*). (*E*) CPR display of occlusive in-stent stenosis (*arrow*) with superior midrenal infarct (*arrow*) in a patient with a proximal left renal arterial (LRA) stent.

do not calcify (**Fig. 6**). The dissecting type often occurs with trauma or may be spontaneous in the setting of atherosclerosis or FMD. The intrarenal type can be seen with the vasculitides, infectious disease, FMD, or atherosclerosis (**Fig. 7**).[10]

Renal artery aneurysms can be accurately portrayed with CT angiography. The use of multiplanar and curved-planar reformatted images improves vessel display when arteries are tortuous. Utilization of thin sections improves sensitivity for small aneurysms; however, small intrarenal aneurysms are often beyond the spatial resolution of systems currently in use.

Mural calcification of renal artery aneurysms is common and even thought to be somewhat protective against rupture.[19] This calcification typically appears as a continuous or partial calcified

rim along the aneurysmal wall on noncontrast CT or even radiographs (**Fig. 8**). Mural thrombus of aneurysms is common, usually only evident as a focal filling defect or nonenhancement at the time of CT angiography.

RENAL ANOMALIES

Renal anomalies including horseshoe kidney and crossed renal ectopia are well characterized on CT angiographic studies that include a nephrographic phase component. Anomalies are usually not of clinical importance unless there are associated disease processes, such as renal tumors or arterial aneurysms that require operative intervention. In these circumstances, high-resolution CT angiography is important in showing anomalous vessels, origin of anomalous renal arteries in

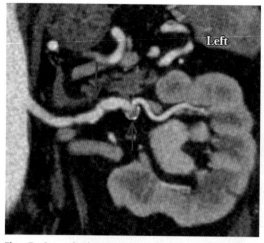

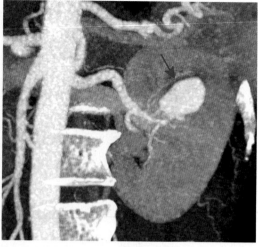

Fig. 5. Curved planar reformat display of saccular aneurysm at the bifurcation of the left renal artery with mural thrombus and calcification (*lateral arrow*). Note the mild luminal irregularity of the mid and distal renal artery secondary to FMD (*medial arrow*), just proximal to the aneurysm.

Fig. 7. Subvolume MIP display of intrarenal saccular aneurysm (*arrow*) in the setting of FMD. Note the subtle luminal irregularity of the mid and distal main renal artery secondary to FMD.

relation to possible aortic aneurysms, and the feeding vessels supplying renal tumor (**Fig. 9**).

Patients with anomalies may also have associated hydronephrosis, and demarcation of the pyelocalyceal system and ureters is important. In these patients, the CT angiographic study is best complimented by a delayed excretory phase study to show the upper tracts.

ACUTE RENAL ARTERY OCCLUSIVE DISEASE: DISSECTION AND THROMBOEMBOLISM

Arterial dissection is the most common cause of acute occlusion of the renal artery. Renal artery thromboembolism is actually uncommon and typically results from a cardiac or aortic source. Even less commonly, acute occlusion can occur

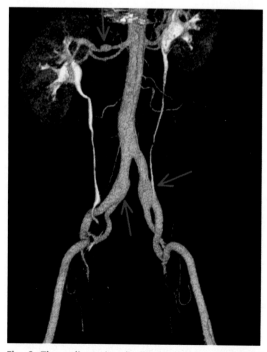

Fig. 6. Three-dimensional volume-rendered display of fusiform ectasia of the common iliac arteries (*inferior 2 arrows*) with fusiform abdominal aortic aneurysm and fusiform aneurysm of the right renal artery (*superiormost arrow*) in the setting of Ehlers-Danlos syndrome.

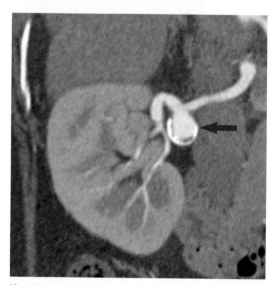

Fig. 8. Curved planar reformat display of another saccular aneurysm with mural thrombus and calcification arising from the distal, perihilar right renal artery.

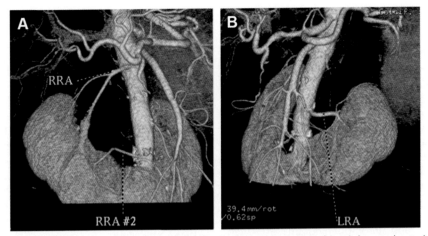

Fig. 9. Three-dimensional volume-rendered display of a horseshoe kidney and its right renal arteries (RRA) (*A*) and left renal artery (LRA) (*B*).

because of hypercoagulability, vasculitis, paraneoplastic syndrome, venous occlusion, and dehydration.[10] Renal infarction or acute loss of renal function caused by acute thrombosis in a chronically stenotic artery is not a frequent occurrence, owing to relative ischemia causing increased recruitment of collateral circulation over time.

Unfortunately, the diagnosis of acute renal artery occlusion can be difficult, as symptoms and clinical findings are often vague or nonspecific, manifesting as nausea and vomiting, back or flank pain, or hematuria, with or without fever or leukocytosis.[10] These symptoms overlap with urolithiasis and retroperitoneal hematoma, which are typically imaged by a noncontrast technique. Although detection can be difficult and often delayed, the window for parenchymal salvage remains narrow (60–90 min), as collateral circulation is virtually nonexistent in the acute setting.[20] Ideally, CT studies for this indication would be tailored to include a noncontrast component, an arterial phase component to delineate the arterial obstruction, and a nephrographic-phase component to better delineate the extent of renal infarction.

Renal artery dissection may be a primary renal artery process limited to the main renal artery or its intrarenal branches or may be from extension of an aortic dissection. In such latter cases of renal artery dissection resulting from an aortic dissection, flow to the involved kidney may be significantly compromised, leading to renal infarction. The primary diagnostic criteria is presence of an intraluminal flap, usually imaged when the process involves a main renal artery, particularly in association with an aortic dissection, but more difficult to detect if the dissection only involves a primary division branch.

Renal artery dissection can also be a manifestation of fibrodysplastic disease, in which case multifocal or bilateral involvement is possible (**Fig. 10**).[21]

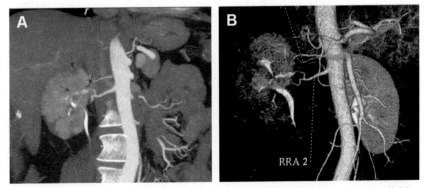

Fig. 10. (*A*) Subvolume MIP display of renal artery dissection involving a superior primary division of the renal artery (*central arrows*) with multifocal renal cortical infarcts (more *peripheral arrows*) in the setting of relatively advanced FMD. (*B*) Three-dimensional volume-rendered display of the same patient in (*A*). The smaller peripheral arrows denote the wedge-shaped defects of the cortical renal infarcts. RRA, right renal arteries.

An unusual cause of abdominal aortic and renal artery dissection is cocaine abuse (**Fig. 11**).

Another uncommon cause of renal artery dissection is a systemic connective disorder, such as Ehlers-Danlos syndrome, which can result in the combination of main artery and branch aneurysms and intrarenal artery dissections.

In the elderly, thromboembolism (typically originating in the heart) in the setting of subtherapeutic international normalized ratio can be a rare cause of acute renal infarct.[22] Renal arterial emboli are often associated with emboli to other abdominal visceral arteries and the extremities (**Fig. 12**).[23] The embolus may involve the main or segmental renal artery and result in complete or partial renal infarction.

Dissection and thromboembolism are often indistinguishable because of the small size of the vessel and rapid thrombosis of dissection. Typically, acute renal artery occlusion appears as abrupt cutoff or luminal nonenhancement at and beyond the level of the occlusion. Depending on the location of occlusion, the only findings may be secondary parenchymal changes/nonvascular findings, including the classic wedge-shaped area, or asymmetric hypoenhancement, asymmetric perinephric fat stranding, or diffuse/segmental swelling (**Fig. 13**).[24] Additionally, because capsular arteries often arise proximal to the occlusion, there can be minimal perfusion to the supplied subcapsular parenchyma that can occur, leading the "capsular rim" sign. This sign results in a thin rim of persistent contrast enhancement relative to the ischemic, deeper tissue. Although this phenomenon can be apparent within hours of ischemic onset, it is more often evident days later.[10,22]

RENAL TRAUMA

Renal injuries most commonly occur after blunt trauma, typically secondary to sudden deceleration during motor vehicle collisions. Blunt renal trauma accounts for 80% to 90% of all renal injuries, with the remainder owing to penetrating

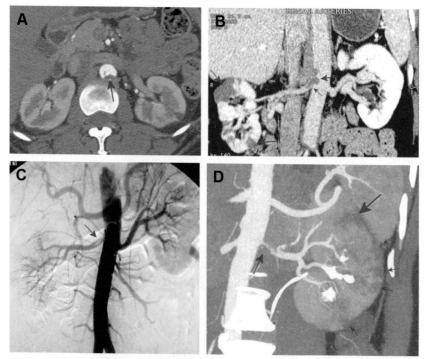

Fig. 11. Cocaine-induced hypertensive aortorenal dissection with multifocal right renal infarcts. (*A*) Axial image shows the aortic component with dissection flap and posterior luminal thrombus (*arrow*). (*B*) Direct extension of the aortic dissection with thrombus into the proximal right renal artery (*medial/central arrows*) and multiple wedge-shaped cortical infarcts of the right kidney (*right lateral/peripheral arrows*) caused by embolic disease. (*C*) Digital subtraction angiographic correlative image obtained for preoperative planning shows the luminal filling defect into the proximal right renal artery (*arrow*). (*D*) A subsequent CT of the same patient was obtained at a later date. A coronal subvolume MIP display shows a second, subsequent cocaine-induced hypertensive dissection, now of the left renal artery (*medial arrow*), with embolic disease causing multiple peripheral wedge-shaped cortical infarcts of the left (*peripheral/lateral arrows*).

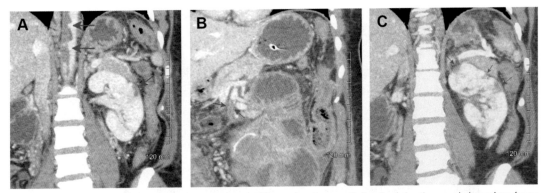

Fig. 12. (*A*) Coronal MPR. Relatively long segment of irregular thoracoabdominal aortic mural thrombus (superior 2 *arrows*) at the level of the aortic hiatus, note the left lateral renal wedge-shaped hypoenhancing infarct secondary to embolism. (*B*) Coronal MPR in the same patient shows embolus in the superior mesenteric artery several centimeters distal to the origin of the artery. The arrows are on either side of the superior mesenteric artery at the level of the linear hypoattenuating luminal thrombus, with the artery surrounded by periarterial fat. (*C*) Note the multifocal left renal infarcts on this coronal MPR in the same patient caused by embolic disease to the left renal artery (*arrows*).

trauma.[25] Like liver and splenic injuries, renal injuries are now commonly classified by a grading system devised by the American Association for the Surgery of Trauma, which takes into account size and location of hematoma, laceration, or contusion and involvement of the vascular pedicle.[26]

Most renal injuries are localized to the renal cortex (grades 1–3) and are treated conservatively. Persistent hemorrhage secondary to pseudoaneurysm, arteriovenous fistula, or arteriocalyceal fistula, is usually manifested clinically by persistent hematuria and is an indication for endovascular intervention (**Fig. 14**).

Severe trauma may result in renal artery occlusion secondary to dissection and thrombosis or to renal artery transection and massive retroperitoneal bleeding. Rarely, severe trauma results in transection or even avulsion of the vascular pedicle. In such cases, rapid exsanguination and cardiovascular collapse may be encountered because of the relatively high cardiac output to the kidneys. As such, immediate operative management may be preferred to CT because of the grave clinical status of these patients.[25]

High-grade renal injuries include collecting system disruption, where distinction of extravasated enhanced blood and urine becomes critical. Any patient with renal trauma examined by CT scanning in the emergency room setting requires physician evaluation after the initial angionephrographic phase acquisition to determine whether delayed

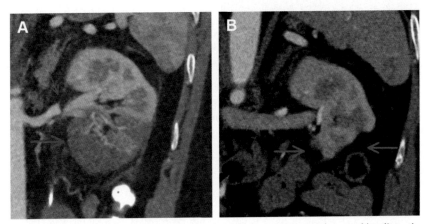

Fig. 13. (*A*) Abrupt cutoff of the prehilar left main renal artery (*superior arrow*) caused by dissection with acute, swollen inferior polar renal infarct (*inferior arrow*). (*B*) Subsequent CT of the same patient as *A* now shows the cortical scarring and retraction from the infarct (*arrows*).

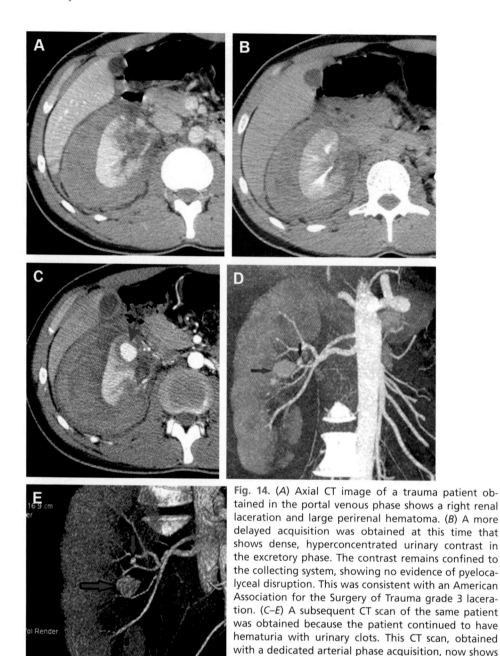

Fig. 14. (A) Axial CT image of a trauma patient obtained in the portal venous phase shows a right renal laceration and large perirenal hematoma. (B) A more delayed acquisition was obtained at this time that shows dense, hyperconcentrated urinary contrast in the excretory phase. The contrast remains confined to the collecting system, showing no evidence of pyelocalyceal disruption. This was consistent with an American Association for the Surgery of Trauma grade 3 laceration. (C–E) A subsequent CT scan of the same patient was obtained because the patient continued to have hematuria with urinary clots. This CT scan, obtained with a dedicated arterial phase acquisition, now shows a relatively large, previously occult pseudoaneurysm (arrow on C). Also displayed as an MIP (D) and volume-rendered (E) reformat. Both of these reformatted images show 2 renal arteries, with the relatively large (larger lateral arrow) and a smaller adjacent pseudoaneurysm (smaller superomedial arrow) arising from branches of the more inferior of the 2 arteries.

imaging is required for satisfactory evaluation of suspected calyceal disruption.

Currently, conventional angiography is reserved for therapeutic intervention or uncertainty at the time of CT angiography rather than for diagnostic purposes.[25]

RENAL TRANSPLANTS

Approximately 15,000 renal transplant procedures are performed annually in the United States. Potential living renal donors now contribute to a large proportion of renal transplant procedures.[27] The potential donors are evaluated for the suitability of their native kidneys with particular emphasis on excluding renal artery pathologic findings including fibrodysplastic disease, demonstrating the first bifurcation point of the main renal artery in relation to the aortic orifice, demonstration of accessory renal arteries, and the presence of single or multiple renal veins (**Fig. 15**). Most living donor kidneys are now harvested laproscopically, and the smaller surgical field of view increases the importance of detailed anatomic information before surgery.

Modern CT angiography is considered the best modality for preoperative evaluation.[28–30] Preoperative CT evaluation typically consists of a precontrast/noncontrast acquisition, arterial phase acquisition, and some combination of parenchymal and pyelographic phases. The noncontrast CT is primarily for the evaluation of vascular calcifications and nephrolithiasis.[28]

An obvious advantage of CT angiography over conventional angiography is that the parenchyma can be evaluated by the same study. Crossed ectopia or horseshoe kidneys are readily apparent at CT and contraindicated for donation. Similarly, other pathologic findings such as neoplasms, polycystic kidney disease, and medullary sponge kidney are also easily identified on CT and are generally considered contraindications.

Presurgical knowledge of multiple renal arteries and their location is critical. Accessory renal arteries arise separately from the aorta or iliac arteries and include arteries directly supplying the poles of the kidney (polar arteries). Prehilar or early bifurcating arteries originate 1.5 to 2 cm from the ostium. Occasionally, these prehilar vessels can prevent adequate arterial anastomosis at the time of transplant. Having more than 2 renal arteries is a relative contraindication for donation,

occurring about 5% of the time.[28] Donation is still possible with 3 arteries provided the third artery supplies a relatively small proportion of renal blood flow and can, therefore, be sacrificed. Important measurements for the surgeon include length of the right main renal artery to its first bifurcation, the distance from the right inferior vena cava (IVC) margin to the right renal artery's first bifurcation and the length of the left renal artery to its first bifurcation. The surgeon also needs to know if there is intra- versus extrahilar segmental bifurcation.[28]

Renal vein anatomy varies less often than arterial anatomy. If there is more than one renal vein, it typically occurs on the right and occurs up to 15% of the time.[31] Generally, the left kidney is preferred for nephrectomy because of the longer renal vein. Circumaortic (6% of donors) and retro-aortic (3% of donors) are the most common of the left renal venous variants and are typically not considered contraindications. Most frequently, there are no tributaries to the right renal vein; however, 30% of right adrenal, 7% of right gonadal, and 3% hemiazygos or lumbar veins drain into the right renal vein. On the other hand, the left renal vein typically receives the left adrenal and left gonadal veins, with the inferior phrenic and capsular veins typically draining directly into the left adrenal vein. Measurements required for the surgeon include length of the right renal vein from the IVC to its segmental confluence, length of the left renal vein from the IVC to its segmental confluence, and the length from the left renal vein segmental confluence to the left margin of the aorta.[28]

Congenital anomalies of the proximal collecting system are also readily apparent on CT, especially opacified systems in the pyelographic phase. Although duplications are not

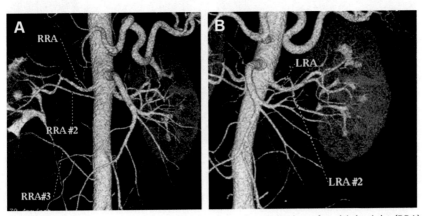

Fig. 15. Potential renal donor. Three-dimensional volume-rendered display of multiple right (RRA) (*A*) and left (LRA) (*B*) renal arteries.

necessarily a contraindication for harvesting, severe hydronephrosis, papillary necrosis, and transitional cell carcinoma are contraindications for transplantation.[28]

Potential renal transplant recipients require imaging of the aortoiliac system to determine a suitable implant site for the donor renal artery to the iliac arteries, most commonly the external iliac artery. In patients without known aneurysm or evident peripheral vascular disease, a noncontrast CT examination is used to determine the extent of iliac artery vascular calcification, providing the transplant surgeon information on the suitability of a likely implant site.

After successful renal transplantation, the most used postoperative imaging study is renal sonography, which can evaluate transplant morphology, hydronephrosis, peritransplant fluid collections, and possible arterial stenosis or venous thrombosis. In patients with suspected transplant arterial anastomotic stenosis, a Doppler ultrasound scan can be followed by a preintervention CT angiographic study with emphasis, as with native kidneys, on the subvolume MIP and curved planar reformations to evaluate for the suspected transplant renal artery stenosis (Fig. 16).

RENAL TUMORS

Renal cell carcinoma (RCC) is believed to represent more than 80% of kidney malignancies. Kidney and renal pelvis malignancies account for 61,500 new cancer diagnoses and more than 14,000 deaths in 2015.[32] More than 60% of newly diagnosed RCCs are discovered incidentally by imaging.[33] Although most renal malignancies are RCC, differentiation between RCC and hypervascular angiomyolipoma (AML) is important. AMLs are benign hamartomas contain varying amounts of abnormal blood vessels, smooth muscle, and adipose tissue. Typically,

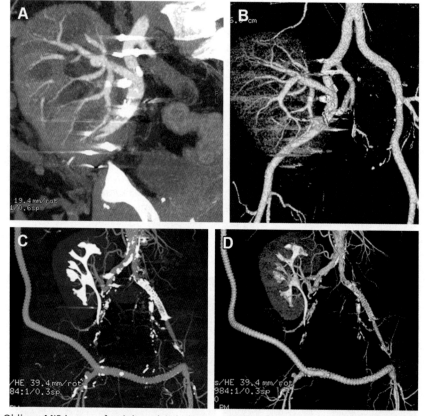

Fig. 16. (A) Oblique MIP image of a right pelvic kidney transplant. Vascular clips cause adjacent metallic artifact without obscuring the normally patent main renal artery. (B) Three-dimensional volume-rendered image of the same transplant in (A). (C) MIP reformatted image of a right pelvic renal transplant shows a normally patent main renal artery and opacification of the collecting system in a patient with patent axillofemoral and femoral-femoral arterial bypass grafts. End-to-side anastomosis of the transplant renal artery to the distal most patent aspect of the more distally occluded right common iliac artery (arrow). A left common iliac arterial stent is also in place. (D) Three-dimensional volume-rendered reformatted image of the same patient in (C).

demonstration of macroscopic adipose tissue within a renal lesion is considered diagnostic of AML (**Figs. 17** and **18**). However, approximately 5% of AML are lipid poor and undetectable by CT, and lipid rich RCCs have been described. In these instances, an imaging overlap exists between the 2 entities. One study suggests that differential enhancement on a multiphasic CT and precontrast appearance of the lesions may differentiate between the various subtypes of RCC and AML.[34,35] Additionally, MRI with fat suppression or chemical shift imaging may increase sensitivity for diagnostic findings of AML.[34] Although there are multiple potential differentiating characteristics using multiphasic CT and MR, ultimately, biopsy or excision may be required for diagnosis.

Isolated hypervascular metastatic disease to the kidney is extremely rare and has been described in patients with metastatic neuroendocrine tumor or even synchronous or metachronous contralateral RCC. Other metastatic lesions including primary lung tumor or melanoma tend to be relatively hypovascular.

Because most RCCs are incidentally discovered, more are found at early stages and smaller sizes allowing for subtotal nephrectomy or nephron-sparing surgery and percutaneous ablation techniques. As such, comprehensive imaging with CT angiography is an important part of preoperative planning at many institutions.

A well-known phenomenon of RCC is its tendency to invade vasculature, with renal vein invasion occurring 25% to 30% of the time and IVC invasion 7% of the time. Therefore, careful evaluation of these structures on CT angiography is critical for RCC staging. Furthermore, the increased surgical complexity introduced with nephron-sparing surgery and introduction of percutaneous ablation techniques have increased the importance of a good 3-dimensional representation of the kidney, tumor, and vascular association. CT can show both bland venous thrombosis and tumor thrombus.[36] Bland thrombosis typically appears as a hypoattenuating filling defect in the vascular system. Tumor thrombus detection may be more difficult, but some enhancement in the filling defect will correctly identify its malignant nature. When there is extension of tumor thrombus into the IVC, description of the cephalad extent of thrombus is important planning information for the surgeon (**Figs. 19** and **20**).

Dual-energy CT may be helpful for the differentiation of RCC subtypes. Clear cell and papillary RCC are the 2 most common subtypes, accounting for 70% to 80% and 14% to 20% of variants, respectively. Differentiation between the 2 is clinically relevant because both prognosis and clinical treatments differ. The clear cell variant is classically described to be a hypervascular lesion, whereas papillary is relatively hypovascular. One dual-energy CT study suggests there is good discrimination between the 2 variants using iodine quantification, with an overall accuracy of 95%. This finding also suggests stratification of tumor grade is possible at the extremes, with some limitation differentiating between grades II and III.[37] Dual energy CT used for staging also provides the benefit of a virtual noncontrast CT, eliminating the radiation dose associated with a separate acquisition (**Fig. 21**).[38]

RENAL VOLUME FLOW DETERMINATIONS

Intravenous angiographic techniques, both CT angiography and MR angiography, provide a morphologic display of the renal arteries and sites of suspected significant stenosis. The hemodynamic significance of a stenosis can be inferred by the degree of luminal diameter reduction and the presence of collateral circulation. Doppler sonography is also valuable if the main renal artery stenosis is associated with a tardus parvus intrarenal arterial flow waveform indicating a significant drop in pulse pressure across the stenosis.

Additional information on the hemodynamic significance of a renal artery stenosis can be obtained by volume flow determinations of

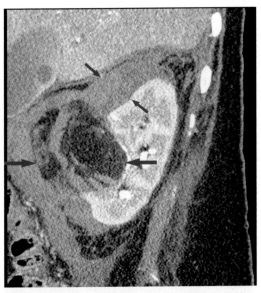

Fig. 17. Large central/hilar angiomyolipoma shows macroscopic fat (larger 2 inferior *arrows*). Note the perirenal hematoma (smaller 2 superior *arrows*); rupture and bleeding is a well-known complication of larger angiomyolipomas.

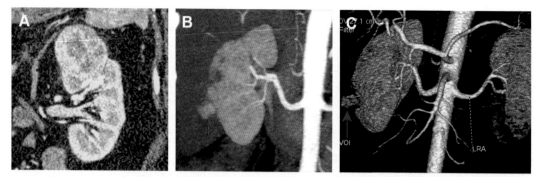

Fig. 18. (A) Large, heterogeneous hypervascular and exophytic superior polar left renal cell carcinoma (arrows). Curved planar reformat (B) and 3-dimensional volume-rendered (C) displays of a small, exophytic right renal cell carcinoma (arrow). LRA, left renal artery.

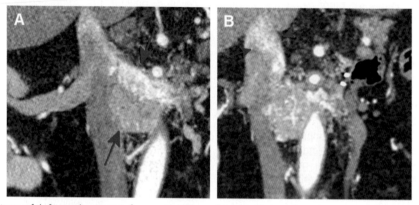

Fig. 19. History of left nephrectomy for renal cell carcinoma. The patient has a vascular/enhancing tumor thrombus expanding the left renal vein (A, arrows) extending into the IVC (B, arrows).

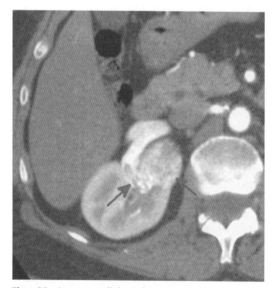

Fig. 20. Anteromedial right renal cell carcinoma (medial arrow) with extension of vascular tumor into the hilar portion of the right renal vein (lateral arrow). This is an arterial phase image (note hyperdense contrast in the aorta) and early filling of the right renal vein, indicative of arteriovenous fistula.

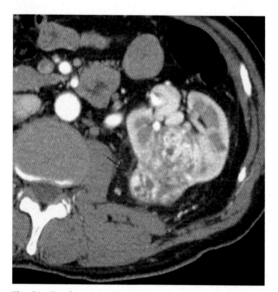

Fig. 21. Dual energy CT. Monoenergetic acquisition of an exophytic, hypervascular posteromedial left renal cell carcinoma (arrow), obtained at 70 keV.

contrast-enhanced CT angiography or MR angiography. Because of increased radiation dose associated with contrast-enhanced multiacquisition CT flow rate determinations (even with radiation-reducing techniques such as iterative reconstruction), MR angiography has been used in selected research settings in comparing volume flow in the normal compared with the suspected abnormal kidney. This information may be useful in determining suitability for endovascular intervention and can be used after interventional procedures to determine volume flow rate improvement.[39]

SUMMARY

High-resolution imaging of vascular and organ anatomy is the primary value of CT angiographic studies and is well illustrated in CT angiography of the renal circulation. From the technical perspective, important aspects are an appropriate choice of injection/acquisition protocol, which exploits the inherent submillimeter high-resolution volumetric acquisition using 64-channel or greater wide detector systems or high-pitched dual tube systems. A standard display of high-resolution images in the axial plane complimented with volume rendering, subvolume MIP, and curved planar reformation provides a suitable template for diagnosis and determining appropriate treatment. It is important for radiologists to understand the technical capabilities of modern CT scanners to effectively use them with appropriate injection/acquisition techniques tailored to the clinical question raised. Not only has the image quality of CT scanners improved over the last decade, but this been accompanied by improvement in 3-dimensional display techniques tailored to potential clinical interventions, achieved with decreasing levels of radiation dose subsequent to the introduction of iterative reconstruction. Several CT angiography applications in the renal circulation have become particularly valuable in routine clinical practice, including evaluation of suspected renal artery stenosis, occlusion, aneurysm, and the pre- postoperative evaluation of renal transplants.

REFERENCES

1. Tuna IS, Tatli S. Contrast-enhanced CT and MR imaging of renal vessels. Abdom Imaging 2014;39(4):875–91.
2. Castelli PK, Dillman JR, Kershaw DB, et al. Renal sonography with doppler for detecting suspected pediatric renin-mediated hypertension – is it adequate? Pediatr Radiol 2013;44(1):42–9.
3. Pei Y, Shen H, Li J, et al. Evaluation of renal artery in hypertensive patients by unenhanced MR angiography using spatial labeling with multiple inversion pulses sequence and by CT Angiography. Am J Roentgenol 2012;199(5):1142–8.
4. Foley WD. Renal MDCT. Eur J Radiol 2003;45(Suppl 1):S73–8.
5. Safian RD, Textor SC. Renal-artery stenosis. N Engl J Med 2001;344(7):431–42.
6. Fauci AS, Harrison TR. Harrison's manual of medicine. 17th edition. New York: McGraw-Hill; 2008.
7. Rountas C, Vlychou M, Vassiou K, et al. Imaging modalities for renal artery stenosis in suspected renovascular hypertension: prospective intraindividual comparison of color Doppler US, CT angiography, GD-enhanced MR angiography, and digital subtraction angiography. Ren Fail 2007;29(3): 295–302.
8. Sabharwal R, Vladica P, Coleman P. Multidetector spiral CT renal angiography in the diagnosis of renal artery fibromuscular dysplasia. Eur J Radiol 2007; 61(3):520–7.
9. Hansen KJ, Edwards MS, Craven TE, et al. Prevalence of renovascular disease in the eldery: a population-based study. J Vasc Surg 2002;36(3): 443–51.
10. Kawashima A, Sandler CM, Ernst RD, et al. CT evaluation of renovascular disease. Radiographics 2000;20(5):1321–40.
11. Pellerin O, Sapoval M, Trinquart L, et al. Accuracy of multidetector computer tomographic angiography assisted by post-processing software for diagnosis atheromatous renal artery stenosis. Diagn Interv Imaging 2013;94:1123.
12. Fraioli F, Catalano C, Bertoletti L, et al. Multidetector-row CT angiography of renal artery stenosis in 50 consecutive patients: prospective interobserver comparison with DSA. Radiol Med 2006;111(3): 459–68.
13. Vasbinder GB, Nelemans PJ, Kessels AG, et al. Renal Artery Diagnostic Imaging Study in Hypertension (RADISH) Study Group. Accuracy of computed tomographic angiography and magnetic resonance angiography for diagnosing renal artery stenosis. Ann Intern Med 2004;141(9):674–82.
14. Modrall JG, Rosero EB, Timaran CH, et al. Assessing outcomes to determine whether symptoms related to hypertension justify renal artery stenting. J Vasc Surg 2012;55(2):413–9.
15. Modrall JG, Timaran CH, Rosero EB, et al. Predictors of outcome for renal artery stenting performed for salvage of renal function. J Vasc Surg 2011; 54(5):1414–21.
16. Bush RL, Martin LG, MacDonald MJ, et al. Endovascular revascularization of renal artery stenosis in the solitary functioning kidney. Ann Vasc Surg 2001; 15(1):60–6.
17. Bulbul MA, Farrow GA. Renal artery aneurysms. Urology 1992;40(2):124–6.

18. Sabharwal R, Vladica P, Law WP, et al. Multidetector spiral CT renal angiography in the diagnosis of giant renal artery aneurysms. Abdom Imaging 2006;31(3): 374–8.

19. Schorn B, Falk V, Dalichau H, et al. Kidney salvage in a case of ruptured renal artery aneurysm: case report and literature review. Cardiovasc Surg 1997; 5(1):134–6.

20. Kaufman JA, Lee MJ. Vascular and interventional radiology: the requisites. 2nd edition. Philadelphia: Mosby; 2014.

21. Olin JW, Froehlich J, Gu X, et al. The United States Registry for fibromuscular dysplasia: results in the first 447 patients. Circulation 2012;125(25):3182–90.

22. Hazanov N, Somin M, Attali M, et al. Acute renal embolism. Forty-four cases of renal infarction in patients with atrial fibrillation. Medicine (Baltimore) 2004;83(5):292–9.

23. Rajkovic Z, Zelic Z, Papes D, et al. Synchronous celiac axis and superior mesenteric artery embolism. Vasa 2011;40(6):495–8.

24. Suzer O, Shirkhoda A, Jafri SZ, et al. CT features of renal infarction. Eur J Radiol 2002;44(1):59–64.

25. Kawashima A, Sandler CM, Corl FM, et al. Imaging of renal trauma: a comprehensive review. Radiographics 2001;21(3):557–74.

26. Santucci RA, McAnich JW, Safir M, et al. Validation of the American Association for the surgery of trauma organ injury severity scale for the kidney. J Trauma 2001;50(2):195–200.

27. Razavizadeh RT, Tabassi KT, Rana TM. Pre-operative evaluation of living kidney donors using computerized tomographic angiography (CTA) and conventional angiography: comparison with intraoperative findings. Saudi J Kidney Dis Transpl 2012; 23(3):471–6.

28. Sebastia C, Peri L, Salvador R. Multidetector CT of living renal donors: lessons learned from surgeons. Radiographics 2010;30(7):1875–90.

29. Asghari B, Babaei M, Pakroshan B, et al. Role of multidetector computed tomography for evaluation of living kidney donors. Nephrourol Mon 2013;5(4): 870–3.

30. Blondin D, Andersen K, Kroepil P, et al. Analysis of 64-row multidetector CT images for preoperative angiographic evaluation of potential living kidney donors. Radiologe 2008;48(7):673–80 [in German].

31. Kawamoto S, Fishman EK. MDCT angiography of living laparoscopic renal donors. Abdom Imaging 2006;31(3):361–73.

32. American Cancer Society. Cancer facts and figures 2015. Atlanta (GA): American Cancer Society; 2015.

33. Jayson M, Sanders H. Increased incidence of serendipitously discovered renal cell carcinoma. Urology 1998;51:203–5.

34. Farrell C, Noyes SL, Tourojman M, et al. Renal angiomyolipoma: preoperative identification of atypical fat-poor AML. Curr Urol Rep 2015;16:12.

35. Pierorazio PM, Hyams ES, Tsai S, et al. Multiphasic enhancement patterns of small renal masses ($\leq$4 cm) on preoperative computed tomography: utility for distinguishing subtypes of renal cell carcinoma, angiomyolipoma, and oncocytoma. Urology 2013;81(6):1265–71.

36. Xu Y, Shao P, Zhu X, et al. Three-dimensional renal CT angiography for guiding segmental renal artery clamping during laparoscopic partial nephrectomy. Clin Radiol 2013;68(11):609–16.

37. Mileto A, Marin D, Alfaro-Cordoba M, et al. Iodine quantification to distinguish clear cell from papillary renal cell carcinoma at dual-energy multidetector CT: a multireader diagnostic performance study. Radiology 2014;273(3):813–20.

38. Graser A, Johnson TR, Hecht EM, et al. Dualenergy CT in patients suspected of having renal masses: can virtual nonenhanced images replace true nonenhanced images? Radiology 2009;252(2): 433–40.

39. Michaely HJ, Schoenberg SO, Oesingmann N, et al. Renal artery stenosis: functional assessment with dynamic MR perfusion measurements- feasibility study. Radiology 2006;238(2):586–96.

Computed Tomography Angiography of the Small Bowel and Mesentery

Siva P. Raman, MD*, Elliot K. Fishman, MD

KEYWORDS

- Computed tomography angiography (CTA) • Small bowel • Mesenteric ischemia
- Acute gastrointestinal bleeding • Median arcuate ligament syndrome • Small bowel vasculitis
- Mesenteric artery dissection

KEY POINTS

- Positive oral contrast media should be avoided in cases in which small bowel disorder is suspected, because high-density contrast within the bowel may result in beam hardening and streak artifact that can obscure the adjacent bowel wall, thereby preventing the accurate delineation of subtle bowel wall thickening or abnormal bowel wall enhancement.
- Computed tomography (CT) can serve as a valuable diagnostic modality in the evaluation of gastrointestinal (GI) bleeding, allowing delineation of active contrast extravasation, as well as the diagnosis of several other disease entities that might result in GI bleeding.
- Mesenteric ischemia has several different causes, each of which can result in different imaging patterns on CT.

INTRODUCTION

Multidetector computed tomography (MDCT) has supplanted fluoroscopic studies as the first-line imaging modality in patients with suspected small bowel or mesenteric disorders. Unlike fluoroscopy, which has always been limited by its inherently nonspecific findings and inability to evaluate extraluminal abnormalities, MDCT provides a range of information about both bowel and mesenteric findings that is much more likely to allow a specific diagnosis. The advantages of MDCT as a small bowel-imaging tool have increased over the last 2 decades, both as a result of improvements in imaging protocols (including the continued refinement of enterography protocols) and because of improvements in scanner technology. In particular, the latest generation of MDCT scanners (including 64-slice, 128-slice, and dual-source scanners) now offer unparalleled improvements in temporal resolution that allow the reliable acquisition of images at peak arterial enhancement, often with associated improvements in spatial resolution as well. Accordingly, it is now possible to acquire exquisite computed tomography angiography (CTA) images of the bowel, mesentery, and mesenteric vasculature (including second-order and third-order branch vessels), as well as create three-dimensional (3D) reconstructions of extraordinary detail.

These technological developments, and the resultant improvements in CTA imaging, have proved particularly valuable in the evaluation of small bowel vascular and inflammatory disorders, diagnoses in which arterial phase images might be able to offer far greater information than standard venous phase imaging. This article details

Disclosures: The authors have no relevant conflicts of interest or financial disclosures.
Department of Radiology, Johns Hopkins University, JHOC 3251, 601 North Caroline Street, Baltimore, MD 21287, USA
* Corresponding author.
E-mail address: srsraman3@gmail.com

Radiol Clin N Am 54 (2016) 87–100
http://dx.doi.org/10.1016/j.rcl.2015.08.002

the MDCT imaging findings of several small bowel vascular and inflammatory disorders, including mesenteric ischemia, median arcuate ligament syndrome, acute gastrointestinal (GI) bleeding, mesenteric artery dissection, superior mesenteric artery (SMA) syndrome, and Crohn disease, with a special emphasis on the role of CTA findings in the diagnosis of each of these entities.

COMPUTED TOMOGRAPHY PROTOCOLS

The imaging protocols used to evaluate suspected small bowel inflammatory and vascular disorders should vary depending on the acuity of the patient's presentation. In the setting of an acute presentation, oral contrast of any kind should typically be avoided: positive oral contrast should not be administered, because the accumulation of high-density contrast within the bowel may result in beam hardening and streak artifact that can obscure the adjacent bowel wall, thereby preventing the accurate delineation of subtle bowel wall thickening or abnormal bowel wall enhancement. Alternatively, although neutral contrast agents (eg, VoLumen) can be helpful in terms of allowing bowel distension and better accentuating abnormalities of the bowel wall (both in term of thickness and enhancement), many acutely ill patients are not able to ingest the requisite contrast, and, moreover, waiting for the ingestion of the contrast agent may delay treatment in the most acutely sick patients. In our own practice, usually in the emergency room setting, we do not routinely administer oral contrast agents for patients with suspected acute small bowel disorders (eg, ischemia), and instead use water as our agent of choice. We also prefer to avoid administering contrast in cases of suspected acute GI bleeding, because the contrast medium can dilute sites of active extravasation, thereby making them more difficult to identify, and may prove a hindrance for the gastroenterologist if endoscopy is required after the computed tomography (CT) scan.[1] When administering water as our only oral contrast agent, we use a short delay of only 20 to 25 minutes before scanning the patient, so as not to delay the patient's treatment.

Alternatively, for patients with a more subacute or chronic presentation, where there is greater importance placed on the need for good bowel distension, we typically perform our standard CT enterography protocol, with the administration of neutral contrast agents to distend the bowel lumen and improve evaluation of the bowel wall. Although several different agents are available and have been described in the literature, the most widely used agent is barium sulfate (eg,

VoLumen, E-Z-EM, New York), which in our experience is probably the most effective contrast medium for this purpose, albeit still providing variable results because of problems with patient compliance. There is a great deal of variability in the literature regarding the manner in which this contrast may be administered, but in our own practice patients are typically instructed to ingest 450 mL of VoLumen slowly over 10 minutes, followed by additional doses of 450 mL of contrast at 10 and 20 minutes after the first dose, for a total of 1350 mL of contrast. In addition, patients are given 500 mL of water immediately before the scan to distend the stomach and duodenum. In our experience, this oral contrast administration schedule maximizes the odds of distending not only the distal small bowel but the stomach and proximal bowel as well.[1,2]

The administration of intravenous (IV) contrast is of critical importance in these cases, with 100 to 120 mL of nonionic contrast typically injected at a rapid rate (4–5 mL/s). Regardless of whether the patient has an acute or chronic presentation, the use of a dual-phase technique is of paramount importance: arterial phase images are acquired using a bolus trigger (usually at roughly 30 seconds), whereas venous phase images are acquired using a fixed scan delay of roughly 60 seconds (**Box 1**). As is discussed throughout

---

Box 1
Imaging protocols

Imaging protocols for small bowel vascular disorders

- Administer 100 to 120 mL of nonionic IV contrast (4–5 mL/s)

- Arterial phase: bolus trigger during inspiration

- Venous phase: fixed delay at 60 seconds during inspiration

- Avoid oral contrast agents (except water) in patients with suspected GI bleeding or acute presentation

- VoLumen (enterography protocol) in patients with subacute or chronic presentation

  o First dose of VoLumen (slow drink over 10 minutes): 450 mL

  o Second dose of VoLumen (10 minutes after first dose)

  o Third dose of VoLumen (10 minutes after second dose)

  o 500 mL of water immediately before scan

this article, arterial phase images are critical for evaluating the mesenteric vasculature, identifying hyperenhancing small bowel tumors, and for assessing subtle abnormalities in small bowel wall enhancement. In contrast, the venous phase images are the most important for assessing the parenchymal organs of the abdomen, identifying hypovascular small bowel tumors, and for assessing small bowel wall thickening. Although the details of scan acquisition vary depending on the scanner generation, source images in our practice are typically acquired with thin collimation (0.625–0.75 mm), with subsequent reconstruction into 3-mm to 5-mm slices for routine axial image review by the radiologist. Coronal and sagittal multiplanar reformations are automatically created at the scanner by the technologists. In our experience, these multiplanar reformations are critical for providing an all-encompassing overview of the bowel, particularly given that the entirety of the small bowel can be difficult to appreciate on the axial images alone. Global abnormalities in bowel wall thickness or enhancement, as well as the distribution of a bowel abnormality, are often much easier to appreciate in the coronal plane. At the same time, isotropic 0.5-mm to 0.75-mm slices are sent to an independent workstation to allow the generation of 3D reconstructions.[1]

In our own experience, 3D reconstruction methods can be invaluable for the assessment of small bowel abnormalities; in particular, the 2 most important reconstruction methods are (1) maximum intensity projection (MIP) imaging, and (2) volume rendering (VR). MIP imaging entails using a computer algorithm to acquire the highest attenuation voxels in a data set and to project these high-attenuation voxels into a 3D display that can be manipulated by the radiologist. These reconstructions are invaluable in the assessment of the mesenteric vasculature (including the small second-order and third-order branch vessels, which can be visualized on the latest generations of scanners), and can accentuate vascular abnormalities that may not be readily appreciated on the source axial images. VR is a much more computationally complex process (it is beyond the scope of this article) but, in simple terms, it involves using a computer algorithm to assign a specific color and transparency to each voxel in a data set based on both its attenuation and its relationship to adjacent voxels, and then using this information to create an interactive 3D display. VR techniques are more valuable for assessing the bowel wall itself (rather than the vasculature), and can nicely show the 3D relationships of adjacent organs and structures.[1,3–8]

ACUTE ABNORMALITIES
Acute Gastrointestinal Bleeding

The assessment of acute small bowel bleeding has always been problematic, and even though the small bowel accounts for up to 5% of all acute GI bleeding, these cases have always proved difficult to diagnose using any modality.[9] From a gastroenterologist's perspective, the diagnosis of small bowel bleeding is often one of exclusion, typically arrived at after negative upper endoscopy and colonoscopy, with a specific site of bleeding never definitively identified. Although there are some endoscopic methods (eg, push enteroscopy) that allow the gastroenterologist to visualize up to 120 cm beyond the ligament of Treitz, this method still misses a significant amount of the small bowel. Moreover, the method is time-consuming, and is unable to identify cases of intermittent bleeding.[10,11]

Traditional radiologic methods for assessment of small bowel bleeding include tagged red blood cell (RBC) scans and angiography, both of which carry their own downsides. Admittedly, tagged RBC scans are sensitive, capable of detecting bleeding as slow as 0.1 mL/min, and the ability to sequentially scan the patient improves the detection of intermittent bleeding. Nevertheless, these studies are inherently limited by their poor spatial resolution, and even if bleeding is detected the exact site of bleeding can be difficult to identify with confidence (particularly in the small bowel). Moreover, these scans provide no information as to the cause of the bleeding. However, although angiography is an effective modality for the treatment of bleeding, is a poor diagnostic modality, with a sensitivity for only rapid bleeding (usually >1 mL/min), an inability to identify intermittent bleeding, and a limited contrast resolution that makes it difficult to identify subtle sites of bleeding (especially with a nonselective SMA injection). Accordingly, CT has now emerged as an important modality for the assessment of this group of patients, providing reasonable sensitivity (bleeding rates as low as 0.35 mL/min) and the ability to provide additional diagnostic information that may show infectious, inflammatory, or ischemic causes of bleeding (eg, ischemia, Crohn). Although the data regarding the efficacy of CT are still in the early stages, there is at least 1 study that has shown CT to have a sensitivity of up to 92% for acute GI bleeding.[1,4,12,13] Another recent study examining the role of CT in the large bowel found that the overall sensitivity for sites of bleeding increased by 15% in patients who underwent CT before endoscopy, and that CT served as a valuable triage tool in determining which patients might benefit from endoscopy.[14] Another study similarly suggested that, in patients with lower GI bleeding and a negative CTA, the risk of rebleeding was low, with only 22.6% requiring further radiologic or surgical intervention, and with virtually all patients with rebleeding showing signs of hemodynamic instability. This study suggests that CTA can be useful as a triage tool, and that patients with negative CTA and no signs of hemodynamic instability may be managed conservatively.[15]

When performing studies for this indication, proper technique is critical: the acquisition of at least 2 phases is necessary, with the inclusion of arterial phase images being critical for the identification of sites of active extravasation (the most important sign of active bleeding) (Fig. 1). Moreover, contrast must be injected rapidly (at least 4–5 mL/s) in order to maximize the chances of identifying contrast extravasation. Notably, the most important pitfall of interpreting these studies is confusing intrinsically hyperdense material in the bowel (eg, suture, old ingested barium) for a site of bleeding, and differentiating this intrinsically hyperdense material from true bleeding requires cross-referencing the arterial phase images with a second phase (either noncontrast images or venous phase images). Noncontrast images are perhaps the easiest to use, because the presence of hyperdense material can be readily identified and compared with sites of suspected bleeding on the arterial phase images. Alternatively, if venous phase images are acquired, a true bleed should change in both size and morphology between the two phases, whereas intrinsically hyperdense material is unchanged in size and morphology between the two contrast phases (Fig. 2). The extent of contrast extravasation can be variable depending on the rapidity of bleeding, with slower bleeds resulting in subtle pooling of

contrast, whereas brisker bleeds may result in a linear jet of contrast or even fill the lumen of a segment of bowel.[4,11,12] However, even in cases in which active extravasation is not visualized, CT offers the opportunity to diagnose a variety of other abnormalities that may explain the patient's bleeding, such as ischemia, inflammatory bowel disease, small bowel tumor, and arteriovenous malformation, and that is perhaps the greatest advantage of CT compared with other radiologic and endoscopic competitors.

Acute Mesenteric Ischemia

Acute mesenteric ischemia represents a life-threatening disorder with extraordinarily high rates of mortality (~60–80%), largely caused by the large percentage of blood flow normally routed to the small bowel and the extreme sensitivity of the small bowel to diminished blood flow.[16] Acute mesenteric ischemia can be broadly divided into 4 major categories. First, acute arterial occlusion, which is reported to be the most common cause of mesenteric ischemia, accounting for up to 70% of cases. There are a large number of different embolic sources possible, although the most common causes tend to be emboli from the heart in patients with atrial fibrillation, ulcerated atherosclerotic plaque in the aorta, and cardiac thrombus in patients with myocardial infarctions.[17] Emboli often lodge in the proximal aspect of the SMA given its acute angulation at its origin from the aorta, and the entirety of the small bowel distribution may be involved in such cases, although smaller emboli can extend more distally into SMA branches and affect just a short segment of bowel.[18] Although most cases of arterial occlusion result from emboli, in rare instances it can also result from SMA thrombosis in patients

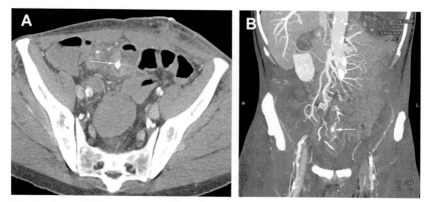

Fig. 1. Axial (A) and coronal MIP reformation (B) in a patient with suspected lower GI bleeding shows a site of active extravasation (arrow) in a small bowel loop located in the deep pelvis. As in this case, MIP reconstructions can be valuable in improving the conspicuity of these often subtle sites of bleeding.

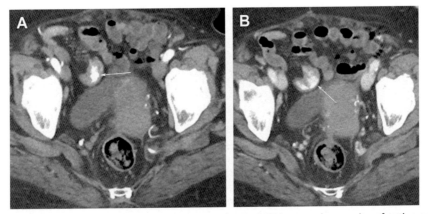

Fig. 2. Axial arterial (*A*) and venous (*B*) phase contrast-enhanced CT images show a site of active extravasation (*arrow*) in a small bowel loop in the right lower quadrant. Note that the extravasation increases in size and changes in shape between the two phases, allowing its differentiation from intrinsically high-attenuation material.

with extensive underlying atherosclerotic disease. Second, acute venous occlusion is an uncommon cause of mesenteric ischemia, accounting for only 10% of all cases, with ischemia typically related to thrombosis of the superior mesenteric vein (SMV). Many of these patients are intrinsically hypercoagulable (with either a known or undiagnosed hypercoagulable syndrome), are using medications that are prothrombotic (eg, oral contraceptives), have undergone complex hepatobiliary surgery that places them at increased risk of SMV thrombosis, or have SMV thrombosis in the setting of septic thrombophlebitis caused by an underlying GI tract infection.[19] Third, nonocclusive mesenteric ischemia (NOMI) results from diminished blood flow to the small bowel in the setting of hypotension secondary to heart failure, cardiogenic shock, renal failure, overly aggressive diuresis, septic shock, and so forth. Some sources suggest that NOMI accounts for roughly 30% of all cases of bowel ischemia, although this is almost certainly an underestimate of this commonly underdiagnosed entity. This entity is almost always diagnosed in critically ill elderly patients in the intensive care unit setting, although can rarely be seen in younger patients using vasoconstrictive drugs (eg, digitalis or cocaine).[1,20] Fourth, complicated bowel obstructions cause ischemia because of strangulation of the arterial and venous blood supply to the bowel, with ischemia most likely in cases of either severe obstructions or closed-loop bowel obstructions with twisting and occlusion of the vascular pedicle supplying the bowel. In such cases, the presence of a bowel obstruction is typically not a diagnostic dilemma, because these patients have acute, severe presentations, but radiologists

must recognize imaging features of superimposed ischemia.[1,21]

Although there is some overlap in the imaging appearance of bowel ischemia resulting from each of these 4 causes, it is important to note that each of these 4 individual causes of bowel ischemia is associated with a unique constellation of imaging findings. Although there is a tendency to equate bowel ischemia with the presence of bowel wall thickening, bowel ischemia caused by arterial occlusion is usually not associated with wall thickening, and the most important imaging finding in such patients is the presence of abnormal hypoenhancement of the bowel wall, often with thinning of the bowel wall over time, especially in the setting of transmural infarction (**Figs. 3** and **4**). In many cases, this hypoenhancement is easier to identify on arterial phase imaging, making dual-phase acquisitions critical in cases of suspected ischemia. These cases can be difficult to diagnose if the abnormal wall enhancement is overlooked, because there is usually a general paucity of adjacent mesenteric fat stranding, edema, and hemorrhage. As the ischemia progresses in these patients, the bowel can dilate, usually suggesting transmural infarction (**Table 1**).

In contrast, ischemia related to venous occlusion is much easier to appreciate, not only because there is usually significant mesenteric edema, fat stranding, and hemorrhage but because the bowel wall is usually markedly thickened with significant mucosal hyperemia. The thickened wall can be hypodense because of submucosal edema or hyperdense as a result of intramural hemorrhage. In cases of venous ischemia (unlike arterial occlusion), the bowel can appear

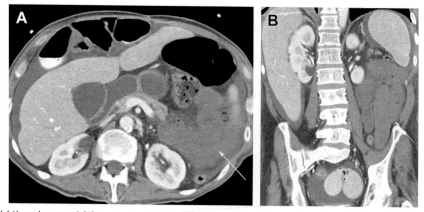

Fig. 3. Axial (*A*) and coronal (*B*) contrast-enhanced images in a patient with an embolus in the SMA (not shown) show diffuse hypoenhancement of the small bowel in the left abdomen (*arrow*), compatible with acute mesenteric ischemia.

dilated even in the absence of true transmural infarction (see **Table 1**).[16,22,23]

However, NOMI does not have a consistent imaging pattern, and can resemble the previously described patterns for either arterial or venous occlusion, or may simply appear as nonspecific bowel wall thickening (**Fig. 5**). However, the diagnosis in these cases is usually strongly suggested by the patient's clinical history. In addition, patients with ischemia caused by complicated bowel obstructions often has features of both arterial and venous occlusion, because the twisting of the vascular pedicle can interrupt both the arterial and venous blood supplies to the bowel (**Figs. 6 and 7**). Some portions of the involved bowel often appear similar to an arterial occlusion, with evidence of bowel wall hypoenhancement but no overt bowel wall thickening, whereas other portions of the involved bowel can appear similar to a venous occlusion, with severe wall thickening and intense mucosal hyperemia. The presence of a closed loop obstruction should always alert the radiologist to the possibility of ischemia, with dilated bowel loops often appearing tethered and radiating to a central point.[16,22,23]

Regardless of the cause of the obstruction, the presence of pneumatosis and portal venous gas is virtually diagnostic of the presence of transmural bowel infarction, with specificities approaching 100% for the presence of ischemia (**Figs. 8**

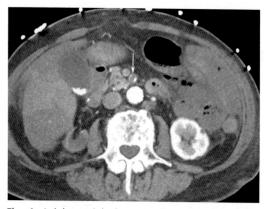

Fig. 4. Axial arterial phase CT shows an embolus in the SMA (*arrow*) with diffuse hypoenhancement of the small bowel in the left abdomen, compatible with acute mesenteric ischemia caused by arterial occlusion.

Table 1 Diagnostic criteria for bowel ischemia: typical imaging findings associated with arterial and venous causes of ischemia	
Arterial Occlusion	**Venous Occlusion**
Typically SMA embolus	SMV thrombosis
No bowel wall thickening	Marked bowel wall thickening
Bowel wall may be paper thin	Bowel wall may be hypodense because of edema or hyperdense because of hemorrhage
No mucosal hyperenhancement	Mucosal hyperenhancement
Bowel dilates only with infarction	Bowel may dilate without infarction
Little mesenteric stranding, hemorrhage, or edema	Usually significant mesenteric inflammation with fluid and hemorrhage

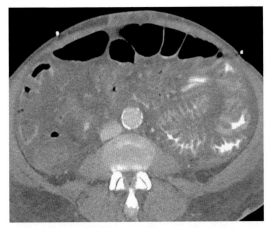

Fig. 5. Axial contrast-enhanced CT in a patient with severe hypotension after myocardial infarction shows diffusely thick-walled small bowel caused by NOMI. This diagnosis should always be suspected when confronted by abnormal-appearing bowel in a patient with a suggestive clinical history.

and 9). However, these findings (particularly pneumatosis) can, in rare cases, be present in nonischemic conditions as well, including in patients who have undergone bowel intervention (eg, a gastrostomy tube or jejunostomy tube), bowel trauma, severe infections, or severe inflammation.[24]

Vasculitis

Vasculitis represents a range of different diseases that result in inflammation and necrosis of the blood vessels, with different types of vasculitis showing involvement of different types of vasculature. In the past, vasculitis has been divided into 3 categories depending on the caliber of vessels involved: large vessel vasculitis, which involves the aorta and its major branches (eg, Takayasu arteritis, giant cell arteritis); medium vessel arteritis (eg, polyarteritis nodosa [PAN], Kawasaki disease); and small vessel vasculitis (eg, lupus vasculitis, Henoch-Schönlein purpura [HSP], Wegner granulomatosis, Behçet disease). Although a detailed discussion of each of these entities is beyond the scope of this article, the entities most likely to involve the small bowel include HSP, lupus vasculitis, Behçet disease, and PAN.[1,25,26]

PAN is a medium vessel vasculitis with a strong tendency to involve the mesenteric arteries (~50% of cases), with the creation of aneurysms at arterial branch points, as well as the development of bowel ischemia, GI hemorrhage, and bowel perforation.[27] HSP is a small vessel vasculitis that is most common in children, but that can affect patients in young adulthood as well, and results in the deposition of immunoglobulin A–predominant complexes on various organs, including the skin, bowel, kidneys, and joints. A sizable percentage of patients with HSP experience bowel involvement (~60%), with the small bowel being most common.[28,29] Imaging findings are typically striking and suggestive of either severe inflammation or ischemia, with evidence of bowel wall thickening, ulceration, mesenteric edema, hemorrhage, ascites, and reactive lymphadenopathy. Young patients with this disorder have a unique tendency to develop intussusceptions in the small bowel caused by hemorrhage and edema in the bowel wall serving as a lead point. Lupus vasculitis is an autoimmune disease that can affect any portion of the bowel because of immune complex deposition, or result in ischemia caused by these patients' hypercoagulability and consequent venous thrombosis. Imaging findings are suggestive of small bowel ischemia or

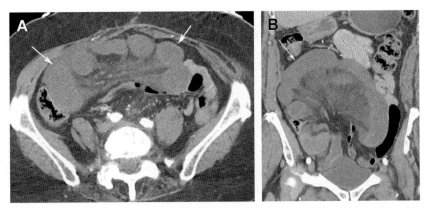

Fig. 6. Axial (*A*) and coronal (*B*) CT images show a closed loop obstruction, with multiple dilated loops of bowel (*arrows*) appearing abnormally tethered and radiating to a central point. Note that the bowel loops appear thickened and abnormally hypoenhancing, compatible with bowel ischemia.

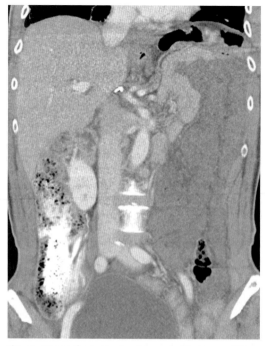

Fig. 7. Coronal contrast-enhanced CT shows diffuse hypoenhancement of the small bowel in the left abdomen, ultimately discovered to represent diffuse bowel ischemia from an internal hernia.

severe inflammation, with bowel wall thickening, mucosal hyperemia, and mesenteric inflammation.[30–32] Behçet disease is a small vessel vasculitis occurring in young men with a strong tendency to involve the distal ileum, and that can mimic the imaging findings of Crohn disease or even malignancy. Bowel wall thickening can be severe, masslike, and irregular, mimicking the appearance of a discrete mass.[1,25,26,33]

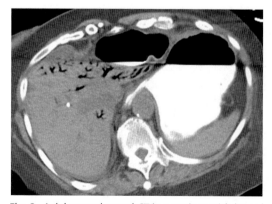

Fig. 8. Axial nonenhanced CT in a patient with bowel ischemia shows extensive portal venous gas, a finding with nearly 100% specificity for ischemia.

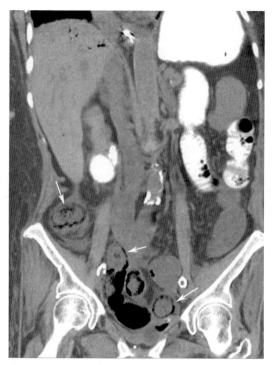

Fig. 9. Coronal nonenhanced CT shows pneumatosis (arrows) in multiple bowel loops in the pelvis, as well as small amounts of portal venous gas, findings that are nearly diagnostic of bowel ischemia.

In general, if a patient does not carry a known diagnosis of vasculitis, a specific diagnosis may not be possible based on imaging alone, and even if vasculitis is suspected the specific type of vasculitis cannot usually be diagnosed based on imaging. However, the presence of severe bowel inflammation or even ischemia in a young person should strongly prompt consideration of this diagnosis, particularly when the patient does not have other known comorbidities to explain possible bowel ischemia (**Figs. 10** and **11**). Careful evaluation of the mesenteric vasculature in such patients is critical, because the presence of aneurysms, dissections, or beading of the vessels should strongly suggest this diagnosis (**Fig. 12**).

Acute Crohn Disease–Related Inflammation

Crohn disease is a form of transmural inflammatory bowel disease that affects an estimated 1.5 million Americans and Europeans. Even despite the growing use of capsule endoscopy, CT enterography still remains the first-line modality for the imaging of patients with Crohn disease, particularly in the acute setting, and can also play a valuable role in excluding the presence of strictures or obstruction before performing capsule endoscopy. CT has proved to be an excellent modality

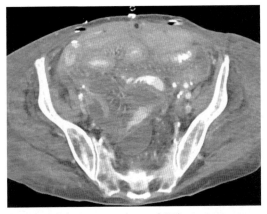

Fig. 10. Axial contrast-enhanced CT in a young person with severe abdominal pain shows diffusely thick-walled, inflamed bowel, some of which shows possible intramural hemorrhage. This finding was found to represent vasculitis.

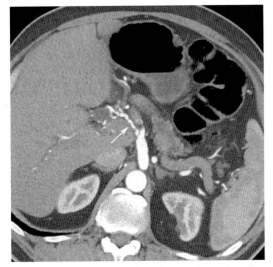

Fig. 12. Axial contrast-enhanced CT shows beading and irregularity of the hepatic artery (*arrow*) in a patient with PAN.

for delineating the presence of active inflammation, which most often involves the distal ileum but can affect any portion of the GI tract from the mouth to the anus. In particular, the addition of arterial phase imaging has proved to be extraordinarily valuable in identifying sites of early inflammation, even in cases in which the venous phase images appear unremarkable.[34]

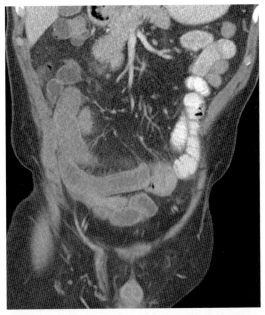

Fig. 11. Coronal contrast-enhanced CT shows severely thick-walled, inflamed small bowel in the right lower quadrant in a young person with lupus vasculitis. As in this case, vasculitis of the small bowel can be indistinguishable from bowel ischemia.

In the earliest stages of active inflammation, venous phase images may appear grossly normal with little or no bowel wall thickening and no significant adjacent mesenteric inflammation. However, in such cases, it is common for arterial phase images, particularly when analyzed in conjunction with 3D MIP techniques, to show subtle hyperemia of the affected bowel wall, as well as subtle engorgement of the vasa recta supplying the affected segment. More severe degrees of involvement tend to be visible regardless of the phase of contrast, with the development of frank bowel wall thickening; mucosal hyperemia on both the arterial and venous phase images; bowel wall mural stratification with submucosal edema and mucosal hyperemia; and extensive surrounding mesenteric fat stranding, fluid, and edema (**Figs. 13 and 14**). CT angiographic images are less important for identifying the chronic stigmata of Crohn disease (eg, mesenteric fatty proliferation or pseudosacculations along the mesenteric margin of the bowel). Moreover, angiographic images probably provide little additional value in identifying acute complications of Crohn-related inflammation, such as sinus tracts, fistulae, or abscesses. Even with the incorporation of dual-phase technique, it can be difficult in some cases to differentiate a chronic fibrotic structure from a stricture caused by active inflammation, particularly in those cases with little surrounding mesenteric inflammation, because both types of strictures can show some degree of arterial hyperenhancement.[34]

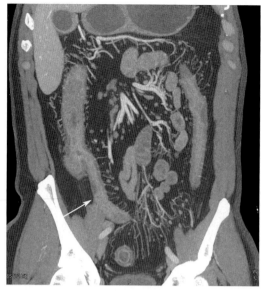

Fig. 13. Coronal volume-rendered contrast-enhanced CT shows extensive thickening and hyperenhancement of the distal ileum (*arrow*) and the colon in a patient with Crohn-related ileitis and colitis. Note the engorgement of the vasa recta supplying these bowel segments and the reactive lymphadenopathy.

CHRONIC DISORDERS
Mesenteric Artery Dissection

The identification of incidental dissections of the visceral arteries, at one time erroneously thought to be extraordinarily rare and possibly uniformly fatal, has become increasingly common with the more frequent acquisition of arterial phase imaging, the improved spatial resolution of modern scanners, and the increasingly common routine reconstruction of multiplanar reformats (given that many dissections are not readily apparent in the axial plane). Although most visceral artery dissections merely reflect the extension of an aortic dissection into a branch vessel, isolated visceral artery dissections are still thought to be rare (despite their increasing diagnosis), and almost always reflect an underlying intrinsic weakness of the vessel wall caused by such entities as fibromuscular dysplasia (FMD), cystic medial necrosis, collagen vascular disease, vasculitis, Marfan, or Ehlers-Danlos. The most commonly involved vessel is the SMA, although any visceral artery can theoretically be involved.[1,35] In most cases, isolated visceral artery dissections occur close to the vessel ostium, possibly as a result of shear stresses to the vessels in this location.[36]

Although less common than asymptomatic, incidental dissections, the presence of edema, stranding, hemorrhage, or inflammation around the vessel, or alternatively acute abdominal pain that is thought to be attributable to the dissection, raise the possibility of an acute dissection, and should precipitate prompt referral of the patient to a vascular surgeon or interventional radiologist (**Figs. 15–17**). Despite this, most acute mesenteric artery dissections have favorable outcomes, and most patients are treated with anticoagulation and close radiographic follow-up, with endovascular treatments reserved for those patients who

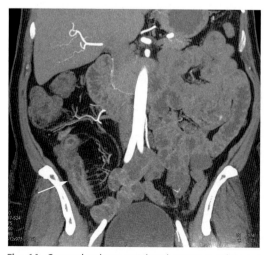

Fig. 14. Coronal volume-rendered contrast-enhanced CT shows extensive thickening and hyperenhancement of the distal ileum (*arrow*), a classic distribution of involvement for Crohn inflammation of the bowel.

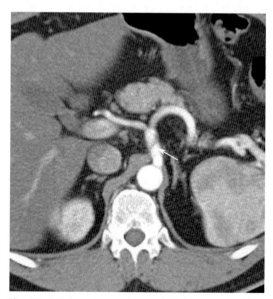

Fig. 15. Axial contrast-enhanced CT shows an incidentally identified dissection (*arrow*) in the celiac artery in an asymptomatic patient.

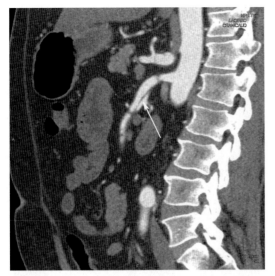

Fig. 16. Sagittal contrast-enhanced CT shows a dissection in the SMA (*arrow*), with a more subtle dissection in the celiac artery, in a patient with FMD.

fail conservative therapy.[36,37] However, in most instances, this is an incidental diagnosis that only requires clinical attention if the dissection is flow limiting or if the vessel is aneurysmal as a result of the dissection.[35,38]

Median Arcuate Ligament Syndrome

The median arcuate ligament is a fibrous arch bridging the right and left diaphragmatic crus

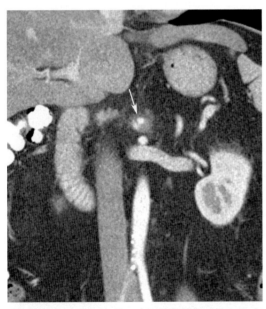

Fig. 17. Coronal contrast-enhanced CT shows an acute celiac artery dissection (*arrow*) in a patient with abdominal pain. Note the stranding around the artery, a feature suggesting acuity.

across the aortic hiatus. In a small percentage of the population, the median arcuate ligament has an abnormally low insertion across the celiac artery origin. This position can result in compression and narrowing of the celiac artery, particularly if the celiac artery is positioned abnormally high. Although uncommon, this compression of the celiac origin can result in a hemodynamically significant stenosis that can be symptomatic. Classically, symptoms are seen in young women or thin individuals who report abdominal pain after eating, exercising, or inspiring; a constellation of symptoms that is like those of chronic mesenteric ischemia.[39]

In patients with median arcuate ligament compression, the characteristic impression on the celiac trunk is described as J shaped (**Fig. 18**). Although compression of the celiac origin by the median arcuate ligament is commonly seen in patients who are asymptomatic and being scanned for other reasons, the presence of collateral vessels between the celiac and SMA or poststenotic dilatation of the celiac artery may suggest the possibility of a hemodynamically significant stenosis and should prompt correlation with patient symptoms. In particular, these collaterals are usually seen surrounding the pancreatic head, and the presence of collaterals in this classic

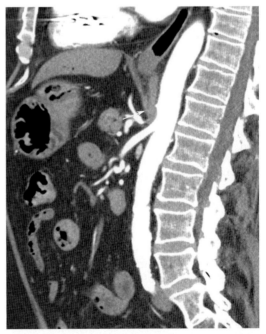

Fig. 18. Sagittal contrast-enhanced CT shows occlusion of the proximal celiac artery caused by compression by the median arcuate ligament (*arrow*). Note the classic J-shaped indentation on the celiac artery.

location should always prompt careful attention to the celiac and SMA origins for the presence of a stenosis. Although not commonly performed in practice, some institutions have described performing separate inspiratory and expiratory acquisitions to better gauge the maximum degree of compression, because compression typically worsens with inspiration.[1,39]

The treatment of median arcuate ligament syndrome is controversial, because the exact cause of pain in these patients is unclear. Notably, symptoms of chronic mesenteric ischemia classically occur in patients with stenosis of at least 2 or 3 major mesenteric arteries, but this group of patients with median arcuate ligament compression usually have a widely patent SMA and inferior mesenteric artery (IMA). Accordingly, some clinicians think that symptoms in these patients are not the result of intestinal ischemia per se, but of compression of the splanchnic nerve plexus, which is located near the diaphragmatic fibers. The most widely used treatment involves dividing the fibers of the median arcuate ligament near the celiac origin, but celiac ganglionectomy has also been proposed by some groups.[40]

Superior Mesenteric Artery Syndrome

SMA syndrome represents a constellation of nonspecific symptoms (eg, anorexia, vomiting, weight loss) caused by compression of the duodenum between the aorta and SMA. The entity is thought to reflect an abnormally small distance between the SMA and aorta, and tends to be seen most often in patients with rapid weight loss or patients who have undergone recent surgery with resultant redistribution of the retroperitoneal fat. The diagnosis is best made using arterial phase images, which should show an abnormally small aortomesenteric distance of less than 8 mm (normally 10–34 mm) and an abnormally small aortomesenteric angle of only 6° to 22° (Fig. 19). In our experience, 3D reconstructions are often more accurate in determining the aortomesenteric angle compared with standard sagittal reformations, because such reconstructions allow the aorta and SMA to be placed in the same plane. However, in order to make this diagnosis accurately, simple numerical cutoffs are not sufficient, because there should be ancillary imaging findings suggesting true duodenal obstruction, such as abrupt narrowing of the duodenum between the aorta and SMA and upstream distension of the stomach and first portion of the duodenum. Another helpful ancillary feature is the presence of dilated left-sided

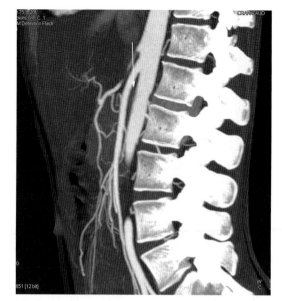

Fig. 19. Sagittal contrast-enhanced arterial phase CT shows marked narrowing of the aortomesenteric angle (*arrow*) in a patient with suspected SMA syndrome.

venous collaterals and a dilated left gonadal vein, reflecting compression of the left renal vein between the aorta and SMA. Treatment of SMA syndrome is typically conservative, although in rare cases patients require surgical bypass to relieve the duodenal obstruction.[41]

Chronic Mesenteric Ischemia

Classically diagnosed in elderly patients who have abdominal pain after meals with signs of anorexia and chronic weight loss, chronic mesenteric ischemia is much less common than acute mesenteric ischemia.[42] Most cases are attributable to atherosclerotic narrowing of the origin of the major mesenteric arteries, and symptoms typically result only in patients who have a significant stenosis in at least 2 of the 3 major mesenteric arteries (celiac, SMA, and IMA). However, given that atherosclerotic disease is widespread in the elderly population, the diagnosis of this entity requires not only correlation with appropriate clinical symptoms but also visualization of collateral pathways (eg, celiac-SMA collaterals via the pancreaticoduodenal arcade and SMA-IMA collaterals via the arc of Riolan and marginal artery of Drummond) (Fig. 20). Although these collateral pathways can compensate for significant stenoses over long periods of time, symptoms usually develop when blood flow via these collaterals is no longer sufficient to supply the bowel.[1,43]

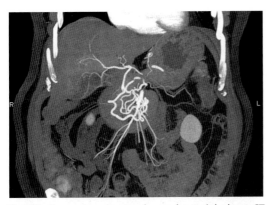

Fig. 20. Coronal contrast-enhanced arterial phase CT with MIP reconstruction shows extensive collaterals around the pancreatic head, a finding strongly suggestive of a critical stenosis of either the celiac artery or SMA.

SUMMARY

CT has largely supplanted other available radiologic modalities in the evaluation of a wide variety of vascular and inflammatory abnormalities of the small bowel, with CT angiography playing a major role in the diagnostic efficacy of MDCT for these diseases. Proper protocol design and appropriate use of multiplanar reformations and 3D reconstructions are critical for obtaining the correct diagnosis in these cases.

REFERENCES

1. Gore RM, Levine MS. Textbook of gastrointestinal radiology. 4th edition. Philadelphia: Saunders; 2014.
2. Barlow JM, Goss BC, Hansel SL, et al. CT enterography: technical and interpretive pitfalls. Abdom Imaging 2015;40(5):1081–96.
3. Raman SP, Horton KM, Fishman EK. Transitional cell carcinoma of the upper urinary tract: optimizing image interpretation with 3D reconstructions. Abdom Imaging 2012;37:1129–40.
4. Raman SP, Horton KM, Fishman EK. MDCT and CT angiography evaluation of rectal bleeding: the role of volume visualization. AJR Am J Roentgenol 2013;201:589–97.
5. Raman SP, Horton KM, Fishman EK. MDCT evaluation of ureteral tumors: advantages of 3D reconstruction and volume visualization. AJR Am J Roentgenol 2013;201:1239–47.
6. Raman SP, Fishman EK. Abnormalities of the distal common bile duct and ampulla: diagnostic approach and differential diagnosis using multiplanar reformations and 3D imaging. AJR Am J Roentgenol 2014;203:17–28.
7. Raman SP, Horton KM, Fishman EK. Multimodality imaging of pancreatic cancer-computed tomography,

magnetic resonance imaging, and positron emission tomography. Cancer J 2012;18:511–22.
8. Raman SP, Chen Y, Fishman EK. Cross-sectional imaging and the role of positron emission tomography in pancreatic cancer evaluation. Semin Oncol 2015; 42:40–58.
9. Stunell H, Buckley O, Lyburn ID, et al. The role of computerized tomography in the evaluation of gastrointestinal bleeding following negative or failed endoscopy: a review of current status. J Postgrad Med 2008;54:126–34.
10. Filippone A, Cianci R, Milano A, et al. Obscure and occult gastrointestinal bleeding: comparison of different imaging modalities. Abdom Imaging 2012; 37:41–52.
11. Artigas JM, Marti M, Soto JA, et al. Multidetector CT angiography for acute gastrointestinal bleeding: technique and findings. Radiographics 2013;33: 1453–70.
12. Geffroy Y, Rodallec MH, Boulay-Coletta I, et al. Multidetector CT angiography in acute gastrointestinal bleeding: why, when, and how. Radiographics 2011;31:E35–46.
13. Horton KM, Jeffrey RB Jr, Federle MP, et al. Acute gastrointestinal bleeding: the potential role of 64 MDCT and 3D imaging in the diagnosis. Emerg Radiol 2009;16:349–56.
14. Nagata N, Niikura R, Aoki T, et al. Role of urgent contrast-enhanced multidetector computed tomography for acute lower gastrointestinal bleeding in patients undergoing early colonoscopy. J Gastroenterol 2015. [Epub ahead of print].
15. Chan V, Tse D, Dixon S, et al. Outcome following a negative CT angiogram for gastrointestinal hemorrhage. Cardiovasc Intervent Radiol 2015;38: 329–35.
16. Horton KM, Fishman EK. Multidetector CT angiography in the diagnosis of mesenteric ischemia. Radiol Clin North Am 2007;45:275–88.
17. McKinsey JF, Gewertz BL. Acute mesenteric ischemia. Surg Clin North Am 1997;77:307–18.
18. Tendler DA. Acute intestinal ischemia and infarction. Semin Gastrointest Dis 2003;14:66–76.
19. Rhee RY, Gloviczki P, Mendonca CT, et al. Mesenteric venous thrombosis: still a lethal disease in the 1990s. J Vasc Surg 1994;20:688–97.
20. Sudhakar CB, Al-Hakeem M, MacArthur JD, et al. Mesenteric ischemia secondary to cocaine abuse: case reports and literature review. Am J Gastroenterol 1997;92:1053–4.
21. Santillan CS. Computed tomography of small bowel obstruction. Radiol Clin North Am 2013;51: 17–27.
22. Aschoff AJ, Stuber G, Becker BW, et al. Evaluation of acute mesenteric ischemia: accuracy of biphasic mesenteric multi-detector CT angiography. Abdom Imaging 2009;34:345–57.

23. Furukawa A, Kanasaki S, Kono N, et al. CT diagnosis of acute mesenteric ischemia from various causes. AJR Am J Roentgenol 2009;192:408–16.

24. Wiesner W, Khurana B, Ji H, et al. CT of acute bowel ischemia. Radiology 2003;226:635–50.

25. Ha HK, Lee SH, Rha SE, et al. Radiologic features of vasculitis involving the gastrointestinal tract. Radiographics 2000;20:779–94.

26. Hokama A, Kishimoto K, Ihama Y, et al. Endoscopic and radiographic features of gastrointestinal involvement in vasculitis. World J Gastrointest Endosc 2012; 4:50–6.

27. Levine SM, Hellmann DB, Stone JH. Gastrointestinal involvement in polyarteritis nodosa (1986-2000): presentation and outcomes in 24 patients. Am J Med 2002;112:386–91.

28. Ebert EC. Gastrointestinal manifestations of Henoch-Schonlein purpura. Dig Dis Sci 2008;53:2011–9.

29. Prathiba Rajalakshmi P, Srinivasan K. Gastrointestinal manifestations of Henoch-Schonlein purpura: a report of two cases. World J Radiol 2015;7:66–9.

30. Lalani TA, Kanne JP, Hatfield GA, et al. Imaging findings in systemic lupus erythematosus. Radiographics 2004;24:1069–86.

31. Huang DF, Chen WS. Images in clinical medicine. Lupus-associated intestinal vasculitis. N Engl J Med 2009;361:e3.

32. Ju JH, Min JK, Jung CK, et al. Lupus mesenteric vasculitis can cause acute abdominal pain in patients with SLE. Nat Rev Rheumatol 2009;5:273–81.

33. Ha HK, Lee HJ, Yang SK, et al. Intestinal Behcet syndrome: CT features of patients with and patients without complications. Radiology 1998;209:449–54.

34. Raman SP, Horton KM, Fishman EK. Computed tomography of Crohn's disease: the role of three dimensional technique. World J Radiol 2013;5: 193–201.

35. Verde F, Bleich KB, Oshmyansky A, et al. Isolated celiac and superior mesenteric artery dissection identified with MDCT: imaging findings and clinical course. J Comput Assist Tomogr 2012;36:539–45.

36. Ko SH, Hye R, Frankel DA. Management of spontaneous isolated visceral artery dissection. Ann Vasc Surg 2015;29:470–4.

37. Satokawa H, Takase S, Seto Y, et al. Management strategy of isolated spontaneous dissection of the superior mesenteric artery. Ann Vasc Dis 2014;7: 232–8.

38. Rong JJ, Qian AM, Sang HF, et al. Immediate and middle term outcome of symptomatic spontaneous isolated dissection of the superior mesenteric artery. Abdom Imaging 2015;40:151–8.

39. Horton KM, Talamini MA, Fishman EK. Median arcuate ligament syndrome: evaluation with CT angiography. Radiographics 2005;25:1177–82.

40. Skeik N, Cooper LT, Duncan AA, et al. Median arcuate ligament syndrome: a nonvascular, vascular diagnosis. Vasc Endovascular Surg 2011;45:433–7.

41. Raman SP, Neyman EG, Horton KM, et al. Superior mesenteric artery syndrome: spectrum of CT findings with multiplanar reconstructions and 3-D imaging. Abdom Imaging 2012;37:1079–88.

42. Moawad J, Gewertz BL. Chronic mesenteric ischemia. Clinical presentation and diagnosis. Surg Clin North Am 1997;77:357–69.

43. Cognet F, Ben Salem D, Dranssart M, et al. Chronic mesenteric ischemia: imaging and percutaneous treatment. Radiographics 2002;22:863–79 [discussion: 879–80].

Computed Tomography Angiography of the Upper Extremities

Radhika B. Dave, MD[a], Dominik Fleischmann, MD[b],*

KEYWORDS

- CTA • Upper extremity • Arterial anatomy • Vasculitis • Penetrating trauma • Dissection
- Vascular malformation • Arteriovenous fistula

KEY POINTS

- Upper extremity CTA is a powerful tool in the evaluation of acute and nonacute arterial pathology; however, certain technical principles including patient positioning, choice of contrast injection site and rate of administration, and physiologic considerations must be optimized to achieve a high-quality angiographic study.
- The utility of CTA in the setting of trauma has been recognized; however, it's less well-known and varied clinical applications in the subacute setting are also important and include presurgical anatomic mapping including identification of variant arterial anatomy, evaluation of connective disorders, vasculitis, overuse syndromes, arteriovenous fistula/grafts, vascular malformations, compression syndromes, and assessment of perivascular pathology.
- Volume-rendered, maximum intensity projection, and multiplanar reformat images are indispensable for evaluating the data set.

INTRODUCTION

In an era where noninvasive imaging has formed the cornerstone of medical triage, computed tomography angiography (CTA) has found its niche. Better-known uses of CTA include evaluation of the central vasculature for aortic dissection, pulmonary embolism, and aortic aneurysm. However, CTA of the upper extremity has been gaining popularity over the last decade with the advent of faster multidetector scanners yielding improved spatial and temporal resolution. In our institution, upper extremity CTA is one of the last territories where CT has replaced conventional angiography because of improvements and increasing availability of high-end scanners that have adequate spatial resolution and anatomic coverage. Compared with MRI or other modalities, CT has widespread availability and fast acquisition times, strengths especially critical in the setting of acute trauma. Several authors have described the role of CTA of the upper extremities in the setting of acute vascular and extravascular injury over recent years.[1–4] We have also have previously illustrated a variety of acute clinical applications of upper extremity CTA.[5] However, the use of CTA in the subacute setting is less well defined. Examples of subacute roles of CTA include presurgical anatomic mapping and delineating the vascular manifestations of connective tissue diseases; vasculitis; overuse syndromes; arteriovenous (AV) dialysis fistulas; AV malformations (AVM); compression syndromes; and perivascular pathology, such as abscesses and neoplasms. CTA can readily identify thromboembolic phenomena, aneurysms, and stenoses associated with these disease entities.

a Department of Radiology, Stanford University Medical Center, 300 Pasteur Drive, S-072, Stanford, CA 94305-5105, USA; b Cardiovascular Imaging Section, Department of Radiology, Stanford University School of Medicine, 300 Pasteur Drive, S-072, Stanford, CA 94305-5105, USA
* Corresponding author.
E-mail address: d.fleischmann@stanford.edu

Radiol Clin N Am 54 (2016) 101–114
http://dx.doi.org/10.1016/j.rcl.2015.08.008
0033-8389/16/$ – see front matter © 2016 Elsevier Inc. All rights reserved.

SCAN PROTOCOLS AND PHYSIOLOGIC CONSIDERATIONS
Patient Positioning

Appropriate patient positioning is critical for upper extremity CTA image quality. The guiding principle is to position the anatomy of interest close to the isocenter of the scanner, unobstructed by nonrelevant anatomy, such as the contralateral arm, shoulders, and abdomen, while keeping the patient comfortable. Patients can be positioned headfirst either in the supine or prone position on the scanner table with the arm to be scanned placed above the patient's head. The fingers should be spread out and taped down. The laser light of the scanner should be used to align the arm and fingers as close as possible with the isocenter of the scanner where spatial resolution is best. Younger and mobile individuals can easily tolerate a prone or oblique prone position with the entire upper extremity, thoracic inlet, and aortic arch close to the isocenter. The contralateral arm is positioned next to the patients' body, which also moves the shoulders out of the same transverse plane. Less mobile patients are typically scanned supine, with tape and pillows supporting the upper extremity.

In immobile patients or in the setting of trauma, the upper extremity is scanned at the side of a patient's body. Again, every attempt should be made to place the anatomy of interest as close to the isocenter as allowed under the circumstances, for instance by adjusting table height or putting the hand and forearm on the patient's abdomen rather than next to the pelvis.

Scanning Parameters

Contrast medium injection

Proper choice of injection site is critical when imaging the upper extremity. Injection of contrast into the extremity contralateral to the side of interest should be chosen whenever possible to avoid masking pathology by streak artifact. However, if radiographic evaluation of both extremities is desired, contrast injection via a central AV catheter is preferred for optimal data acquisition. This is typically the case in preprocedure imaging obtained for dialysis fistula planning purposes.

Injection protocols at our institution are based on patient weight and injection of contrast is typically performed in a biphasic manner. Table 1 lists our institution's upper extremity contrast injection protocol based on patient weight.

Scan time plus the diagnostic delay should equal the injection duration. It is critical to select the scanning range first and then set the scan time to 30 seconds in all patients. Additionally, the injection duration is set to 30 seconds for all patients assuming the diagnostic delay is essentially zero. This is done to avoid outrunning the contrast bolus. Automated bolus tracking is performed at the ascending aorta, with the trigger set at the 100 HU level with a minimum user delay of 2 seconds. A normal monitoring delay is 8 seconds with injection of the upper extremity. If injection is performed via the foot, the monitoring delay is set to 15 seconds. The scan time should be chosen based on the injection duration to avoid outrunning the contrast bolus. Scan times are chosen with the assumption that upper extremity scan times can be extrapolated from known lower extremity scan times. A saline flush of 40 mL is performed after injection of contrast, set at the same flow rate as the phase 2 contrast injection. Of note, slower acquisition/scanning protocols allow for adequate filling of small peripheral arteries.

Physiologic considerations that affect contrast injection include blood flow at rest; presence of inflow obstruction as can be seen in the setting of atherosclerosis; physiologic states with increased blood flow, such as with activity or during reperfusion after an ischemic event; and presence of high-flow lesions or conduits, such as AVM

Table 1
Weight-based upper extremity CTA injection protocol

Body Weight (lb)	Body Weight (kg)	Phase I	Phase II	Total Contrast Medium Volume (mL)
<121	<55	20 mL @ 4.0 mL/s	80 mL @ 3.2 mL/s	100
121–143	<65	23 mL @ 4.5 mL/s	90 mL @ 3.6 mL/s	113
143–187	~75	25 mL @ 5.0 mL/s	100 mL @ 4.0 mL/s	125
187–209	>85	28 mL @ 5.5 mL/s	110 mL @ 4.4 mL/s	138
>209	>95	30 mL @ 6.0 mL/s	120 mL @ 4.8 mL/s	150

Adapted from Lippert H, Pabst R. Arterial variations in man: classification and frequency. Wurzburg (Germany): J. F. Bergmann Verlag Munchen; 1985.

or AV fistulas or grafts in dialysis patients. The upper extremity arterial system is typically a high-resistance vascular bed characterized by high-resistance arterial waveforms as evident on spectral Doppler imaging with minimal forward flow during diastole.

By making use of physiologic principles, several maneuvers can be performed to improve arterial inflow into the extremity of interest for the purposes of acquiring a higher-quality examination. For instance, blood flow is improved by compressing a major artery temporarily, which results in physiologic hyperemia to its tributary. To make use of this principle, a blood pressure cuff is inflated for 1 minute and immediately released before injection. A 1-minute exercise of squeezing a ball or object before taping down the patient's fingers can also result in improved visualization of small vessels making use of physiologic hyperemia of exercise. In addition, warming the hand or extremity before scanning results in physiologic vasodilation, which helps differentiate vasoconstriction from true arterial stenoses. Additionally, vasodilation can improve visualization of smaller arteries and is particularly useful in imaging trauma patients and those with Raynaud phenomenon.

Image Postprocessing

Powerful postprocessing software is required to visualize and interpret high-resolution upper extremity CTA datasets and for communicating findings to referring physicians. A detailed discussion of image processing for upper extremity CTA is beyond the scope of this article and is found elsewhere. We routinely use thin-slab volume rendering, thin-slab maximum intensity projection images, and multiplanar reformats to interrogate the datasets interactively in the reading room. Real-time interactive adjustment of the opacity transfer function is performed when creating volume-rendered images and is chosen based on the given anatomy, vessel size, and degree of contrast opacification. Curved planar reformations are particularly helpful to display luminal pathology, such as webs, stenosis, or aneurysms, and are routinely generated by our 3D laboratory.

NORMAL ANATOMY

Volume rendering is particularly useful in displaying upper extremity arterial anatomy in conjunction with the anatomic landmarks that define the transitions between vascular structures. Conventional upper extremity vascular anatomy is delineated in **Fig. 1**.

Examples of anatomic landmarks include the lateral margin of the first rib that demarcates the boundary between the subclavian artery and the axillary artery, and the inferior margin of the tendons of the latissimus dorsi and teres major muscles that delineate the transition between the axillary artery and brachial artery.[6] The normal location of the branch point of the brachial artery into the radial and ulnar arteries is at the level of the antecubital fossa near the coronoid process of the ulna.[6] Conventional branching anatomy is seen in approximately 70% of individuals.[7] Understanding these normal anatomic relationships can serve to alert one to the presence of a high bifurcation of the brachial artery or lack of regression of the median artery. These examples of variant anatomy are discussed in a separate section.

Normal arterial anatomy of the hand is appreciated in **Fig. 2**. The arterial supply to the hand is redundant. The ulnar artery is the larger of the

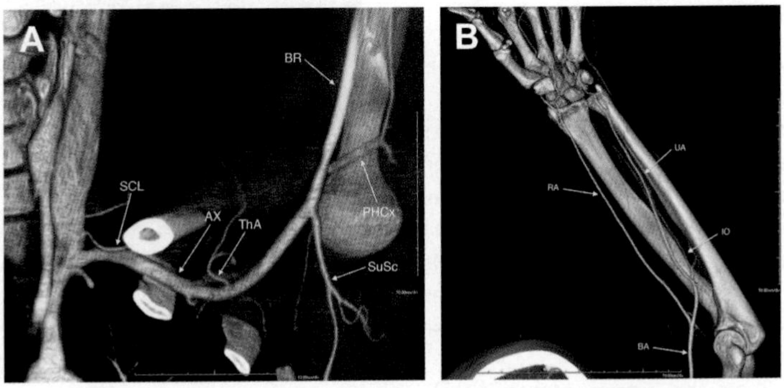

Fig. 1. Normal arterial anatomy of the upper extremity. Volume-rendered (VR) CTA images of the proximal left upper extremity (*A*) and forearm (*B*) demonstrate major branches of the subclavian (SCL), axillary (AX), and brachial arteries (BR). Major branches include the thoracoacromial (ThA), subscapular (SuSc), and posterior humeral circumflex (PHCx) arteries. Major arteries of the forearm are identified distal to the bifurcation of the brachial artery (BA). Branches include the radial artery (RA), ulnar artery (UA), and interosseous artery (IO).

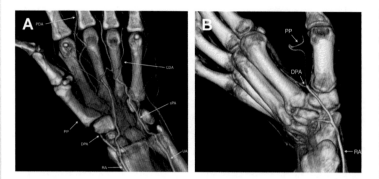

Fig. 2. VR CTA images (A,B) of the left wrist demonstrate the major arteries of the hand and wrist. The ulnar artery (UA) is noted medially and is seen to supply the superficial palmar arch (sPA), the common palmar digital artery (CDA), and proper palmar digital arteries (PDA) more distally. The RA is seen to better advantage on this sagittal oblique VR image (B) supplying the princeps pollicis artery (PP) and the deep palmar arch (DPA) that is partially visualized.

two subdivisions of the brachial artery and thus the dominant vascular supply to the hand is via the ulnar artery.[6]

The superficial palmar arch is primarily supplied by the ulnar artery and is located superficial to the flexor tendons of the forearm. The major tributaries of the superficial palmar arch include the common palmar digital arteries and the proper palmar digital arteries more distally. The superficial palmar arch is located distal to the deep palmar arch. The radial artery primarily supplies the deep palmar arch. The distal radial artery is seen coursing dorsal to the trapezium and the base of the first metacarpal piercing the first metacarpal interosseous space in 96% of individuals.[7] The major tributaries of the deep palmar arch include the princeps pollicis artery that supplies the thumb and several palmar metacarpal arteries that supply the metacarpals and digits. The arterial supply to the hand is redundant via the palmar arches. Understanding this normal anatomy is useful, such as in the setting of trauma or evaluating the vascular manifestations of collagen vascular disease.

VARIANT ANATOMY

Identification of variants in arterial anatomy is particularly important in preoperative planning for skin flaps, muscle transfer, or carpal tunnel release. **Fig. 3** illustrates normally persisting forearm vessels including the radial, ulnar, and interosseous arteries and normally regressing vessels, such as the median and superficial brachial arteries.[7] Of note, several variant arteries of the forearm are vessels that normally regress in utero.

Anatomic variants of the upper extremity arteries are common and explained by the complex embryology of the human upper extremity as demonstrated in **Fig. 3**. An example of a persistent median artery is shown in **Fig. 4**.

In humans, the median artery is normally present in early embryonic development but typically regresses in utero from the second month of gestation.[7] The superficial course of this vessel in relation to the flexor tendons should be noted for identification purposes, and its close proximity to the flexor retinaculum. Failure to identify variant anatomy can also have surgical implications in the setting of carpal tunnel release, because this vessel could be encountered and be inadvertently severed.

Identification of variant anatomy is also important in the setting of trauma, where clinical findings may underestimate the severity of injury if variant anatomy is not suspected. **Fig. 5** demonstrates a case where a brachial artery injury was missed clinically because variant origin of the radial artery proximal to the level of injury resulted in a preserved radial pulse.

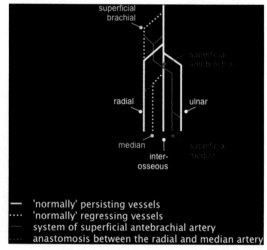

superficial brachial

superficial antebrachial

radial   ulnar

median   superficial median
inter-
osseous

— 'normally' persisting vessels
···· 'normally' regressing vessels
  system of superficial antebrachial artery
···· anastomosis between the radial and median artery

Fig. 3. Schematic of the evolution of upper extremity vascular anatomy. (*Modified from* Lippert H, Pabst R. Arterial variations in man: classification and frequency. Wurzburg (Germany): J. F. Bergmann Verlag Munchen; 1985.)

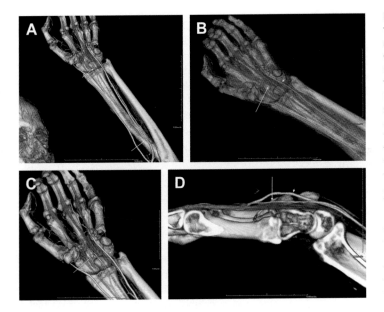

Fig. 4. A 27-year-old man presents for preoperative evaluation for microvascular muscle transfer. VR CTA images demonstrate a persistent median artery (*arrow*) originating from the ulnar artery (*A*, *B*) coursing in parallel to the median nerve (not shown). The median artery and nerve are located just superficial to the flexor tendons of the wrist but deep to the flexor retinaculum and traverse the carpal tunnel. In this case, the median artery terminates as the arterial supply to the third digit (*C*). The ulnar artery (*arrowhead*) is noted medial to this variant artery (*C*) and is seen supplying an incomplete superficial palmar arch. The close anatomic relationship of this variant vessel with the flexor tendons within the carpal tunnel is appreciated with this profile view (*D*) of the wrist in extension.

The brachioradial artery can originate from either the brachial artery or axillary artery but most commonly originates from the upper third of the brachial artery.[8] To review, the brachial artery bifurcates conventionally into the radial and ulnar arteries at the level of the antecubital fossa in approximately 70% of individuals.[7] Therefore, the location of this patient's injury would normally jeopardize perfusion to the radial artery and render a nonpalpable or weak radial artery pulse. The presence of variant anatomy explains the palpable radial artery pulse at the level of the wrist on physical examination despite traumatic injury to the brachial artery. The extent of this patient's injury was underestimated clinically resulting in massive blood loss requiring multiple transfusions. The patient's brachial artery and radial nerve injury were surgically repaired and forearm fasciotomy and carpal tunnel release were also performed. Of note, a high origin of the radial artery or brachioradial artery is the most common arterial variant in the arm and forearm and is most commonly unilateral.[8]

Trauma

CTA is also useful in the setting of penetrating trauma including gunshot wounds, stab wounds, and foreign bodies. CTA is used not only to assess vascular injuries, but also is used to assess the

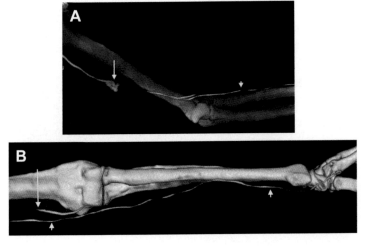

Fig. 5. A 35-year-old man status post stab wound to the left upper extremity during a fight. VR CTA images demonstrate laceration of the brachial artery (*A*) with puddling of extravasated contrast (*arrow*). Variant arterial anatomy is noted (*B*) with a high origin of the radial artery (*arrowhead*) otherwise known as the brachioradial artery. This vessel is unperturbed in contradistinction to the lacerated brachial artery.

integrity of extravascular structures, such as the musculoskeletal system and the expected location of major nerves. An example of this is illustrated in **Fig. 6**, the case of a 25-year-old man status post two-story fall from a height. This patient was working on a telephone pole along the highway when the pole was struck by a motor vehicle. He presented with severe sensory and motor deficits in the left upper extremity.

This injury was treated by anterograde arterial access via a right common femoral artery approach and retrograde access via the left brachial artery. A guidewire was used to traverse the site of arterial injury and snaring of the wire was performed to obtain through and through access. Initial digital subtraction angiography image demonstrates a wire traversing the site of arterial injury. A catheter was placed proximal to the site of injury and injection of contrast demonstrated no significant egress of contrast distal to the site of dissection/occlusion. Spot fluoroscopic image shows placement of an 8 mm × 5 cm GORE VIA-BAHN stent graft (W. L. Gore & associates, Inc, Newark, DE) at the site of arterial injury. Completion digital subtraction angiography image demonstrates minimal residual luminal irregularity at the site of injury with an otherwise patent axillary artery after stent graft placement.

Rheumatologic/Connective Tissue Disorders

CTA can also be used to evaluate vascular involvement in connective tissue disorders. **Fig. 7** illustrates the example of a 51-year-old woman with history of scleroderma.

These patients typically exhibit Raynaud phenomenon resulting in excessive vasoconstriction of peripheral vessels when exposed to cold temperatures. Warming of the hands in this patient population is useful to delineate true arterial occlusion or stenosis from vasoconstriction. CT in addition to plain radiography can also be used for the evaluation of extravascular manifestations of systemic sclerosis including the identification of acro-osteolysis, calcinosis cutis, sclerodactyly, contractures, and ulcerations and pits of the digits.[9–12] The patient in **Fig. 7** demonstrates several of the stigmata of systemic sclerosis including arterial occlusion with collateral formation and a flexion contracture of the third distal interphalangeal joint.

Vasculitis

CTA is useful in the evaluation of large and medium vessel vasculitis given its ability to demonstrate homogeneous circumferential wall thickening and smoothly tapered luminal narrowing as is seen in

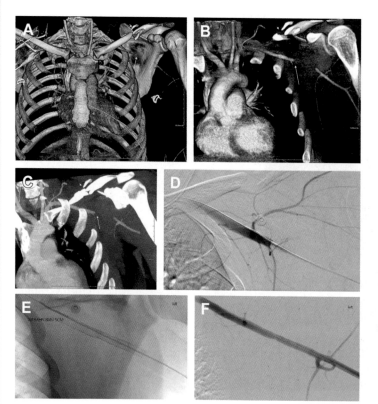

Fig. 6. A 25-year-old man status post two-story fall from a telephone pole. VR (*A*, *B*) and maximum intensity projection (MIP) and multiplanar reformat (MPR) (*C*) CTA images demonstrate traumatic dissection/occlusion of the axillary artery (*arrow*), a comminuted displaced fracture of the mid left clavicle (*arrowhead*), and fat stranding in the region of the brachial plexus. Spot fluoroscopic image (*D*) confirms traumatic dissection/occlusion of the axillary artery after injection of contrast via a catheter located proximal to the site of injury. Spot fluoroscopic image (*E*) shows placement of an 8 mm × 5 cm stent graft at the level of the injury. Postprocedural spot digital subtraction angiography (DSA) image after injection of contrast (*F*) demonstrates a patent axillary artery with minimal residual luminal irregularity at the site of injury.

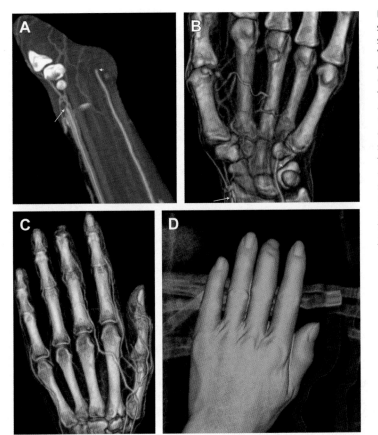

Fig. 7. A 51-year-old woman with scleroderma and multiple digital skin ulcerations. MPR MIP (A) and VR (B) images demonstrate abrupt change in caliber of the distal radial (arrow) and ulnar (arrowhead) arteries with incomplete superficial and deep palmar arches. A few common palmar digital arteries are evident arising from the incomplete superficial palmar arch. VR image of the dorsal aspect of the hand (C) demonstrates several collateral vessels supplying the first to third digits. VR image of the skin (D) demonstrates a flexion contracture of the third distal interphalangeal joint.

large vessel vasculitis. CTA also affords noninvasive evaluation of aneurysms, considered hallmarks of medium vessel vasculitis; the proximal arm vessels; aorta; and extravascular structures, such as the lungs, that can also be involved in vasculitis. However, some authors have suggested that ultrasound and MRI are superior to CT in the evaluation of vessel wall thickening. The sonographic threshold for wall thickening considered diagnostic of large vessel giant cell arteritis is 1.5 cm.[13] A few studies have suggested that color Doppler ultrasound and MRI are more sensitive and specific in the diagnosis of giant cell arteritis compared with temporal artery biopsy, previously considered the gold standard for diagnosis.[14] Consider this example of a 68-year-old woman with symptoms of upper extremity numbness and coolness with episodes of bilateral upper extremity discoloration.

The patient was treated with high-dose steroids and subsequent temporal artery biopsy demonstrated intimal fibrosis without active arteritis. However, a few studies have suggested that temporal artery biopsy is less sensitive in the setting of patients with large vessel giant cell arteritis whose temporal arteries may be unaffected.[13] In addition, the sensitivity of imaging modalities, such as color Doppler ultrasound and MRI, is decreased with corticosteroid treatment and imaging should be performed early within days of initiating therapy.[15] This patient was treated with balloon angioplasty of the left subclavian and axillary arteries with improvement in symptoms.

Fig. 8 demonstrates left subclavian artery wall thickening resulting in smoothly tapered luminal narrowing and a 1-cm left axillary artery aneurysm. High-grade stenosis was identified of the contralateral axillary artery (not shown). Of note, bilateral involvement has been seen in some studies in up to 79% of patients.[16] Subsequent CTA of the chest, abdomen, and pelvis (not shown) demonstrated diffuse wall thickening of the aorta throughout its entire extent and narrowing of the origins of the mesenteric arteries consistent with history diagnosis of large vessel giant cell arteritis. With regards to the upper extremities in patients with large vessel giant cell arteritis, the axillary arteries are involved more commonly than other large vessels, such as the subclavian or brachial arteries.[13]

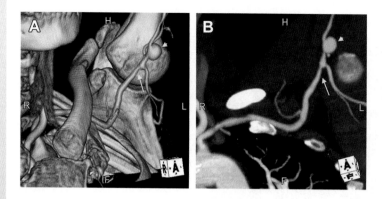

Fig. 8. A 68-year-old woman with history of giant cell arteritis. VR (*A*) and MIP MPR (*B*) images demonstrate irregularity of the left subclavian and axillary arteries, smooth tapered narrowing of the left axillary artery (*arrow*), and a 1-cm aneurysm of the axillary artery (*arrowhead*).

Overuse Syndromes

Manifestations of repetitive traumatic injury can also be identified by CTA. One notable condition includes hypothenar hammer syndrome as diagnosed in this 43-year-old male maintenance worker shown in **Fig. 9**. This patient presented with numbness and color changes of the third and fourth digits with burning pain in the same distribution.

Thrombosis, dissection, or pseudoaneurysm formation of the ulnar artery and resulting digital ischemia is caused by repetitive traumatic injury to the ulnar artery typically caused by repeated impaction of the hypothenar eminence, such as

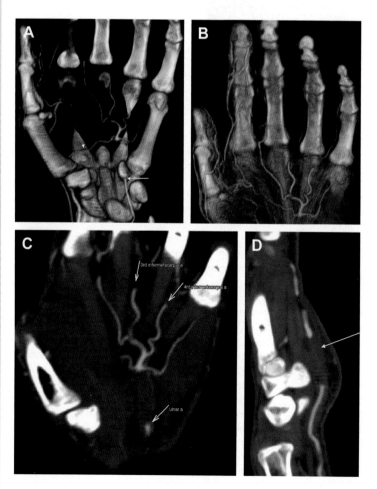

Fig. 9. A 43-year-old male maintenance worker with hypothenar hammer syndrome. VR (*A, B*) and MIP MPR images (*C, D*) demonstrate occlusion of a 2.6-cm segment of the ulnar artery (*arrow*) with collateral perfusion via a near completely intact deep palmar arch (*B*) (*arrowhead*). There is occlusion of the third and fourth palmar metacarpal arteries (*B, C*) with numerous collateral vessels from the radial artery distribution. The ulnar artery (*arrow*) is occluded superficial to the hook of the hammate, best appreciated on sagittal MIP image (*D*).

by the use of a hammer. The ulnar artery is particularly vulnerable because it traverses over the hook of the hamate. In this condition, conventional angiography has demonstrated ulnar artery occlusion, digital emboli, irregularity, and tortuosity in descending order of occurrence and similar findings are seen on CTA. Pathology of excised specimens has shown intimal thickening, fibrosis, and neovascularization. Common symptoms experienced by patients with this syndrome include digital pain, cold intolerance, and cyanosis.[17]

Arteriovenous Fistulae/Grafts

The integrity of vascular grafts and AV fistulae can also be assessed by CTA including for the presence of arterial or venous anastomotic stenosis, graft thrombosis, central venous stenosis, or steal syndrome. **Fig. 10** illustrates the case of a 43-year-old patient with history of IgA nephropathy, end-stage renal disease, and malfunctioning AV fistula that presented with left hand pain in the setting of distal digital ischemia.

The patient had developed a left-sided central venous outflow obstruction treated percutaneously via angioplasty and stent placement and began to develop ischemic changes in the tips of the fingers of her left hand after treatment. Prior arteriogram showed no inflow obstruction to the wrist but severe palmar and digital arterial occlusive disease bilaterally. This patient was shown to have multilobar pulmonary emboli on a separate

study (not shown) caused by distal embolization of thrombus within the enlarged AV fistula.

In addition to other modalities, CTA is used to evaluate for dialysis-associated steal syndrome. This can occur secondary to arterial stenosis or occlusion located either proximal or distal to the arterial anastomosis of the fistula; increased blood flow through the fistula; lack of collateralization; or decreased collateral flow reserve, such as in the setting of atherosclerosis.[18] Patients with this condition can present with a painful, cool, and possibly ischemic extremity distal to the fistula.

Vascular Malformations

Preprocedural CTA can be used for the purposes of anatomic mapping of vascular malformations before intervention. CTA can demonstrate the vascular nidus, enlarged feeding arteries, and draining veins typical of AVM. Additionally, subfascial and intramuscular components of these malformations can be identified. Compared with MRI, CTA features better spatial resolution in the evaluation of high-flow lesions, such as AVMs. However, MRI can provide superior dynamic information, temporal resolution, and tissue contrast. Consider **Fig. 11**, an example of a 16-year-old boy with remote history of trauma to the hand.

These patients can present with redness, warmth, ischemia, palpable thrill, or extremity pain. Treatment options include compression dressings, embolization (single procedure or

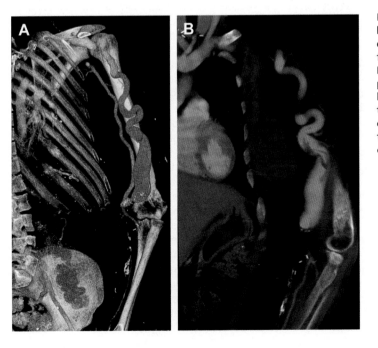

Fig. 10. A 43-year-old woman with history of IgA nephropathy and end-stage renal disease with malfunctioning AV fistula. VR (*A*) and MIP MPR (*B*) images of the left upper extremity demonstrate a dilated brachicephalic AV fistula that contains nonocclusive filling defects concerning for thrombus. This patient was noted to have pulmonary emboli (not shown).

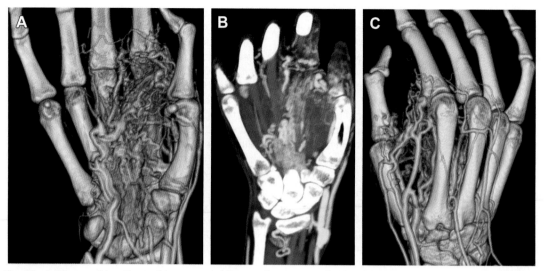

Fig. 11. A 16-year-old patient with a remote history of trauma to the hand. VR (*A, C*) and MIP MPR (*B*) images demonstrate a large arteriovenous malformation with arterial supply from the ulnar and radial arteries and numerous draining veins.

staged), surgical resection, or even amputation in extreme circumstances.[19] Performing CTA before surgical intervention is beneficial in determining the extent of disease, because incomplete resection can lead to recurrence. Transcatheter treatment of vascular malformations includes sclerotherapy of venous malformations with ethanol. Injection of arterial or AV lesions with cyanoacrylate has been found to be successful in the treatment of extremity malformations. Up to 92% of patients in a single series demonstrated an improvement in symptoms or remained asymptomatic after an average of 4 to 5 years of follow-up.[20]

Compression Syndromes

CTA can be used to evaluate for extrinsic compression of arteries. **Fig. 12** demonstrates extrinsic compression of the left subclavian artery between the clavicle and a cervical rib with associated poststenotic dilation in this 24-year-old graduate student with thoracic outlet syndrome that presented with symptoms of neck fullness.

The patient in this example was an active rock climber and noted a mass on the left side of his neck. After an initial work-up for more ominous entities was performed, imaging was obtained, and the bony mass was subsequently attributed to a cervical rib that was palpable on physical examination. The patient did not endorse any neurogenic symptoms. Physical examination demonstrated reduction of the left radial artery pulse with abduction and external rotation of his

left arm. Imaging the patient with the arms in different positions, such as in abduction, can also facilitate the diagnosis of thoracic outlet syndrome.[21] The thoracic outlet boundaries include the interscalene triangle (space bounded posteriorly by the middle/posterior scalene muscles, anteriorly by the anterior scalene muscle, and inferiorly by the first rib), costoclavicular space, and the space posterior to the pectoralis minor.[22] Extrinsic compression of neurovascular structures is exacerbated with the ipsilateral arm in extreme abduction, because this results in further narrowing of the thoracic outlet. This can be noted when comparing the caliber of the subclavian artery in **Fig. 12**C with the arm in abduction compared with **Fig. 12**B with the arm at the patient's side. Evaluation for associated subclavian artery aneurysm must be performed because this can influence treatment planning. Additionally, compression of the subclavian vein and nerve roots of the brachial plexus can also occur because these structures normally traverse the thoracic outlet. This patient was diagnosed with thoracic outlet syndrome and was treated with conservative therapy because he was asymptomatic. There was no significant aneurysmal degeneration or thrombus formation within the subclavian artery or deep venous thrombosis of the subclavian vein identified to indicate surgical management. Of note, this particular patient had osseous fusion of his left cervical rib to the left first rib. This particular configuration has been implicated in clinically symptomatic cervical ribs. In a single series, 74% of patients

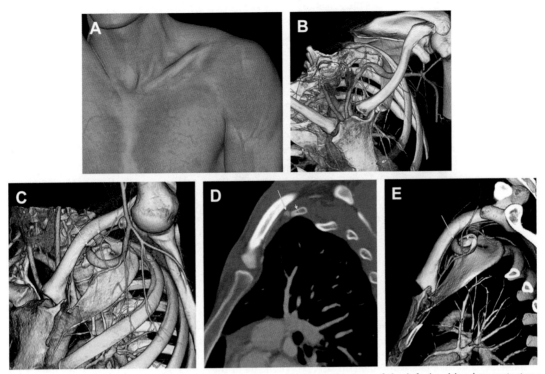

Fig. 12. A 24-year-old man with thoracic outlet syndrome. (A) Skin VR image of the left shoulder demonstrates a prominent vascular structure in the left supraclavicular fossa. VR images with the left arm in adduction (B) and abduction (C) demonstrate compression of the left subclavian artery (arrow) between a cervical rib (arrowhead) and the left clavicle. Narrowing of the costoclavicular space leading to compression of the axillary artery (arrow) is best appreciated on sagittal MPR (D) and VR (E) images.

with clinically symptomatic cervical ribs demonstrated osseous fusion of the cervical and first ribs.[23] Surgical treatment of thoracic outlet syndrome includes resection of the cervical rib if present, first rib, and scalenectomy.[24]

In addition to thoracic outlet syndrome, symptomatic compression of the axillary artery can also occur in throwing athletes. Throwing athletes have been described to develop aneurysms of the axillary artery and axillary artery branches that can thrombose. These patients can develop symptomatic distal arterial embolization into the digital arteries of the hand.[25] Conventional angiography in these patients and in our patient can identify filling defects in the digital arteries. Fig. 13 demonstrates an axillary artery branch pseudoaneurysm in a 19-year-old male quarterback with abrupt onset of right fingertip discoloration, pain, and altered sensation over the thumb and first digit, and a healing wound with scab formation on the tip of the thumb covered in gauze.

In addition to axillary artery aneurysms and distal thromboembolism, axillary artery dissection with positional occlusion can occur in these patients. Some patients have been shown to develop occlusion of the axillary artery adjacent to the humeral head at rest or with abduction of the arm. Patients can present with arterial insufficiency and may endorse symptoms of arm fatigue, numbness of the digits, hypersensitivity to cold, rest pain, or cutaneous manifestations of fingertip embolism. Treatment includes surgical repair with saphenous vein grafts, interposition bypass grafts, patch angioplasty, and ligation or excision of branch aneurysms.[26]

Perivascular Pathology

In addition to extrinsic compression syndromes, CTA can evaluate for extrinsic compression or occlusion of arterial or venous structures caused by adjacent neoplastic processes. For instance, Fig. 14 demonstrates a 62-year-old woman with a large left infraclavicular fossa leiomyosarcoma.

Multiplanar reformat images are particularly useful in the evaluation of vascular structures in the setting of large adjacent tumor burden, because mass effect results in significant distortion of normal anatomy.

Finally, CTA can identify perivascular fluid collections and their relationships to nearby arteries. Fig. 15 illustrates the case of a 33-year-old man

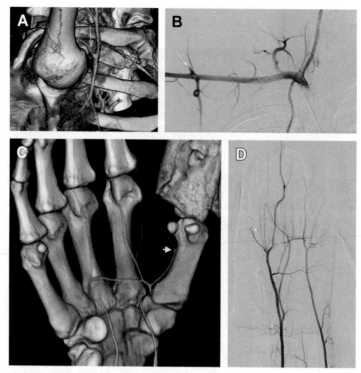

Fig. 13. A 19-year-old quarterback with abrupt onset of right fingertip discoloration, pain, and numbness. VR image (*A*) with the right arm in abduction demonstrates an axillary artery branch (posterior circumflex humeral artery) aneurysm (*arrow*) later confirmed on DSA (*B*). VR image of the right hand shows nonopacification of the distal princeps pollicis artery (*arrowhead*) concerning for distal embolization. A subtle filling defect (*arrowhead*) is seen in a similar location on DSA and VR images of the hand (*C, D*).

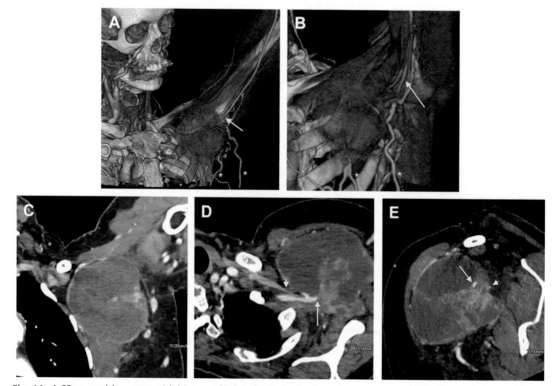

Fig. 14. A 62-year-old woman with history of left infraclavicular fossa leiomyosarcoma. VR images (*A, B*) of the left upper extremity demonstrate a large left anterior chest wall soft tissue mass located inferior to the clavicle. Coronal, axial, and sagittal oblique MPR images (*C–E*) demonstrate the left axillary artery (*arrow*) is encased within the posterior aspect of the mass and appears mildly attenuated but is otherwise patent. However, the axillary vein (*arrowhead*) is occluded posterior to the mass and several large chest wall collateral veins (*asterisks*) are identified.

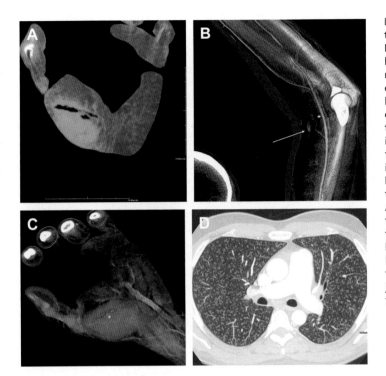

Fig. 15. A 33-year-old man with history of intravenous drug abuse. MPR (*A*) and VR (*B*) images of the left upper extremity demonstrate a rim-enhancing fluid collection compatible with an abscess (*arrow*) located in the antecubital fossa in close proximity to the brachial artery (*arrowhead*). VR image of the ipsilateral hand (*C*) demonstrates foci of subcutaneous air (*asterisk*) in the thenar eminence of the hand from recent intravenous injection into the distal radial artery. Axial MIP (*D*) image of the lungs at the level of the main pulmonary artery demonstrates diffuse tree-in-bud opacities throughout both lungs from end arteriole embolization of crushed enteral narcotics injected intravenously and resulting foreign body granulomatosis.

with history of intravenous drug abuse. This patient had been crushing up tablets of Dilaudid (Purdue Pharma LP, Stamford, CT) and had been injecting the medication intravenously. This study was acquired after the patient inadvertently injected the solution into the radial artery at the level of the wrist resulting in immediate pain and change in color of the hand. A CTA of the upper extremity was obtained secondary to concern for hand ischemia.

Later in the patient's hospital course, he experienced shortness of breath and a CTA of the thorax was obtained because of clinical concern for pulmonary embolism. **Fig. 15** demonstrates diffuse tree-in-bud opacities throughout the bilateral lungs. These findings are presumably secondary to distal embolization of crushed particles of oral narcotic into the terminal arterioles of the pulmonary arterial system ultimately resulting in foreign body granulomatosis. A few case reports of intravenous drug abusers that have intravenously injected crushed oral medications have shown scattered and miliary patterns of pulmonary nodules. Similar to our case, patients have demonstrated symptoms clinically overlapping with that of pulmonary embolism. Endobronchial biopsy of one such patient subsequent to intravenous injection of crushed extended-release oxymorphone (OpanaTM; Endo Pharmaceuticals, Chadds Ford, PA) revealed giant cell formation and perivascular

granulomas adjacent to pulmonary arterioles obstructed by microcrystalline cellulose particles.[27] In another patient with a history of crushing and intravenously injecting tablets of diphenhydramine, a miliary pattern of pulmonary nodules was seen on chest imaging.[28] Although foreign body granulomatosis is a diagnosis of exclusion, identifying secondary signs, such as subcutaneous air or subcutaneous abscesses, from intravenous injection attempts can alert the clinician to consider this rare diagnosis in the differential.

SUMMARY

Upper extremity CTA is a powerful tool in the evaluation of acute and nonacute arterial pathology. However, certain technical principles including patient positioning, choice of contrast injection site and rate of administration, and physiologic considerations must be optimized to achieve a high-quality angiographic study. The utility of CTA in the setting of trauma has been recognized. However, it's less well-known and varied clinical applications in the subacute setting are also important and include presurgical anatomic mapping including identification of variant arterial anatomy, evaluation of connective disorders, vasculitis, overuse syndromes, AV fistula/grafts, vascular malformations, compression syndromes, and assessment of perivascular pathology. Volume-rendered, maximum intensity projection, and multiplanar reformat images are indispensable for evaluating the data set.

REFERENCES

1. Anderson SW, Foster BR, Soto JA. Upper extremity CT angiography in penetrating trauma: use of 64-section multidetector CT. Radiology 2008; 249(3):1064–73.
2. Fishman EK, Horton KM, Johnson PT. Multidetector CT and three-dimensional CT angiography for suspected vascular trauma of the extremities. Radiographics 2008;28(3):653–65 [discussion: 665–6].
3. Pieroni S, Foster BR, Anderson SW, et al. Use of 64-row multidetector CT angiography in blunt and penetrating trauma of the upper and lower extremities. Radiographics 2009;29(3):863–76.
4. Soto JA, Munera F, Morales C, et al. Focal arterial injuries of the proximal extremities: helical CT arteriography as the initial method of diagnosis. Radiology 2001;218(1):188–94.
5. Dave RB, Fleischmann D. Upper extremity CTA: acute clinical applications. Presented at the Radiological Society of North America, 98th Scientific Assembly and Annual Meeting. Chicago, IL, November 25, 2012.
6. Gray H. Anatomy descriptive and surgical. London: J. W. Parker and Son; 1858.
7. Lippert H, Pabst R. Arterial variations in man: classification and frequency. Wurzburg (Germany): J. F. Bergmann Verlag Munchen; 1985.
8. Rodriguez-Niedenfuhr M, Vazquez T, Nearn L, et al. Variations of the arterial pattern in the upper limb revisited: a morphological and statistical study, with a review of the literature. J Anat 2001;199(Pt 5):547–66.
9. Hudson M, Fritzler MJ. Diagnostic criteria of systemic sclerosis. J Autoimmun 2014;48-49:38–41.
10. Johnstone EM, Hutchinson CE, Vail A, et al. Acroosteolysis in systemic sclerosis is associated with digital ischaemia and severe calcinosis. Rheumatology (Oxford) 2012;51(12):2234–8.
11. Shahi V, Wetter DA, Howe BM, et al. Plain radiography is effective for the detection of calcinosis cutis occurring in association with autoimmune connective tissue disease. Br J Dermatol 2013;170(5): 1073–9.
12. Avouac J, Guerini H, Wipff J, et al. Radiological hand involvement in systemic sclerosis. Ann Rheum Dis 2006;65(8):1088–92.
13. Schmidt WA. Imaging in vasculitis. Best Pract Res Clin Rheumatol 2013;27(1):107–18.
14. Bley TA, Reinhard M, Hauenstein C, et al. Comparison of duplex sonography and high-resolution magnetic resonance imaging in the diagnosis of giant cell (temporal) arteritis. Arthritis Rheum 2008;58(8): 2574–8.
15. Hauenstein C, Reinhard M, Geiger J, et al. Effects of early corticosteroid treatment on magnetic resonance imaging and ultrasonography findings in giant cell arteritis. Rheumatology (Oxford) 2012; 51(11):1999–2003.
16. Schmidt WA, Seifert A, Gromnica-Ihle E, et al. Ultrasound of proximal upper extremity arteries to increase the diagnostic yield in large-vessel giant cell arteritis. Rheumatology (Oxford) 2008;47(1): 96–101.
17. Larsen BT, Edwards WD, Jensen MH, et al. Surgical pathology of hypothenar hammer syndrome with new pathogenetic insights: a 25-year institutional experience with clinical and pathologic review of 67 cases. Am J Surg Pathol 2013;37(11):1700–8.
18. Malik J, Tuka V, Kasalova Z, et al. Understanding the dialysis access steal syndrome. A review of the etiologies, diagnosis, prevention and treatment strategies. J Vasc Access 2008;9(3):155–66.
19. Jacobs BJ, Anzarut A, Guerra S, et al. Vascular anomalies of the upper extremity. J Hand Surg Am 2010;35(10):1703–9 [quiz: 1709].
20. Rockman CB, Rosen RJ, Jacobowitz GR, et al. Transcatheter embolization of extremity vascular malformations: the long-term success of multiple interventions. Ann Vasc Surg 2003;17(4):417–23.
21. Remy-Jardin M, Remy J, Masson P, et al. Helical CT angiography of thoracic outlet syndrome: functional anatomy. AJR Am J Roentgenol 2000;174(6): 1667–74.
22. Demondion X, Herbinet P, Van Sint Jan S, et al. Imaging assessment of thoracic outlet syndrome. Radiographics 2006;26(6):1735–50.
23. Chang KZ, Likes K, Davis K, et al. The significance of cervical ribs in thoracic outlet syndrome. J Vasc Surg 2013;57(3):771–5.
24. Rochlin DH, Orlando MS, Likes KC, et al. Bilateral first rib resection and scalenectomy is effective for treatment of thoracic outlet syndrome. J Vasc Surg 2014;60(1):185–90.
25. Kee ST, Dake MD, Wolfe-Johnson B, et al. Ischemia of the throwing hand in major league baseball pitchers: embolic occlusion from aneurysms of axillary artery branches. J Vasc Interv Radiol 1995;6(6): 979–82.
26. Duwayri YM, Emery VB, Driskill MR, et al. Positional compression of the axillary artery causing upper extremity thrombosis and embolism in the elite overhead throwing athlete. J Vasc Surg 2011;53(5): 1329–40.
27. Klochan SA, Taleb M, Hoover MJ, et al. Illicit narcotic injection masquerading as acute pulmonary embolism. Vasc Med 2013;18(2):92–4.
28. Altraja A, Jurgenson K, Roosipuu R, et al. Pulmonary intravascular talcosis mimicking miliary tuberculosis in an intravenous drug addict. BMJ Case Rep 2014; 2014. http://dx.doi.org/10.1136/bcr-2014-203908.

Computed Tomography Angiography of the Lower Extremities

Tessa Sundaram Cook, MD, PhD

KEYWORDS

- CT angiography • Lower extremity imaging • 3-D postprocessing • Peripheral arterial disease
- Lower extremity vascular trauma • Lower extremity bypass

KEY POINTS

- Lower extremity CT angiography (CTA) is indicate in peripheral artery disease, trauma, assessment of variant anatomy and congenital malformations, vasculitis, and surgical planning.
- Arterial variants in the lower extremities most commonly involve the branching of the profunda femoris, popliteal, and calf arteries; characterization is important for surgical planning before perforator flap harvest.
- Patients over the age of 50 are primarily affected by peripheral arterial disease, and undergo CTA for anatomic localization of disease and surgical or endovascular treatment planning.
- Young patients are most commonly affected by nonatherosclerotic disease of the lower extremity arteries, such as trauma, popliteal artery entrapment syndrome, congenital vascular malformations, or vasculitides.

INTRODUCTION

Vascular diseases of the arteries of the lower extremities fall into many categories. The most common of these is peripheral vascular disease secondary to atherosclerosis, which is typically a disease of older adults, and associated with risk factors such as smoking, diabetes mellitus, hypertension, hyperlipidemia, and obesity. Younger patients most commonly suffer trauma to the lower extremities that may be associated with acute vascular injury. In younger patients, less common causes for nonatherosclerotic limb ischemia also exist.

In this article, we discuss the clinical indications for lower extremity computed tomography angiography (CTA) as well as CT scanner settings and other protocol considerations. In addition, we review the normal and variant anatomy of the arterial circulation of the extremities, the effects of ischemic and nonischemic peripheral arterial disease (PAD), congenital vascular malformations, and applications for surgical planning and intervention that directly and indirectly involve the lower extremity vasculature.

CLINICAL INDICATIONS FOR LOWER EXTREMITY COMPUTED TOMOGRAPHY ANGIOGRAPHY

Lower extremity CTA is performed for a number of clinical indications, including peripheral artery disease, trauma, assessment of variant anatomy and congenital malformations, vasculitis, and surgical planning.[1,2]

PAD is defined as atherosclerosis of the aorta, iliac, and lower extremity arteries.[3] It is rare in patients under the age of 50, but prevalence increases to 20% to 30% in patients over the age of 80, and even more in some ethnic subgroups.[4]

Disclosure Statement: The authors have nothing to disclose.
Perelman School of Medicine at the University of Pennsylvania, 3400 Spruce Street, 1 Silverstein Radiology, Philadelphia, PA 19104, USA
E-mail address: Tessa.Cook@uphs.upenn.edu

Radiol Clin N Am 54 (2016) 115–130
http://dx.doi.org/10.1016/j.rcl.2015.08.001
0033-8389/16/$ – see front matter Published by Elsevier Inc.

There is a strong association between PAD and cardiovascular risk factors, such as smoking, hypertension, hypercholesterolemia, and diabetes.[5] In addition, PAD serves as a marker for systemic atherosclerotic burden, and is associated with an increased risk of adverse cardiovascular events such as stroke and myocardial infarction.[6–8]

Early in the course of the disease, patients with PAD may be asymptomatic. Subsequently, they begin to develop claudication—leg pain with varying degrees of activity and exertion—that is typically intermittent and secondary to a single diseased arterial segment.[9] As the disease progresses, they report chronic pain even at rest. Some patients develop skin changes and nonhealing wounds of the ankles and feet, as a result of insufficient arterial circulation reaching the distal extremities. Acute and critical limb ischemia may also occur, warranting more emergent management.[10] Accurate anatomic mapping of disease plays an important role in characterizing the location and extent of lesions and planning of interventions. Treatment options include endovascular repair with angioplasty and stenting, surgical bypass and in severe, intractable cases, limb amputation.[10]

Acute thromboembolic disease may occur as a result of embolism originating in the heart or in a more proximal diseased segment of vessel, or thrombosis of a vessel, bypass graft, or lower extremity aneurysm.[11–13] Patients present with symptoms of acute limb ischemia that can progress over hours to days, and include pain, paresthesias, pallor, pulselessness, and paralysis.[13] The goal of treatment is reperfusion of the affected limb, which is usually achieved with a combination of anticoagulation and either surgery or endovascular intervention; in rare cases, anticoagulation alone is used.[14]

Younger patients (<50 years of age) rarely present with conventional PAD. Instead, they may suffer from nonischemic stenosis associated with medium- and large-vessel vasculitides (such as Takayasu arteritis or Behçet disease) and Buerger disease (also known as thrombangiitis obliterans).[15–18] Takayasu arteritis is more common in female patients than males, and although the aorta, arch vessels, and visceral arteries are typically affected, some patients may also experience lower limb ischemia.[19] Behçet disease is a vasculitis of both arteries and veins, and typically involves vessels above and below the pelvis.[16] Buerger disease preferentially affects smaller arteries in male patients over females, and is seen particularly in heavy smokers.[16,17]

Finally, variant anatomy and congenital vascular malformations can be evaluated with lower extremity CTA. Variant anatomy is typically incidentally identified during imaging for symptom evaluation or in the setting of acute trauma, and can be detected in patients of all ages.[20–25] On the other hand, imaging for vascular malformations such as Klippel–Trenaunay syndrome, Parkes Weber syndrome, and port wine stain with or without hypertrophy is usually targeted to characterization of the malformation and associated complications.[26]

NORMAL AND VARIANT LOWER EXTREMITY VASCULAR ANATOMY ON COMPUTED TOMOGRAPHY ANGIOGRAPHY

The normal arterial anatomy of the lower extremities is shown in **Fig. 1**, using a combination of curved multiplanar reformats and 3-dimensional volume-rendered (3-D VR) images. There is typically little variation in the branching of the aorta into the iliac and femoral arteries. The branching patterns of the profunda femoris artery can vary, specifically with respect to the origin and branching of the medial and lateral circumflex arteries as well as the course of the profunda femoris artery and its branches with respect to the position of the superficial femoral artery (SFA).[23]

Caudal to the pelvis, there is increased potential for variation, typically related to persistence of embryologic arterial segments that normally regress. These variants include persistence of the sciatic artery in the thigh as well as different patterns of branching of the popliteal artery and calf arteries that supply the ankle and foot. The normal branching pattern involves the popliteal artery bifurcating into the anterior tibial artery and the tibioperoneal trunk below the knee, followed by bifurcation of the tibioperoneal trunk into the posterior tibial artery medially and peroneal artery laterally (see **Fig. 1**). However, variant patterns of branching of the popliteal artery can be observed, including a complete trifurcation of the popliteal artery without a tibioperoneal trunk, high takeoff of the anterior tibial artery above the knee, or the posterior tibial artery arising as the first branch of the popliteal artery.[20–22,27] At the ankle, the anterior tibial artery typically gives rise to the dorsalis pedis, which supplies the dorsum of the foot, and the posterior tibial artery gives rise to the plantar arch. However, in cases where either of these calf arteries is hypoplastic, another artery (often the peroneal artery) can supply the dorsalis pedis or plantar arch. **Fig. 2** illustrates the variant patterns of branching of the popliteal artery, as well as of the calf arteries that supply the ankle and foot. **Fig. 3** illustrates high takeoff of the anterior tibial artery above the knee, with a long

A

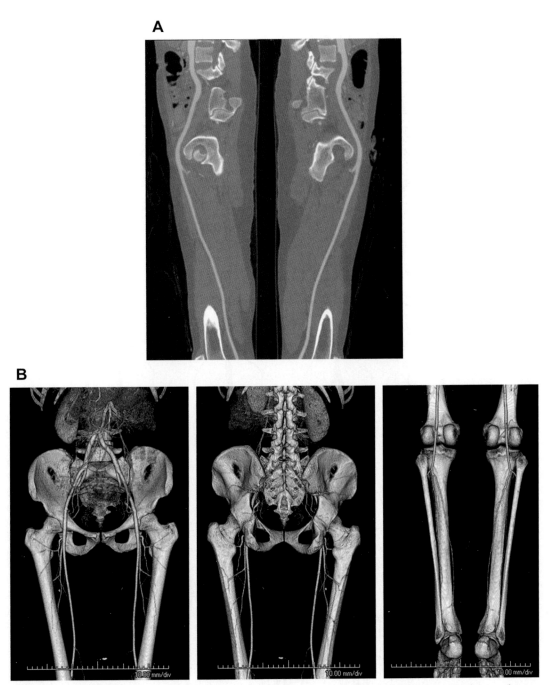

B

Fig. 1. Normal anatomy of the lower extremity arteries depicted using (A) bilateral curved multiplanar reformats from the pelvis to the knees and (B) anterior and posterior 3-dimensional (3-D) volume-rendered images through the thighs and posterior 3-D volume-rendered images through the legs.

tibioperoneal trunk that bifurcates below the knee into the peroneal and posterior tibial arteries.

In addition to variant branching, the anatomic relationship between the popliteal artery and the muscles of the posterior knee joint can produce abnormal findings on angiographic imaging. Most commonly, this involves compression of the popliteal artery by the medial head of the gastrocnemius, although in some cases, an accessory slip of gastrocnemius muscle or even the popliteus muscle can compress the vessel. Collectively, these variants can result in popliteal artery entrapment syndrome (PAES) (Fig. 4), whereby the popliteal artery becomes occluded during plantar

118

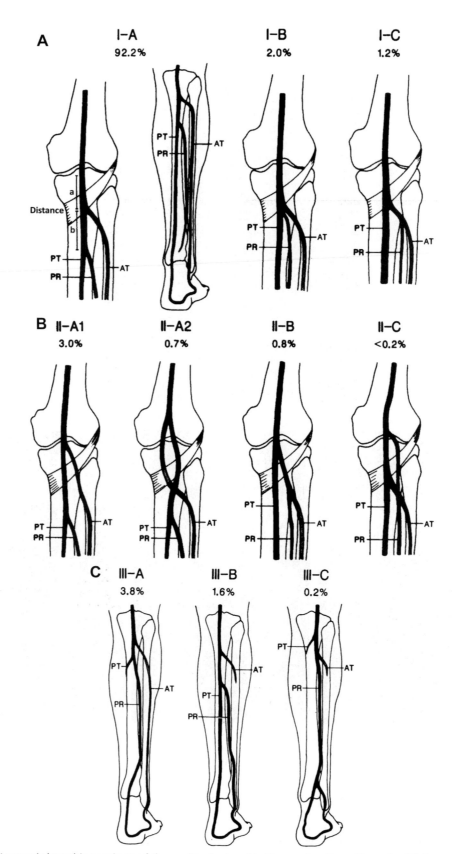

Fig. 2. Anatomic branching variants of the popliteal artery (*A*, *B*) as well as the calf arteries (*C*) that perfuse the ankle and foot. AT, anterior tibial; PR, peroneal; PT, posterior tibial. (*From* Kim D, Orron DE, Skillman JJ. Surgical significance of popliteal arterial variants. A unified angiographic classification. Ann Surg 1989;210(6):777; with permission.)

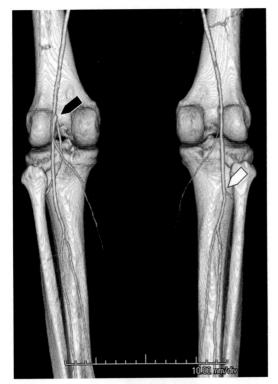

Fig. 3. 3-Dimensional (3-D) volume-rendered image showing high takeoff of the left anterior tibial artery above the knee (*black arrowhead*). By comparison, the right anterior tibial artery arises from a more typical location below the knee (*white arrowhead*).

flexion and/or dorsiflexion of the foot.[24,28] Popliteal artery entrapment typically affects teenagers and young adults, and symptoms often occur in athletic individuals after strenuous activity.[17] Symptoms include calf claudication after exercise or sports, and, in some cases, popliteal artery thrombosis. Vessel stenosis or occlusion can be elicited during dynamic imaging by asking the patient to repeatedly plantarflex and dorsiflex during the imaging study. In some instances, vessel narrowing can be observed during static imaging (**Fig. 5**).

In some patients, a persistent sciatic artery (PSA) can cause intermittent claudication.[29] The embryologic sciatic artery is a continuation of the internal iliac artery, and perfuses the lower extremity during development.[30] As gestation progresses and the SFA develops, it replaces some segments of the sciatic artery. When the sciatic artery persists, the SFA may be normal, hypoplastic, or entirely aplastic.[31–33] A PSA may be clinically silent or present with claudication, rest pain, or a pulsatile gluteal mass.[34] **Fig. 6** demonstrates bilateral persistent sciatic arteries arising from the internal iliac arteries, with decreased caliber of the left SFA with a dilated ipsilateral PSA coursing to the

left lower extremity. In this patient, both the right PSA and the right SFA are normal in caliber.

COMPUTED TOMOGRAPHY ANGIOGRAPHY PROTOCOLS FOR LOWER EXTREMITY IMAGING

CTA imaging protocols for the lower extremity vary depending on the clinical indication. Three phases of imaging are generally performed: precontrast imaging, arterial phase imaging, and venous/delayed phase imaging. The scan regions, injection rates and delay times may be adjusted according to the clinical scenario, to maximize opacification of the relevant vascular beds.[35] Considerations include the presence or absence of atherosclerotic disease, arterial occlusion, trauma, and arteriovenous malformation.

Arterial phase imaging is performed typically using either a fixed scan delay or bolus tracking. When a fixed scan delay (eg, 40 s) is used, imaging automatically commences after the delay elapses from the start of the contrast injection, but does not take into account possible variations in rates of extremity blood flow between patients.[36] By contrast, bolus tracking relies on achieving a predetermined attenuation (usually 100–120 Hounsfield units) within a region of interest in the infrarenal abdominal aorta, and imaging is initiated after a fixed time delay has subsequently elapsed. However, in patients with diminished cardiac output or severe inflow (ie, iliofemoral) disease, the delay may be increased to allow for sufficient opacification of the peripheral vasculature. Similar adjustments may be considered in patients with trauma and suspected vascular injury. Alternatively, immediate delayed imaging from the knees to the toes can also be performed to account for potential scan speed outpacing the contrast bolus. This is particularly important when imaging with modern scanners that offer as much as 320-detector array configurations and rapid table speeds.

The contrast injection may also require adjustment based on the clinical scenario.[37] Typically, 100 mL of iodinated contrast is used, but this quantity may be adjusted upward to image larger patients, or downward if the patient is scanned on newer equipment with faster table speeds. In addition, the choice of iodine concentration may influence other aspects of the injection, such as rate and volume; at our institution, we routinely use 370 mg/mL and adjust the other parameters according to factors such as patient size and intravenous access.

In the current era of increasing awareness of radiation exposure from medical imaging, efforts to decrease exposure associated with CTA of the

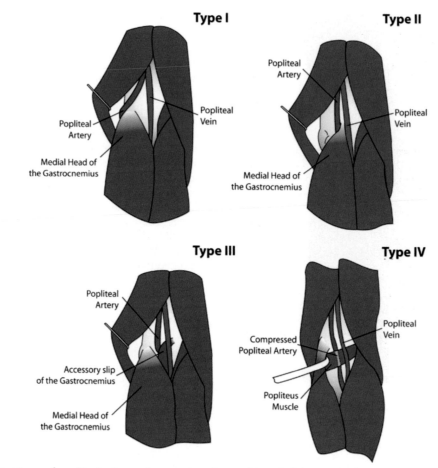

Type I

Popliteal Artery

Popliteal Vein

Popliteal Artery

Medial Head of the Gastrocnemius

Type II

Popliteal Artery

Popliteal Vein

Medial Head of the Gastrocnemius

Type III

Popliteal Artery

Accessory slip of the Gastrocnemius

Medial Head of the Gastrocnemius

Type IV

Popliteal Vein

Compressed Popliteal Artery

Popliteus Muscle

Fig. 4. Four types of popliteal artery entrapment syndrome. (*From* Wright LB, Matchett WJ, Cruz CP, et al. Popliteal artery disease: diagnosis and treatment. Radiographics 2004;24(2):476; with permission.)

lower extremities have been successful. Choosing an x-ray tube peak voltage close to the k-edge of iodine increases the observed attenuation of iodinated contrast; as a result, lowering the x-ray tube voltage to 70 to 80 kVp not only decreases the energy of emitted photons—and by extension—the radiation exposure to the patient, but also improves image quality.[38,39] Increasing the pitch when scanning the extremities with helical CT has also been shown to decrease radiation exposure without sacrificing image quality.[40] Dual-energy CTA has also been used to decrease radiation exposure to patients while maintaining or improving contrast-to-noise ratio.[41,42]

POSTPROCESSING AND INTERPRETATION OF LOWER EXTREMITY COMPUTED TOMOGRAPHY ANGIOGRAPHY

Three-dimensional postprocessing is a critical step in the interpretation of lower extremity CTA.[43,44] Maximum intensity projections (MIPs), oblique or curved multiplanar reformats, 3-D VR images, and shaded surface displays can be used to augment analysis of the reconstructed cross-sectional axial images.[1,36] Curved multiplanar reformats, which use the central axis of a vessel (also known as the centerline) to flatten and project the entire course of a vessel in a single plane, are particularly useful for evaluating vascular patency (see **Fig. 1**).

In the setting of atherosclerotic calcification, the original reconstructed data must be analyzed to avoid overestimation of the degree of stenosis that may occur owing to "blooming" of the calcification on the MIPs.[2,42,45] For similar reasons, 3-D VR images, although useful for overall evaluation of the vascular tree and localization/visualization of possible abnormalities (see **Fig. 15**), should not be used exclusively to quantify the degree of stenosis. However, both 3-D VR images and MIPs can be useful for measuring craniocaudal extent of arterial occlusions, evaluating collateral vessels, and characterizing traumatic vascular injuries.

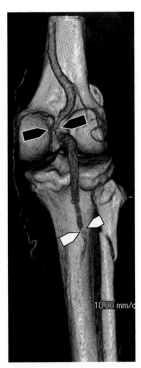

Fig. 5. Popliteal artery entrapment syndrome incidentally detected in a young patient status post trauma. The 3-dimensional volume-rendered image shows medial displacement of the popliteal artery (by the medial head of the gastrocnemius muscle) and resulting effacement of the lumen (*black arrowheads*). Also note the oblique fracture through the proximal femur and the narrowing and abrupt cutoff of the distal popliteal artery, in keeping with vascular injury (*white arrowheads*).

ALTERNATIVES TO COMPUTED TOMOGRAPHY ANGIOGRAPHY FOR THE DIAGNOSIS OF LOWER EXTREMITY VASCULAR DISEASE

The ankle-to-brachial index (ABI), reported as the ratio of systolic blood pressures measured at the ankle and in the brachial artery, is most commonly used to diagnose PAD in an inexpensive, noninvasive fashion.[46] Identifying an ABI of 0.9 or less usually leads to a cross-sectional imaging study to characterize the specific location and severity of the suspected PAD.[47,48] Some studies have shown that ABI correlates with risk factors for cerebrovascular disease as well as PAD.[49] However, wide variability in the literature as to the sensitivity and specificity of ABI testing has led the American Heart Association to issue a scientific statement on the measurement and interpretation of the test.[50] Interestingly, the US Preventative Services Task Force concluded that there was insufficient evidence to recommend ABI as a screening test for PAD in asymptomatic individuals.[51]

Imaging of the lower extremities can be performed with other modalities, including digital subtraction angiography (DSA) and MR angiography (MRA). Before the advent of cross-sectional imaging, DSA served as the gold standard for both diagnostic and interventional techniques.[52] However, since the introduction and maturation of CTA and MRA, both modalities have been and continue to be validated against DSA. Although there was early reluctance on the part of both radiologists and vascular surgeons to transition from

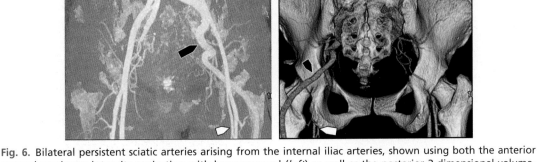

Fig. 6. Bilateral persistent sciatic arteries arising from the internal iliac arteries, shown using both the anterior coronal maximum intensity projection with bone removal (*left*) as well as the posterior 3-dimensional volume-rendered image (*right*). The left-sided persistent sciatic artery (*black arrowhead*) is dilated and the ipsilateral superficial femoral artery (*white arrowhead*) is diminutive.

the invasive to the noninvasive modality,[53] numerous studies have subsequently demonstrated the accuracy of CTA compared with DSA and the added benefit of the noninvasive examination.[38,39,54,55] CTA has also superseded duplex ultrasonography of the lower extremities in the surgical planning workup.[56,57] Both multistation gadolinium-enhanced MRA at 1.5 T and 3.0 T and noncontrast MRA have also been validated against DSA.[58–60] In the past decade, CTA and MRA have largely replaced DSA for diagnostic imaging, although DSA continues to play a role in providing real-time visualization during vascular interventions.[61]

LOWER EXTREMITY ATHEROSCLEROSIS AND ISCHEMIA

Symptoms of PAD are the most common clinical indications for which CTA of the lower extremities is performed.[2] Intermittent claudication, rest pain, critical limb ischemia and nonhealing ulcers are often reasons to consider imaging the lower extremity vasculature.[35,39,42,62–65] **Fig. 7**

demonstrates diffuse iliofemoral atherosclerosis with abrupt cutoff of the distal left SFA in this patient presenting with critical limb ischemia. PAD can increase the friability of lower extremity arteries (**Fig. 8**) by the large pseudoaneurysm arising from the common femoral artery in this patient status post groin access for placement of a percutaneous aortic valve.

The Inter-Society Consensus for the Management of Peripheral Arterial Disease (TASC II) provides a classification system for PAD that can be used to determine the most appropriate treatment. Aortoiliac and femoropopliteal lesions are classified according to the vessels involved, the length of the stenosis, the presence or absence of complete occlusion, as well as the number of lesions (**Figs. 9** and **10**). In both vascular beds, endovascular treatment is preferred for type A and type B lesions, whereas surgical repair is recommended for type C and type D lesions if the patients are good surgical candidates.[66]

In patients for whom surgical repair is preferred to endovascular therapy, a bypass graft must be selected from the choice of autologous saphenous

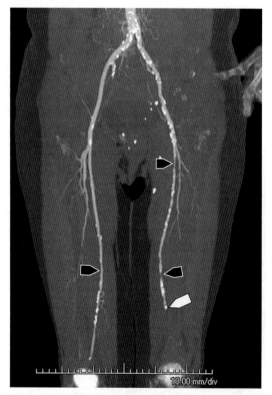

Fig. 7. Coronal maximum intensity projection with bone removal demonstrating diffuse calcified plaque involving the iliac and femoral arteries with multisegment stenoses (examples indicated by *black arrowheads*) and abrupt occlusion of the distal left superficial femoral artery (*white arrowhead*).

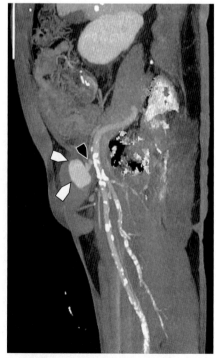

Fig. 8. Oblique sagittal maximum intensity projection in a patient status post groin endovascular access demonstrates a pseudoaneurysm (*white arrowheads*) with a narrow neck (*black arrowhead*) arising from the heavily diseased common femoral artery.

Type A lesions

- Unilateral or bilateral stenoses of CIA
- Unilateral or bilateral single short (≤3 cm) stenosis of EIA

Type B lesions:

- Short (≤3 cm) stenosis of infrarenal aorta
- Unilateral CIA occlusion
- Single or multiple stenosis totaling 3–10 cm involving the EIA not extending into the CFA
- Unilateral EIA occlusion not involving the origins of internal iliac or CFA

Type C lesions

- Bilateral CIA occlusions
- Bilateral EIA stenoses 3–10 cm long not extending into the CFA
- Unilateral EIA stenosis extending into the CFA
- Unilateral EIA occlusion that involves the origins of internal iliac and/or CFA
- Heavily calcified unilateral EIA occlusion with or without involvement of origins of internal iliac and/or CFA

Type D lesions

- Infra-renal aortoiliac occlusion
- Diffuse disease involving the aorta and both iliac arteries requiring treatment
- Diffuse multiple stenoses involving the unilateral CIA, EIA, and CFA
- Unilateral occlusions of both CIA and EIA
- Bilateral occlusions of EIA
- Iliac stenoses in patients with AAA requiring treatment and not amenable to endograft placement or other lesions requiring open aortic or iliac surgery

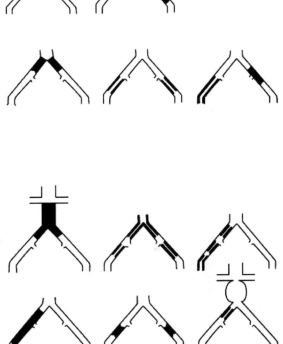

Fig. 9. Inter-Society Consensus for the Management of Peripheral Arterial Disease (TASC) classification of aortoiliac lesions. AAA, abdominal aortic aneurysm; CFA, common femoral artery; CIA, common iliac artery; EIA, external iliac artery. (*From* Norgren L, Hiatt WR, Dormandy JA, et al. Inter-Society Consensus for the management of peripheral arterial disease (TASC II). Int Angiol 2007;45(1 Suppl):S49A; with permission.)

vein grafts or synthetic graft conduits.[64,67] Alternatively, in patients for whom endovascular therapy is preferred, bare metal stents, drug-eluting stents, or covered stents would be candidate choices.[68] **Fig. 11** illustrates a patent right femoropopliteal bypass graft in a patient with bilateral long segment SFA occlusions and small collateral vessels in both thighs. Unusual collaterals involving the bilateral inferior epigastric arteries and additional small abdominal wall vessels have formed in the patient in **Fig. 12**, who was treated originally for aortoiliac occlusion (Leriche syndrome,[62]) with

bilateral axillofemoral bypass grafts that subsequently occluded.

LOWER EXTREMITY VASCULAR TRAUMA

Trauma to the lower extremities can occur from blunt or penetrating causes.[69,70] Blunt trauma includes motor vehicle collisions, falls, athletic injuries, and occupational injuries, and is often associated with severe pelvic, femoral, and/or tibial fractures. Penetrating trauma may occur secondary to ballistics, shrapnel, or low-velocity sharp

Type A lesions

- Single stenosis ≤10 cm in length
- Single occlusion ≤5 cm in length

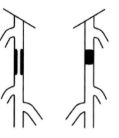

Type B lesions:

- Multiple lesions (stenoses or occlusions), each ≤5 cm
- Single stenosis or occlusion ≤15 cm not involving the infrageniculate popliteal artery
- Single or multiple lesions in the absence of continuous tibial vessels to improve inflow for a distal bypass
- Heavily calcified occlusion ≤5 cm in length
- Single popliteal stenosis

Type C lesions

- Multiple stenoses or occlusions totaling >15 cm with or without heavy calcification
- Recurrent stenoses or occlusions that need treatment after two endovascular interventions

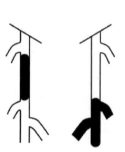

Type D lesions

- Chronic total occlusions of CFA or SFA (>20 cm, involving the popliteal artery)
- Chronic total occlusion of popliteal artery and proximal trifurcation vessels

Fig. 10. Inter-Society Consensus for the Management of Peripheral Arterial Disease (TASC) classification of femoropopliteal lesions. CFA; SFA, superficial femoral artery. (*From* Norgren L, Hiatt WR, Dormandy JA, et al. Inter-Society Consensus for the management of peripheral arterial disease (TASC II). Int Angiol 2007;45(1 Suppl):S51A; with permission.)

objects, and may or may not affect the bones of the extremity depending on the trajectory of the ballistic missile.[71]

Arterial injury in the setting of trauma may result in active extravasation, subcutaneous or intramuscular hematoma, pseudoaneurysm, vessel narrowing/stretching, occlusion, or arteriovenous fistula.[25] Fig. 13 demonstrates abrupt cutoff of the popliteal artery below the knee in this young patient status post through-and-through gunshot wound to the calf. The sagittal oblique thin MIP demonstrates the relationship of 2 branching foci

of extraluminal contrast at the inferiormost aspect of the popliteal artery, representing active extravasation, to the rest of the vessel. The popliteal artery does not opacify distal to these foci of extraluminal contrast. In some cases of trauma, vasospasm may be observed within segments of vessels adjacent to a nonvascular injury, such as a fracture or penetrating trauma, without actual injury to the vessel itself (Fig. 14). As shown in Fig. 15, in the absence of injury to the artery itself, the vasospasm eventually resolves and the normal caliber of the vessel is restored. In some cases, intraluminal vasodilators

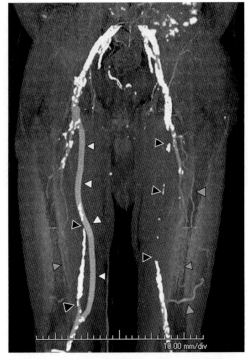

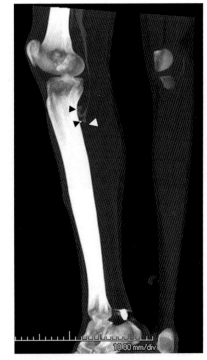

Fig. 11. Coronal maximum intensity projection with bone removal depicts bilateral superficial femoral artery (SFA) occlusions (*black arrowheads*) with small surrounding collateral vessels (*gray arrowheads*), and a patent femoropopliteal bypass graft (*white arrowheads*) connecting the right proximal SFA to the right popliteal artery.

Fig. 13. Oblique sagittal maximum intensity projection demonstrates abrupt cutoff of the popliteal artery below the knee (*white arrowhead*) with 2 branching foci of extraluminal contrast (*black arrowheads*) in keeping with injury to the vessel status post through-and-through gunshot wound.

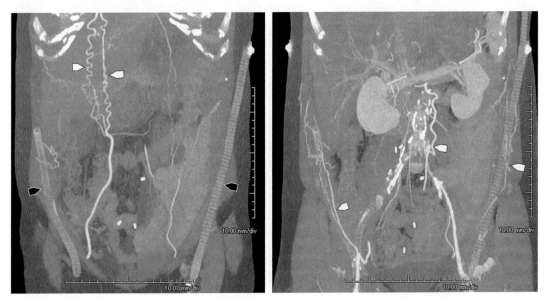

Fig. 12. Coronal thin maximum intensity projections centered at the anterior abdominal wall (*left*) and the kidneys (*right*) demonstrate bilateral occluded axillofemoral bypass grafts (*black arrowheads*) with unusual collateralization involving the bilateral inferior epigastric arteries as well as additional abdominal wall collaterals (*white arrowheads*). The bilateral bypass grafts were placed initially to treat the aortoiliac occlusion, demonstrated by lack of typical opacification in the image to the right.

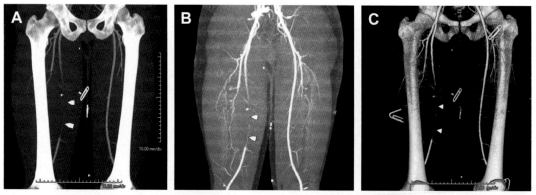

Fig. 14. Coronal (*A*) thin maximum intensity projection (MIP), (*B*) thick MIP with bone removal, and a (*C*) 3-dimensional volume-rendered image demonstrate a long segment of vasospasm of the superficial femoral artery (SFA) in the right thigh (*white arrowheads*) in this young male patient status post gunshot wound. The SFA lumen gradually tapers between the hip and mid thigh on the MIPs, almost completely disappears, and then gradually becomes normal in caliber above the knee.

such as nitroglycerin or papaverine can be administered to reverse vasospasm.

NONATHEROSCLEROTIC DISEASES OF THE LOWER EXTREMITY ARTERIES

During embryologic development, disruption of the evolution of capillary plexuses into arteries, veins and lymphatic channels may result in the formation of arteriovenous malformations.[72] These malformations are typically divided into 2 types: high flow, which contain arterial flow, and low flow, which are more common overall and typically contain venous flow. Although MRA is used more commonly to evaluate arteriovenous malformations because of the potential for dynamic

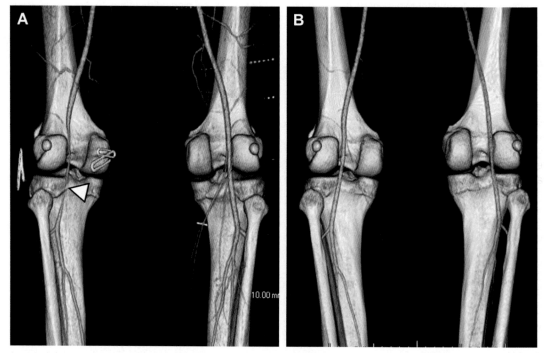

Fig. 15. (*A*) Posterior view of a coronal 3-dimensional volume-rendered (3-D VR) image demonstrates acute vasospasm of the popliteal artery behind the left knee (*white arrowhead*) status post gunshot wound, without active extravasation or other findings to suggest direct vascular injury. The right popliteal artery seems to be normal. (*B*) A 3-D VR from the same patient 48 hours after the initial trauma demonstrates normal caliber of both popliteal arteries in keeping with spontaneous resolution of vasospasm.

contrast-enhanced imaging and the avoidance of radiation exposure in young patients, CTA can also be useful for identifying calcifications.

Fibromuscular dysplasia is seen most commonly in the renal arteries and the extracranial carotid arteries; it is the second most common cause of renal artery stenosis.[34] However, it can also involve the iliofemoral vessels. It is characterized by segmental beading of the affected arteries and may necessitate anticoagulation or even surgery or endovascular repair in the setting of complications.[16]

Certain vasculitides can affect the lower extremity arteries and sometimes cause limb ischemia.[17,18] Takayasu arteritis is a large vessel vasculitis with a preponderance for female patients of childbearing age.[73] Owing to lower extremity involvement, patients experience claudication at a young age. During periods of vascular inflammation, CTA can detect arterial wall thickening and enhancement in addition to stenosis and occlusion. Buerger disease, also known as thrombangiitis obliterans, is a systemic vasculitis of small and medium vessels typically seen in young male patients, particularly in heavy smokers.[16] When the lower extremities are involved, patients again experience claudication. CTA typically reveals normal proximal arteries and progressive lack of opacification of the distal arteries owing to inflammation.

Aneurysms of the lower extremity arteries can also occur owing to both atherosclerotic and non-atherosclerotic causes. Patients with PAD may present with concomitant thrombosis or even occlusion of the affected vessel.[12] Although rare in young patients, aneurysms of the lower extremity arteries are typically congenital in origin and associated either with connective tissue disorders (Marfan, Ehlers–Danlos, and Loeys–Dietz syndromes) or vasculitis (Takayasu or Kawasaki disease, polyarteritis nodosa).[74] Popliteal artery aneurysms may occur in conjunction with popliteal artery entrapment syndrome (PAES), cystic adventitial disease, or trauma.[24] In all instances, CTA plays a role in the evaluation and anatomic characterization of the lesions.

Cystic adventitial disease is a rare cause of intermittent claudication that primarily affects the popliteal artery, but has been also been characterized in small numbers in the femoral arteries.[75,76] It causes mucin production within the adventitia of the artery and subsequent effacement or occlusion of the lumen.[16] The mucinous collections are typically more effectively visualized using T2-weighted MR imaging, but appear as hypodense foci within the arterial wall that compress the lumen on CTA. Endovascular repair has shown to be successful in these patients.[77]

LOWER EXTREMITY COMPUTED TOMOGRAPHY ANGIOGRAPHY FOR TREATMENT PLANNING

CTA of the lower extremities often plays a dual role in the management of patients with suspected lower extremity vascular disease, whether atherosclerotic or otherwise. In patients with PAD, it is often performed both to characterize the extent and severity of atherosclerotic lesions as well as to plan surgical or endovascular interventions.[2,35,57,78,79] Despite increasing comorbidities, fewer patients now undergo amputation to treat complications of PAD, thanks in part to more accurate disease characterization enabling earlier intervention.[79] Similarly, in the trauma setting, CTA helps to rapidly distinguish patients who need emergent intervention from those who can be treated conservatively.[25,70,80,81]

In addition to possible interventions on the lower extremity vasculature, however, CTA also plays a valuable role in surgical planning elsewhere in the body. Perforator flaps—skin, underlying adipose tissue, and an associated vascular pedicle—can be harvested from many different anatomic locations to replace tissue resected for the treatment of cancer, postablation changes, trauma, or burns.[82] Potential harvest locations include the rectus abdominis musculature and multiple sites in the lower extremities (eg, deep inferior epigastric, transverse upper gracilis, superior gluteal, fibular). Candidates for fibular free flap reconstruction after mastectomy or resection of head and neck carcinomas often undergo CTA or MRA of the lower extremities in the course of their surgical planning.[34,78,83,84] During this process, it is particularly important to identify variant popliteal branching anatomy that can affect the perfusion of the extremity from which the fibular flap would be harvested (see **Fig. 2**).[84]

SUMMARY

CTA of the lower extremities is an important and versatile noninvasive tool for diagnosis as well as surgical or endovascular interventional planning. Although lower extremity CTA is most commonly performed in patients who suffer from PAD or trauma affecting the lower extremities, it also plays a role in the workup of nonischemic etiologies and congenital vascular malformations. CT scanner protocols should adjust bolus timing and multiphasic imaging to account for the clinical question of interest, and 3-dimensional postprocessing plays an important role in the visualization and interpretation of these high-resolution imaging examinations.

REFERENCES

1. Algazzar MAA. Role of multi-detector computed tomography angiography in the evaluation of lower limb ischemia. Int J Med Imaging 2014;2(5):125–30.

2. Walls MC, Thavendiranathan P, Rajagopalan S. Advances in CT angiography for peripheral arterial disease. Cardiol Clin 2011;29(3):331–40.

3. Lau JF, Weinberg MD, Olin JW. Peripheral artery disease. Part 1: clinical evaluation and noninvasive diagnosis. Nat Rev Cardiol 2011;8(7):405–18.

4. Criqui MH. The epidemiology of peripheral artery disease. Vasc Med A Companion Braunwald's Hear Dis 2013;211–22.

5. Joosten MM, Pai JK, Bertoia ML, et al. Associations between conventional cardiovascular risk factors and risk of peripheral artery disease in men. JAMA 2012;308:1660–7.

6. Subherwal S, Patel MR, Kober L, et al. Peripheral artery disease is a coronary heart disease risk equivalent among both men and women: results from a nationwide study. Eur J Prev Cardiol 2014;22(3):317–25.

7. Grenon SM, Vittinghoff E, Owens CD, et al. Peripheral artery disease and risk of cardiovascular events in patients with coronary artery disease: insights from the Heart and Soul Study. Vasc Med 2013; 18(4):176–84.

8. O'Neal WT, Efird JT, Nazarian S, et al. Peripheral arterial disease and risk of atrial fibrillation and stroke: the multi-ethnic study of atherosclerosis. J Am Heart Assoc 2014;3:1–7.

9. Peach G, Griffin M, Jones KG, et al. Diagnosis and management of peripheral arterial disease. BMJ 2012;345:1–8.

10. Rooke TW, Hirsch AT, Misra S, et al. Management of patients with peripheral artery disease (compilation of 2005 and 2011 ACCF/AHA guideline recommendations): a report of the American College of Cardiology Foundation/American Heart Association Task Force on Practice Guidelines. J Am Coll Cardiol 2013;61(14):1555–70.

11. Korabathina R, Weintraub AR, Price LL, et al. Twenty-year analysis of trends in the incidence and in-hospital mortality for lower-extremity arterial thromboembolism. Circulation 2013;128(2):115–21.

12. Harbuzariu C, Duncan AA, Bower TC, et al. Profunda femoris artery aneurysms: association with aneurysmal disease and limb ischemia. J Vasc Surg 2008;47(1):31–5.

13. Dormandy J, Heeck L, Vig S. Acute limb ischemia. Semin Vasc Surg 1999;12(2):148–53.

14. O'Connell JB, Quiñones-Baldrich WJ. Proper evaluation and management of acute embolic versus thrombotic limb ischemia. Semin Vasc Surg 2009; 22(1):10–6.

15. Sigl M, Hsu E, Scheffel H, et al. Lower extremity vasculitis in giant cell arteritis: important differential diagnosis in patients with lower limb claudication. Vasa 2014;43(5):326–36.

16. Weinberg I, Jaff MR. Nonatherosclerotic arterial disorders of the lower extremities. Circulation 2012; 126(2):213–22.

17. Morbi A, Gohel MS, Hamady M, et al. Lower-limb ischemia in the young patient: management strategies in an endovascular era. Ann Vasc Surg 2012; 26(4):591–9.

18. Peach G, Loftus IM. Acute and chronic lower limb ischaemia. Surg 2013;31(5):229–35.

19. Zhu FP, Luo S, Wang ZJ, et al. Takayasu arteritis: imaging spectrum at multidetector CT angiography. Br J Radiol 2012;85(1020):e1282–92.

20. Yanik B, Bulbul E, Demirpolat G. Variations of the popliteal artery branching with multidetector CT angiography. Surg Radiol Anat 2014;37(3):223–30.

21. Mauro M, Jaques PF, Moore M. The popliteal artery and its branches: embryologic basis of normal and variant anatomy. Am J Roentgenol 1987;150(2):435–7.

22. Kim D, Orron DE, Skillman JJ. Surgical significance of popliteal arterial variants. A unified angiographic classification. Ann Surg 1989;210(6):776–81.

23. Massoud T, Fletcher E. Anatomical variants of the profunda femoris artery: an angiographic study. Surg Radiol Anat 1997;19:99–103.

24. Wright LB, Matchett WJ, Cruz CP, et al. Popliteal artery disease: diagnosis and treatment. Radiographics 2004;24(2):467–79.

25. Foster BR, Anderson SW, Uyeda JW, et al. Integration of 64-detector lower extremity CT angiography into whole-body trauma imaging: feasibility and early experience. Radiology 2011;261(3):787–95.

26. Redondo P, Aguado L, Martínez-Cuesta A. Diagnosis and management of extensive vascular malformations of the lower limb: part I. Clinical diagnosis. J Am Acad Dermatol 2011;65(5):893–906.

27. Day CP, Orme R. Popliteal artery branching patterns-an angiographic study. Clin Radiol 2006; 61(8):696–9.

28. Lambert AW, Wilkins DC. Popliteal artery entrapment syndrome. Blood Vessel 1972;3(1):53–4.

29. Yamaguchi M, Mii S, Kai T, et al. Intermittent claudication associated with persistent sciatic artery: report of two cases. Surg Today 1997;27(9):863–7.

30. Van Hooft IM, Zeebregts CJ, van Sterkenburg SMM, et al. The persistent sciatic artery. Eur J Vasc Endovasc Surg 2009;37(5):585–91.

31. Mandell VS, Jaques PF, Delany DJ, et al. Persistent sciatic artery: clinical, embryologic and angiographic features. Am J Roentgenol 1985;144:245–9.

32. McLellan GL, Morettin LB. Persistent sciatic artery: clinical, surgical and angiographic aspects. Arch Surg 1982;117:817–22.

33. Santaolalla V, Bernabe MH, Hipola Ulecia JM, et al. Persistent sciatic artery. Ann Vasc Surg 2010;24(5): 691.e7–10.

34. Liu PS, Platt JF. CT angiography in the abdomen: a pictorial review and update. Abdom Imaging 2014; 39(1):196–214.

35. Fleischmann D, Hallett RL, Rubin GD. CT angiography of peripheral arterial disease. J Vasc Interv Radiol 2006;17(1):3–26.

36. Keeling AN, Farrelly C, Carr JC, et al. Technical considerations for lower limb multidetector computed tomographic angiography. Vasc Med 2011;16(2): 131–43.

37. Cademartiri F, van der Lugt A, Luccichenti G, et al. Parameters affecting bolus geometry in CTA: a review. J Comput Assist Tomogr 2002;26(4):598–607.

38. Duan Y, Wang X, Yang X, et al. Diagnostic efficiency of low-dose CT angiography compared with conventional angiography in peripheral arterial occlusions. Am J Roentgenol 2013;201:906–14.

39. Iezzi R, Santoro M, Marano R, et al. Low-Dose Multidetector CT angiography in the evaluation of infrarenal aorta and peripheral arterial occlusive disease. Radiology 2012;263(1):287–98.

40. Park JH, Choo KS, Jeon UB, et al. Image quality and radiation dose of lower extremity CT angiography in 128 slice dual-source CT: comparison of high pitch and low pitch. J Korean Soc Radiol 2014;71(3): 120–7. Available at: http://synapse.koreamed.org/Synapse/Data/PDFData/2016JKSR/jksr-71-120.pdf.

41. Sudarski S, Apfaltrer P, Nance JW Jr, et al. Optimization of keV-settings in abdominal and lower extremity dual-source dual-energy CT angiography determined with virtual monoenergetic imaging. Eur J Radiol 2013;82:e574–81.

42. Kau T, Eicher W, Reiterer C, et al. Dual-energy CT angiography in peripheral arterial occlusive disease-accuracy of maximum intensity projections in clinical routine and subgroup analysis. Eur Radiol 2011;21:1677–86.

43. Sobocinski J, Chenorhokian H, Maurel B, et al. The benefits of EVAR planning using a 3D workstation. Eur J Vasc Endovasc Surg 2013;46(4):418–23.

44. Sun Z. Multislice computed tomography angiography in the diagnosis of cardiovascular disease: 3D visualizations. Front Med 2011;5(3):254–70.

45. Otal H, Takasel K, Igarashi K, et al. MDCT compared with digital subtraction angiography for assessment of lower extremity arterial occlusive disease: importance of reviewing cross-sectional images. Am J Roentgenol 2004;182(1):201–9.

46. Doobay AV, Anand SS. Sensitivity and specificity of the ankle-brachial index to predict future cardiovascular outcomes: a systematic review. Arterioscler Thromb Vasc Biol 2005;25(7):1463–9.

47. Fowkes FG, Housley E, Macintyre CC, et al. Variability of ankle and brachial systolic pressures in the measurement of atherosclerotic peripheral arterial disease. J Epidemiol Community Health 1988; 42(2):128–33.

48. Yao ST, Hobbs JT, Irvine WT. Ankle pressure measurement in arterial disease of the lower extremities. Br J Surg 1968;55(11):859–60.

49. Gronewold J, Hermann DM, Lehmann N, et al. Ankle-brachial index predicts stroke in the general population in addition to classical risk factors. Atherosclerosis 2014;233(2):545–50.

50. Aboyans V, Criqui MH, Abraham P, et al. Measurement and interpretation of the ankle-brachial index: a scientific statement from the American Heart Association. Circulation 2012;126(24):2890–909.

51. Moyer V, US Preventive Services Task Force. Screening for peripheral artery disease and cardiovascular disease risk assessment with the ankle – brachial index in adults: U.S. Preventive Services Task Force Recommendation Statement. Ann Intern Med 2014;159(5):342–9.

52. Guthaner F, Wexler L, Enzmann D, et al. Evaluation of peripheral vascular disease using digital subtraction angiography. Radiology 1983;147:393–8.

53. Adriaensen ME, Kock MC, Stijnen T, et al. Peripheral arterial disease: therapeutic confidence of CT versus digital subtraction angiography and effects on additional imaging recommendations. Radiology 2004;233(2):385–91.

54. Martin ML, Tay KH, Flak B, et al. Multidetector CT angiography of the aortoiliac system and lower extremities: a prospective comparison with digital subtraction angiography. AJR Am J Roentgenol 2003; 180:1085–91.

55. Willmann JK, Baumert B, Schertler T, et al. Aortoiliac and lower extremity arteries assessed with 16-detector row CT angiography: prospective comparison with digital subtraction angiography. Radiology 2005;236(3):1083–93.

56. Kayhan A, Palabiyik F, Serinsöz S, et al. Multidetector CT angiography versus arterial duplex USG in diagnosis of mild lower extremity peripheral arterial disease: is multidetector CT a valuable screening tool? Eur J Radiol 2012;81(3):542–6.

57. De Vos MS, Bol BJ, Gravereaux EC, et al. Treatment planning for peripheral arterial disease based on duplex ultrasonography and computed tomography angiography: Consistency, confidence and the value of additional imaging. Surgery 2014;156(2): 492–502.

58. Hodnett PA, Koktzoglou I, Davarpanah AH, et al. Evaluation of peripheral arterial disease with nonenhanced quiescent-interval single-shot MR angiography. Radiology 2011;260(1):282–93.

59. Burbelko M, Augsten M, Kalinowski MO, et al. Comparison of contrast-enhanced multi-station MR angiography and digital subtraction angiography of the lower extremity arterial disease. J Magn Reson Imaging 2013;37(6):1427–35.

60. Van den Bosch HCM, Westenberg JJM, Caris R, et al. Peripheral arterial occlusive angiography

compared with digital subtraction angiography. Radiology 2013;266(1):337–46.

61. Reekers JA. Interventional radiology in the diabetic lower extremity. Med Clin North Am 2013;97(5):836–45.

62. Catalano C, Fraioli F, Laghi A, et al. Infrarenal aortic and lower-extremity arterial disease: diagnostic performance of multi-detector row CT angiography. Radiology 2004;231:555–63.

63. Huang SY, Nelson RC, Miller MJ, et al. Assessment of vascular contrast and depiction of stenoses in abdominopelvic and lower extremity vasculature. Comparison of dual-energy MDCT with digital subtraction angiography. Acad Radiol 2012;19(9):1149–57.

64. Pollak AW, Norton PT, Kramer CM. Multimodality imaging of lower extremity peripheral arterial disease current role and future directions. Circ Cardiovasc Imaging 2012;5(6):797–807.

65. Sommer WH, Bamberg F, Johnson TRC, et al. Diagnostic accuracy of dynamic computed tomographic angiographic of the lower leg in patients with critical limb ischemia. Invest Radiol 2012;47(6):325–31.

66. Norgren L, Hiatt WR, Dormandy JA, et al. Inter-Society Consensus for the management of peripheral arterial disease (TASC II). Int Angiol 2007;45(1 Suppl):S5A–67A.

67. Defreitas DJ, Love TP, Kasirajan K, et al. Computed tomography angiography-based evaluation of great saphenous vein conduit for lower extremity bypass. J Vasc Surg 2013;57(1):50–5.

68. Kakkar AM, Abbott JD. Percutaneous versus surgical management of lower extremity peripheral artery disease. Curr Atheroscler Rep 2015;17(2):1–9.

69. Guermazi A, Hayashi D, Smith SE, et al. Imaging of blast injuries to the lower extremities sustained in the Boston Marathon bombing. Arthritis Care Res 2013; 65(12):1893–8.

70. Watchorn J, Miles R, Moore N. The role of CT angiography in military trauma. Clin Radiol 2013; 68(1):39–46.

71. Adibi A, Krishnam MS, Dissanayake S, et al. Computed tomography angiography of lower extremities in the emergency room for evaluation of patients with gunshot wounds. Eur Radiol 2014;24: 1586–93.

72. Nozaki T, Nosaka S, Miyazaki O, et al. Syndromes associated with vascular tumors and malformations: a pictorial review. Radiographics 2013;33(1):175–95.

73. Mavrogeni S, Dimitroulas T, Chatziioannou SN, et al. The role of multimodality imaging in the evaluation of Takayasu arteritis. Semin Arthritis Rheum 2013; 42(4):401–12.

74. Lopez-Gutierrez JC, Rodríguez LC, Bret Zurita M, et al. Multiple congenital ectatic and fusiform arterial aneurysms associated with lower limb hypoplasia. J Vasc Surg 2012;56(2):496–9.

75. Patel SD, Guessoum M, Matheiken S. Cystic adventitial disease of the common femoral artery presenting with acute limb ischemia. Ann Vasc Surg 2014; 28(8):1937.e9–11.

76. Wu X, Lun Y, Jiang H, et al. Cystic adventitial disease of the common femoral vessels: report of 2 cases and literature review. Vasc Endovascular Surg 2014;48(4):325–8.

77. Mertens R, Bergoeing M, Mariné L, et al. Endovascular treatment of cystic adventitial disease of the popliteal artery. Ann Vasc Surg 2013;27(8):1185. e1–3.

78. Higueras Suñé MC, López Ojeda A, Narváez García JA, et al. Use of angioscanning in the surgical planning of perforator flaps in the lower extremities. J Plast Reconstr Aesthet Surg 2011;64:1207–15.

79. Egorova NN, Guillerme S, Gelijns A, et al. An analysis of the outcomes of a decade of experience with lower extremity revascularization including limb salvage, lengths of stay, and safety. J Vasc Surg 2010;51(4):878–85.e1.

80. Wallin D, Yaghoubian A, Rosing D, et al. Computed tomographic angiography as the primary diagnostic modality in penetrating lower extremity vascular injuries: a level I trauma experience. Ann Vasc Surg 2011;25(5):620–3.

81. Fox N, Rajani RR, Bokhari F, et al. Evaluation and management of penetrating lower extremity arterial trauma. J Trauma Acute Care Surg 2012;73(5): S315–20.

82. Kagen A, Hossain R, Dayan E, et al. Modern perforator flap imaging with high-resolution blood pool MR angiography. RadioGraphics 2015;35(3): 1–15.

83. Jin KN, Lee W, Yin YH, et al. Preoperative evaluation of lower extremity arteries for free fibula transfer using MDCT angiography. J Comput Assist Tomogr 2007;31(5):820–5.

84. Chow LC, Napoli A, Klein MB, et al. Vascular mapping of the leg with multi-detector row CT angiography prior to free-flap transplantation. Radiology 2005;237(1):353–60.

Computed Tomography Angiography for Preoperative Thoracoabdominal Flap Planning

Ryan B. O'Malley, MD[a],*, Tracy J. Robinson, MD, MS[b],
Jeffrey H. Kozlow, MD, MS[c], Peter S. Liu, MD[d]

KEYWORDS

- Computed tomography angiography • Breast cancer • Deep inferior epigastric perforator (DIEP) flap
- Perforator-based flap • Breast reconstruction

KEY POINTS

- Evolution of breast reconstruction has led to complex muscle-sparing techniques that require microvascular anastomoses and considerable surgical expertise.
- The deep inferior epigastric perforator (DIEP) flap preserves the rectus muscle and anterior rectus sheath, using only subcutaneous fat and skin with perforating vessels.
- Preoperative CTA provides accuracy for perforator identification, resulting in improved operative performance and clinical outcomes.
- CTA can help to select perforators with optimal characteristics, allowing plastic surgeons to improve flap design and plan a targeted dissection strategy.
- In select cases, CTA is also used to evaluate thoracic anatomy and recipient vasculature, which allows for additional preoperative planning and customization.

BACKGROUND

Breast cancer is the second most common cancer in the United States with an estimated 232,670 new cases and 40,000 deaths in 2014 (National Cancer Institute. Surveillance, Epidemiology, and End Results (SEER); available from: http://www.seer.cancer.gov/about). However, comprehensive treatment is increasingly effective as death rates have fallen on average 1.9% each year over 2002 to 2011 with a 5-year relative survival of 90.6% (SEER 9 incidence and U.S. mortality 1975–2011, all races, females; rates are age adjusted). Additionally, the vast majority of patients (93%) are diagnosed with curable localized or regional disease and thus are potential surgical

Disclosure Statement: The authors have nothing to disclose.
[a] Department of Radiology, University of Washington Medical Center, 1959 Northeast Pacific Street, Box 357115, Seattle, WA 98195-7117, USA; [b] Seattle Radiologists, 1229 Madison Street, Suite 900, Seattle, WA 98104, USA; [c] Section of Plastic Surgery, Department of Surgery, University of Michigan Health System, 1500 East Medical Center Drive, Ann Arbor, MI 48109-0340, USA; [d] Cleveland Clinic, 9500 Euclid Avenue, L10-413, Cleveland, OH 44195, USA
* Corresponding author.
E-mail address: ryanomal@uw.edu

Radiol Clin N Am 54 (2016) 131–145
http://dx.doi.org/10.1016/j.rcl.2015.08.007
0033-8389/16/$ – see front matter © 2016 Elsevier Inc. All rights reserved.

candidates (SEER 18 2004–2010, all races, females by SEER summary stage 2000). Since 1990, breast-conserving therapy (lumpectomy plus radiation therapy) has been recommended by the National Institutes of Health as the preferred management for appropriately selected patients with early stage breast cancer.[1] Mastectomy rates subsequently declined, reaching a nadir in 2005. However, since 2005, mastectomy rates in the United States have risen among all demographic groups, but most significantly among younger women.[1] Moreover, as lumpectomy rates decrease, more women are also choosing to undergo contralateral prophylactic mastectomy, particularly women 45 years or younger.[2] The exact cause for these trends is undoubtedly multifactorial, but advances in surgical technique and access to breast reconstruction likely play a role in decision making. The reconstruction options now available make mastectomy a more appealing option that it was previously.[3] Postmastectomy breast reconstruction is typically performed using either a breast implant placed under the pectoralis major muscle or by transferring the localized adiposity of the lower abdomen in an autologous reconstruction. For women opting to undergo an autologous reconstruction, the deep inferior epigastric perforator (DIEP) flap has emerged as a state-of-the-art option by allowing preservation of the rectus abdominis muscle compared with other techniques. Successful transfer of the lower abdominal skin and adipose tissue is based on selecting and then dissecting out intramuscular perforator blood vessels that originate from the deep inferior epigastric artery (DIEA), traverse through the rectus abdominis muscle, and then pierce the anterior abdominal fascia to supply the overlying skin and fat. Performing a DIEP flap is an intensive, time-consuming process that relies heavily on surgical expertise and careful evaluation of the vascular anatomy. However, preoperative imaging with computed tomography angiography (CTA) is an effective tool for optimizing patient selection and guiding operative dissection.

SURGICAL EVOLUTION

Breast reconstruction is an essential component of a comprehensive breast cancer treatment plan and has been federally mandated since 1998. Reconstruction options have become increasingly innovative, with multiple options available for all patients and body types. All reconstruction plans seek to ensure an adequate skin envelope and then filling of the breast volume and shape. Multiple studies have demonstrated the quality

of life and body image benefits for women undergoing breast reconstruction. Although breast reconstruction can be performed with silicone or saline-filled implants, these types of reconstruction may not feel or look "natural" and carry the long-term risks of implantable mechanical devices. Autologous reconstruction uses a patient's own subcutaneous fat and skin to reconstruct the breast and often provides improved appearance, feel, and durability. However, these reconstructions require a second donor site for flap harvest with associated donor site morbidity.

In many women, the lower abdomen (between the umbilicus and the pubic hair line) has sufficient excess adipose tissue for breast reconstruction that can be harvested and closed with a low transverse scar similar to a "tummy tuck." Initially described in 1982 by Hartrampf, the transverse rectus abdominus myocutaneous (TRAM) flap was the first major option for autologous reconstruction, serving as the standard for breast reconstruction for nearly 10 years. Initially, the TRAM flap was a pedicled flap using the superior epigastric vessels, wherein the entire rectus abdominis muscle, subcutaneous fat, overlying skin, and the native vascular pedicle were rotated on the vascular stalk to the reconstruction site. The TRAM flap then evolved into a free flap using the inferior epigastric vessels where, using microdissection, the flap is detached completely from the donor site vasculature and anastomosed to the reconstruction site.

Although TRAM flaps were widely used and provided effective natural breast reconstruction, they also resulted in substantial donor site morbidity, including pain, cosmetic defect or laxity, hernia, nerve injury, and postoperative loss of function.[4] As a result, surgical techniques continued to evolve, striving to minimize donor site morbidity by minimizing disruption of the rectus muscle and maintaining vascularity and innervation.[5] Because the rectus muscle and anterior rectus sheath are the primary determinants of abdominal contour and strength, the muscle-sparing TRAM uses only a small muscle segment with a small portion of the anterior rectus sheath, rather than the entire muscle.

Continued evolution led to even more extreme muscle-sparing techniques where no rectus muscle is used in the flap. The DIEP flap is a free flap that preserves the rectus muscle and anterior rectus sheath, using only subcutaneous fat and skin with 1 to 3 perforating vessels (**Fig. 1**).[6] Compared with a TRAM flap, the DIEP flap provides the same excellent tissue for breast reconstruction, but has distinct advantages at the

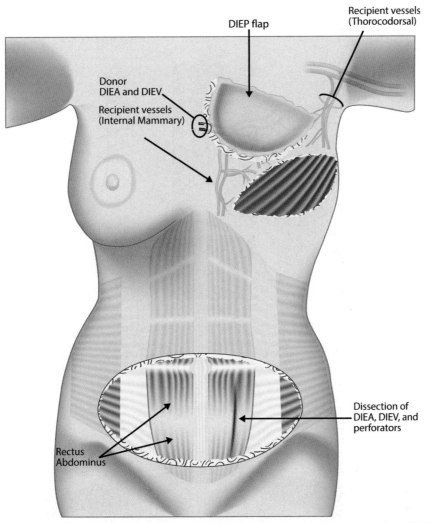

Fig. 1. Coronal illustration of deep inferior epigastric perforator (DIEP) flap reconstruction. The DIEP flap is a free flap that does not incorporate any portion of the rectus muscle, solely using the overlying skin and subcutaneous fat for the reconstruction. During the microdissection, rectus muscle fibers are spread longitudinally to minimize disruption. DIEA, deep inferior epigastric artery; DIEV, deep inferior epigastric vein.

donor site. Because the rectus abdominis muscle is preserved, patients undergoing DIEP flap reconstruction have lower abdominal wall hernia and bulge rates, better sensation recovery, and return to baseline rectus and oblique muscle function.[7–13] However, advantages at the donor site come at the expense of increased flap complications when compared with TRAM and other muscle-sparing techniques with increased rates of fat necrosis, venous congestion, and flap loss.[8–11,14,15] DIEP flaps are also more time consuming, requiring considerable surgical expertise and experience. As such, the choice of breast construction is an individual decision for both patient and surgeon, which must balance preservation of abdominal musculature

and donor site morbidity with long-term flap viability.

ANATOMY

The DIEA is the dominant vascular supply of the anterior abdominal wall, arising from the distal external iliac artery, just above the inguinal ligament.[16] After arising from the external iliac artery, the DIEA ascends with the deep inferior epigastric vein between the posterior border of the rectus muscle and posterior rectus sheath, often with some intramuscular course (**Fig. 2**). There are 3 distinct branching patterns of the DIEA (**Fig. 3**): a single trunk (type I), bifurcation with 2 major intramuscular branches above the arcuate line (type II),

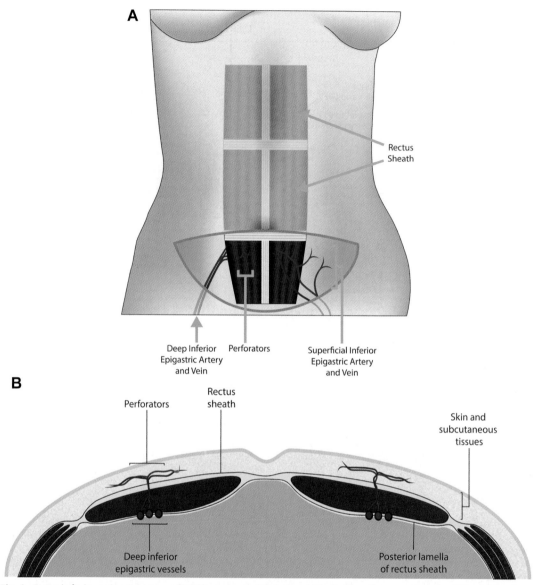

Fig. 2. Deep inferior epigastric artery (DIEA) anatomy. (*A*) Coronal illustration demonstrates the DIEA arising from the distal external iliac artery just above the inguinal ligament, then ascending to provide most of the vascular supply of the anterior abdominal wall. (*B*) Axial illustration of the anterior abdominal wall shows the deep inferior epigastric artery and vein coursing together between the posterior aspect of the rectus muscle and posterior rectus sheath. Perforators arise from the DIEA, traverse the rectus muscle, then supply the overlying skin and subcutaneous fat.

and division into 3 or more branches (type III).[17] As it ascends, the DIEA gives rise to a variable number of perforating arteries that penetrate the rectus muscle, traverse the muscle anteriorly, and supply a segment of overlying skin and fat. These perforator arteries (and veins) are the basis for microdissection when performing a DIEP flap.

DIEA perforators have 3 distinct anatomic segments, as defined by the anatomic spaces through which they proceed (**Fig. 4**).[18] The intramuscular

segment refers to a perforator's course through the rectus muscle and is a key consideration for surgical dissection because a longer, more oblique intramuscular course results in more complex microdissection. Some perforators penetrate a musculotendinous intersection and have no intramuscular segment, which is preferred by some surgeons. As it exits the rectus muscle, a perforator may have a subfascial course between the anterior border of the rectus muscle and anterior

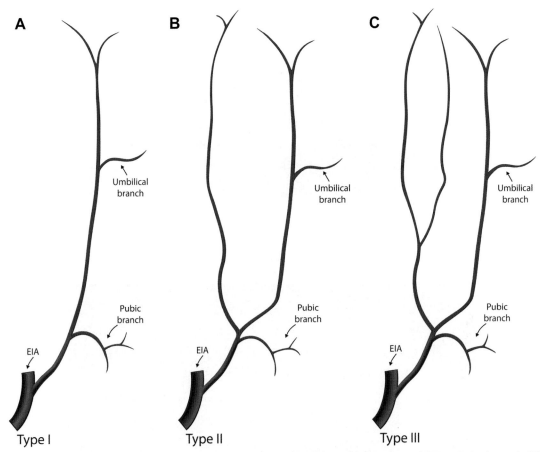

Fig. 3. Coronal illustration of deep inferior epigastric artery (DIEA) branching patterns. (*A*) Type I, single trunk. (*B*) Type II, bifurcation with 2 major intramuscular branches above the arcuate line. Note that this configuration typically has medial and lateral rows of perforators corresponding to the medial and lateral branches. (*C*) Type III, division into 3 (or more) branches.

rectus sheath. A longer subfascial course is also disadvantageous because it requires more careful dissection when incising the rectus sheath. Finally, the perforator penetrates the anterior rectus sheath and terminates in its subcutaneous segment with branching and anastomoses with the superficial inferior epigastric artery.

OPERATIVE TECHNIQUE

The proposed flap is outlined on the patient's skin marked with a "road map" of the preoperatively identified perforators (**Fig. 5**). A 2-team approach is typically used, allowing for simultaneous dissection of both the abdominal flap and recipient vessels. An ellipsoid flap is raised lateral to medial and perforators are carefully evaluated as they are encountered (**Fig. 6**). Perforators deemed unsuitable are sacrificed. Suitable perforators are chosen based on caliber and location (preferably a single dominant perforator or 2–3 small perforators

in the same row), then dissected to their origin at the DIEA. While dissecting, the anterior rectus sheath is opened around the perforator(s), taking care not to damage the subfascial segment. As dissection continues along the intramuscular segment, the rectus muscle is spread longitudinally in the direction of its fibers to minimize disruption. Dissection continues until the pedicle is deemed to be of sufficient length and caliber for anastomosis with the recipient vessels, then the artery and vein are ligated (**Fig. 7**). Microvascular anastomosis is performed to the recipient vessels, typically the internal mammary vessels, although the thoracodorsal vessels may also be used.

ROLE OF PREOPERATIVE COMPUTED TOMOGRAPHY ANGIOGRAPHY

CTA has become the gold standard in preoperative imaging for DIEP flaps, allowing surgeons to

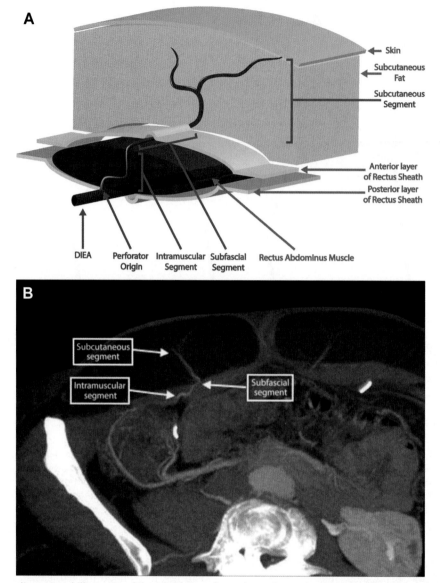

Fig. 4. Three-dimensional illustration (*A*) and axial maximum intensity projection (*B*) of the deep inferior epigastric artery (DIEA) perforator segments. After arising from the DIEA, perforators first traverse the rectus muscle (intramuscular segment), then course between the anterior aspect of the rectus muscle and anterior recuts sheath (subfascial segment) before terminating and branching in the overlying subcutaneous fat (subcutaneous segment). During microdissection, the length and location of the subfascial segment is of particular importance to avoid damaging the vessel while incising the fascia.

improve flap design and plan a targeted dissection strategy. In addition to the steep learning curve already present when harvesting perforator flaps, DIEA anatomy is highly variable with varying perforator size, number, location, and course. Moreover, perforators vary significantly between patients and even within a single patient's hemi-abdomen, which makes for complex surgical dissection and affects flap planning.[19] By identifying perforators preoperatively, CTA provides localization relative to the umbilicus to expedite and simplify intraoperative identification. CTA can also help select perforators with optimal characteristics, thus allowing for perforator(s) and hemiabdomen of choice to be chosen preoperatively, facilitating a more targeted microdissection, minimal rectus disruption, shorter operative times, and less of a learning curve, all of which may help to decrease flap-related complications. Additionally, patients with unsuitable anatomy can be

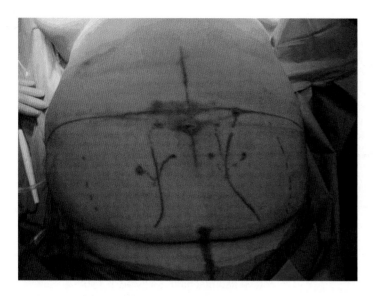

Fig. 5. Intraoperative photograph before the deep inferior epigastric perforator flap is cut. Using preoperative CT angiography, the perforators are marked on the patient's skin and the proposed flap is outlined.

identified preoperatively. In some patients, the inferior epigastric artery is congenitally absent or occluded from prior surgery. There is also a small subset of patients that have no suitable perforators. For these patients, CTA identifies these findings preoperatively, thus preventing unnecessary surgery and allowing for an alternate reconstruction plan.

CTA has been shown to be highly accurate for identifying perforators with reported sensitivities and positive predictive values approaching 100% for identifying perforators greater than 1 mm.[20] Beyond simply identifying the perforators, CTA also provides multiplanar 3-dimensional assessment of the intramuscular, subfascial, and subcutaneous segments and can use volume-rendered,

grid-based localization, all of which can aid in surgical planning. Postprocessed images generated by CTA can be tailored to each surgeon's preferences, and then viewed in the clinic with the patient and in the operating room.

Before the advent of CTA, duplex ultrasonography was the mainstay for perforator mapping because it is inexpensive, widely available, and provides both perforator diameter and flow velocity.[19] However, CTA has been shown to be less operator dependent and less time consuming compared with ultrasonography.[20] CTA also demonstrates the entire course of the perforators, as well as the DIEA anatomy, which is not feasible sonographically. A metaanalysis has also shown better outcomes in patients undergoing preoperative

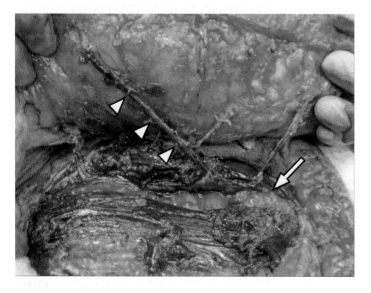

Fig. 6. Intraoperative photograph as the deep inferior epigastric perforator flap is harvested. An ellipsoid flap is raised lateral-to-medial and the perforators are carefully dissected (arrowheads). As the perforator is dissected along its intramuscular segment, the rectus muscle fibers are spread longitudinally (arrow) to minimized disruption.

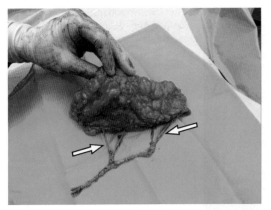

Fig. 7. Intraoperative photograph after deep inferior epigastric perforator (DIEP) flap harvest, before anastomosis. Microdissection of the perforators (*arrows*) continues until the vascular pedicle is deemed to be sufficient length and size, then the artery and vein are ligated. The DIEP flap is then mobilized to the recipient site and microvascular anastomosis is performed.

planning CTA compared with ultrasonography, with decreased rates of flap loss and donor site morbidity.[21] More recently, MR angiography has emerged as an alternative to CTA and has been shown to be equally effective identifying arterial anatomy, without the risk of ionizing radiation.[22] However, CTA remains faster, more widely available, and superior in identifying intramuscular course and branching type.[23]

Using CTA before DIEP flap has been shown to result in excellent clinical outcomes. DIEP flaps performed after preoperative CTA report decreased operative time, operative stress for the surgeon, intraoperative blood loss requiring transfusion, hernia rates, and duration of inpatient hospital stay.[17,24–28] By identifying the optimal perforators and decreasing operative time, CTA also results in decreased rates of fat necrosis and flap loss, thus mitigating many of the disadvantages associated with performing a DIEP flap.[20] Although performing a CTA is inherently more expensive than its historical comparison (ultrasonography), using CTA can decrease overall costs by decreasing operative times and hospital duration of stay, which is a major consideration in today's health care landscape.[29]

The main limitation of CTA is the exposure to ionizing radiation, particularly because many breast cancer patients considering mastectomy are younger and potentially at higher risk for radiation-related effects. By modifying the technique and scanning only the area of interest, the radiation dose can be diminished and remains low compared with other routine examinations.[30]

Use of iodinated contrast carries the risk of contrast-induced nephropathy and allergic-like reactions that also must be considered. Incidental findings discovered on CTA may require additional workup or imaging, thus delaying surgery.[31] Compared with duplex ultrasonography, CTA also cannot provide functional information, such as flow velocity.

COMPUTED TOMOGRAPHY ANGIOGRAPHY TECHNIQUE

From a technical perspective, a CTA performed for preoperative DIEP flap imaging is essentially a modified version of a standard aortic CTA protocol, in which opacification of the inferior epigastric circulation is prioritized. The scan parameters from the CTA protocol used at our institution for preoperative flap planning are listed in **Table 1**. Several aspects are discussed in greater detail elsewhere in this article.

Patient preparation for scanning is similar to other aortic imaging protocols, including the necessity for large-bore intravenous access for high contrast rate injections. Oral contrast material is not used because bowel detail is irrelevant to the primary scan purpose and greater attenuation bowel content would adversely affect 3-dimensional (3D) reformatted images. Patients are asked to remove any clothing in the infraumbilical region (particularly tight-fighting items) so as to replicate similar skin contours with what would be expected in the operating room.

As with standard aortic CTA, a helical/volumetric scan technique is used for DIEP flap planning CTA studies. At our institution, thin section isotropic 0.625 mm imaging is obtained through the abdomen and pelvis because the technologists are familiar with the scout image anatomic markers for such a standard scan range. Some authors advocate use of a more targeted scan range in flap-planning CTA studies, which extends from approximately 4 cm above the umbilicus through the common femoral artery.[18] The field of view is adjusted to fit patient size, but it is mandatory to cover the entire skin surface. For intravenous contrast, 100 mL of a high iodine-concentration contrast material (370 mg iodine/mL) is given at 5 mL/s, followed by a normal saline chaser via a dual-head injector system. Other scan parameters from our institution include: pitch 1.375:1; speed 55; kVp 100 to 120 kVp based on patient weight; automatic mA with lower and higher constraints of 100 and 575, respectively; and noise index 34.5. For noise reduction, we routinely use a 30% blended iterative reconstruction method with filtered back projection (adaptive statistical

Table 1
Acquisition parameters for preoperative flap planning CT angiography

Scan Type	Helical
Gantry rotation time	0.5 s
Detector coverage	40 mm
Slice thickness	0.625 mm
Interval	0.625 mm
Pitch	1.375:1
Speed	55
kVp	100 (if <165 lbs); 120 (if >165 lbs)
mA	Auto (minimum 100/maximum 575)
Noise index	34.5
ASIR%	30
FOV	Fit to body habitus, include anterior skin
Start scan	Lesser trochanters
End scan	2 cm above the celiac axis (if abdomen and pelvis coverage); above the clavicles/acromioclavicular joints (if chest, abdomen, and pelvis coverage)
Contrast	100 mL of high iodine concentration contrast material (370 mg I/mL) at 5 mL/s, follow with 100 mL of normal saline flush
Timing	Bolus tracking software with region of interest placed at level of celiac axis in descending aorta, threshold 150 HU, diagnostic delay 5 seconds

Abbreviations: ASIR, adaptive statistical iterative reconstruction; FOV, field of view.

iterative reconstruction; GE Healthcare, Wauke-sha, WI). This is particularly useful when paired with a low kVp technique, leading to improved angiographic enhancement per unit of iodinated contrast material.[32]

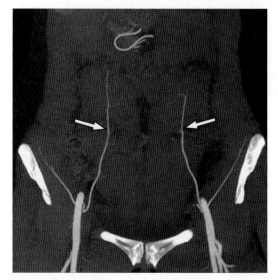

Fig. 8. Oblique coronal maximum intensity projection image of anterior abdominal wall. This postprocessed view is obtained to give an overview of the deep inferior epigastric artery (DIEA) branching pattern, which is type I bilaterally in this example. Arrows = DIEA.

CTA studies for DIEP flap planning differ from standard aorta CTA studies with regard to scan direction and bolus timing; these parameters are altered specifically to optimize contrast opacification of the DIEA system. Scan direction should be performed caudal to cranial, reverse of the normal scan direction for aortic imaging. This scanning direction pairs with the physiologic upward direction of blood flow within the DIEA system from the external iliac artery.[33] Scan timing is generally accomplished using a bolus tracking technique, although the exact timing should be adjusted to achieve peak opacification in the DIEA system. This can be accomplished by elongating the scan delay after threshold attenuation is reached in a standard abdominal location, such as near the celiac axis.[34] Alternatively, the bolus tracking region of interest can be centered over the common femoral arteries and a minimum scan delay can be used because opacification at this vascular site is more temporally congruent with good DIEA opacification.[18] With modern scanner technology (ie, 64 detector elements or greater), scan duration is usually less than 30 seconds.

POSTPROCESSING

Several standard postprocessed image sets are generated from the original thin-section axial data and aid in radiologist interpretation and communicating relevant results to the plastic surgeon. At our institution, the standard reformatted series includes 3 specific items. The first reformatted image is an oblique coronal maximum intensity projection (MIP) image that depicts the branching pattern of the DIEA system (**Fig. 8**). This is often performed using a subvolume of the axial dataset, rather than a full-volume MIP, thereby avoiding erroneous incorporation of vascular detail from other body wall or retroperitoneal vessels into the field of view. Next, stacks of thick overlapping MIP images are reconstructed in axial (10 mm/ 2.5 mm) and sagittal (30–40 mm/5 mm) planes. These are particularly useful in identifying and characterizing the entire course of a DIEA perforator, because the thicker volume allows better depiction of the multiple segments as a perforator passes through the rectus musculature (**Fig. 9**). Finally, volume-rendered images are created, which depict the anterior view of the patient's abdomen and demarcate the physical location of relevant perforator vessels (**Fig. 10**). The locations may be reported using a superimposed grid system or by using Cartesian coordinates/distances reported from a fixed location, such as the umbilicus.[16] Several rendering methods or a combination of techniques can be used, with the goal of depicting the location of a specific perforator artery and its relevant course through the abdominal wall. At our institution, this is accomplished using a combination of a targeted MIP image of the perforator to demonstrate the vascular course and a complimentary volume-rendered image with opaque surface shading algorithm to demonstrate the spatial location/coordinates. Other groups have suggested that using volume-rendered images with transparent subcutaneous fat can be used to simultaneously demonstrate the location of a perforator artery and its relevant subfascial course.[18]

At one of our author's institutions, much of the postprocessing work is performed by a skilled 3D technologist in a dedicated 3D laboratory, with supervision and final decision making given to the interpreting radiologist. Each 3D technologist has been trained in relevant anatomy and clinical rationale for doing CTA studies in potential DIEP flap patients. We do not specifically assess postprocessing time for individual studies at our institution; however, anecdotal comments from experienced technologists suggest that processing times are similar to other vascular CTA studies. One group that uses a similar model of 3D technologist preprocessing and radiologist

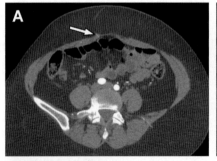
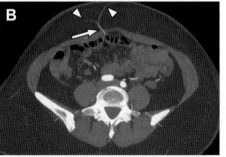
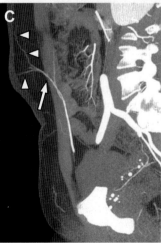

Fig. 9. Value of thick overlapping reformatted images. Thin section axial CT source image (*A*), thick overlapping axial maximum intensity projection (MIP) image (*B*), and thick overlapping sagittal MIP image (*C*) demonstrate right abdominal wall perforator vessel (*arrow*). However, the overall conspicuity of the vessel and the extent of subcutaneous branching (*arrowheads*) are much better depicted on the overlapping MIP images. Thick overlapping MIP images are superior in depicting the oblique course of small vessels compared with the thin section axial CT source images.

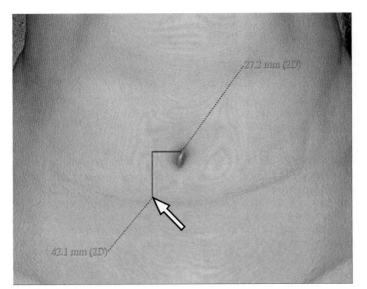

Fig. 10. Volume-rendered image demonstrates the perforator location (*arrow*) relative to umbilicus using Cartesian coordinate system/distances. Depending on site preferences, many perforators may be marked, although different perforator locations are generally depicted on separate images to avoid confusion as to location.

oversight stated that approximate time spent on postprocessing such studies were approximately 10 and 7 minutes, respectively.[18]

REPORTING

Reporting structure varies by individual and institution, but certain elements should be present in most reports. At our institution, the right and

left sides of the abdominal wall are discussed independently, with several anatomic features described (including patency of the inferior epigastric artery and branching anatomy type), and multiple individual perforators listed in a tabulated format. Based on discussions with our plastic surgeons, a comprehensive listing of all perforators identified is usually presented, including small caliber vessels or those that have limited subcutaneous branching. An effort is made to demonstrate the larger perforators by labeling such vessels as "large" or "dominant" in the report. Perforators located greater than 3 cm above the umbilicus are generally ignored, particularly if their continuity with the DIEA system is ambiguous. With this inclusive list of perforators, the plastic surgeon is afforded the maximum latitude in designing a robust flap. However, this comprehensive listing method can be tedious for identification and reporting purposes.

There is evolving literature suggesting that radiologists can adopt a more focused or targeted approach for identifying potential perforators on CTA studies.[34] To do this, radiologists must become more familiar with the relevant surgical principles that guide flap design. A good perforator should provide sufficient blood supply for the flap while also minimizing intramuscular dissection. Ideally, these perforators are centrally located within the flap, have broad subcutaneous branching, and have a short intramuscular course, which allows for a shorter intraoperative dissection. In type II branching patterns, medial row perforators are preferred because motor nerves that innervate the rectus muscle typically course with the most

---

Box 1

"Navarra meeting" criteria optimized for flap-planning CT angiography

1. Large-caliber deep inferior epigastric artery with associated vascular pedicle

2. Large-caliber perforator vessel, including both artery and vein

3. Perforator located in infraumbilical or periumbilical region, ≤3 cm above the umbilicus

4. Short intramuscular course

5. Perforating veins communicate with superficial venous system/network

6. Broad vascular branching pattern in subcutaneous tissue/planned flap

7. Longer subfascial course

8. Avoid tendinous intersections and abdominal wall scars

Adapted from Casares Santiago M, Garcia-Tutor E, Rodriguez Caravaca G, et al. Optimising the preoperative planning of deep inferior epigastric perforator flaps for breast reconstruction. Eur Radiol 2014;24(9):2100; with permission.

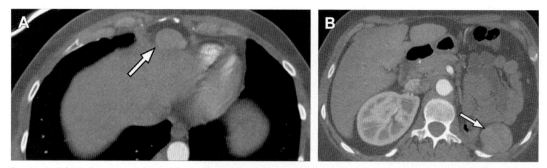

Fig. 11. Incidental mass near xiphoid process/cardiophrenic space, confirmed to represent splenosis. Axial CT angiography images from preoperative flap planning study in 47-year-old woman at level of xiphoid process (A) and interpolar region of right kidney (B) demonstrate nodular masses near the cardiophrenic space and in the left abdomen, respectively (arrows in A, B). The patient had a history of prior trauma necessitating splenectomy and these foci were suspected to represent splenosis, although lymphadenopathy was also considered. A follow-up damaged red blood cell scan demonstrated uptake in both lesions, as well as other smaller foci scattered around the abdomen and pelvis, corroborating a diagnosis of splenosis.

lateral branch of the DIEA and perforators.[20] One recent study suggests that recent consensus discussion on ideal flap design criteria, also referred to as the "Navarra meeting criteria," can be translated successfully into radiologic criteria (**Box 1**) that permit choosing only the best 2 perforators (main and secondary/alternative) on a single examination.[34] In 100 of 105 cases (95%), the actual vascular perforator used in surgery was concordant with the perforator selection identified using the radiologic criteria, yielding a very high concordance (kappa index = 0.93).

Finally, any incidental findings in the abdomen and pelvis should be reported, particularly if a finding may alter the surgical plan. There is limited published work on the rate of clinically significant incidental findings in patients undergoing CTA for potential DIEP flap creation. One study found a

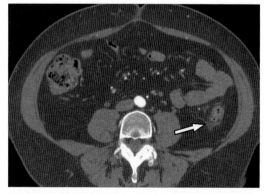

Fig. 12. Incidental diverticulitis. Axial CT angiography image from preoperative flap planning study in a 57-year-old woman demonstrates inflammatory stranding around the descending colon with some adjacent fascial thickening and fluid (arrow) compatible with diverticulitis. Clinically significant nonvascular findings may be evident in patients presenting for preoperative flap planning, which can delay or alter the treatment plan. This patient was treated with antibiotics and underwent successful deep inferior epigastric perforator flap harvesting several weeks later.

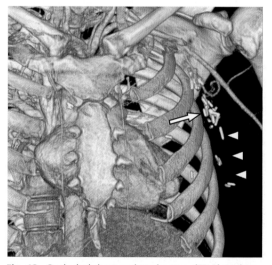

Fig. 13. Occluded thoracodorsal artery (TDA). Volume rendered image from preoperative flap planning study in a 45-year-old woman demonstrates numerous surgical clips (arrow) in axilla from prior lymph node dissection. There is an absence of the normal expected TDA along the left thoracic wall (arrowheads indicate expected location of vessel). The findings of occluded TDA were corroborated by focused Doppler examination, and subsequent breast reconstruction was performed using the internal mammary artery as a recipient site for vascular anastomosis.

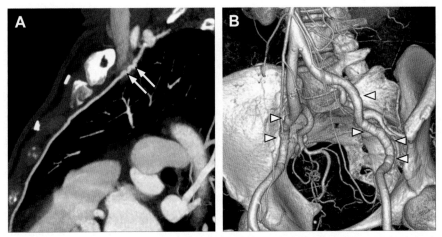

Fig. 14. Fibromuscular dysplasia involving the internal mammary artery (IMA). Oblique sagittal maximum intensity projection image of chest (*A*) and volume-rendered image of pelvis (*B*) taken from preoperative flap planning study in a 71-year-old woman. In the chest, there are several irregular areas of narrowing and dilation along the cephalad aspect of the left IMA (*arrows* in *A*). More pronounced areas of multifocal narrowing are noted in the bilateral iliac artery circulation (*arrowheads* in *B*), resulting in a beaded appearance of the pelvic arterial circulation.

13% rate of incidental findings, with 6% receiving additional imaging to confirm a benign finding, and 2% requiring a delay in breast reconstruction surgery while an incidental finding/process was worked up or treated.[31] Importantly, there were zero cases of unexpected malignancy or progression of disease. These results are similar to our own experience, including several cases that simulated malignancy and required further imaging, as well as unexpected secondary processes that required treatment, thereby delaying surgery in either case (**Figs. 11** and **12**).

ADDITIONAL IMAGING CONSIDERATIONS

Recent literature has debated the utility of preoperative imaging of potential recipient vascular sites in the chest, with several groups suggesting a more proactive approach to concomitant preoperative thoracic imaging.[35–37] Preoperative imaging in the chest can be useful for assessing internal mammary artery (IMA) size, location, and anatomy; all of these factors may influence the surgical approach, such as site for microvascular anastomosis and ability to perform a rib-sparing operation. Novel IMA perforator-based donor vascular anastomoses are increasingly considered because of several benefits, including decreased size of donor site vascular pedicle (ie, shorter length of DIEA) and improved flap geometry in reconstruction bed owing to closer anastomosis.[36] Preoperative thoracic CTA can also identify intrinsic or acquired vascular disease in recipient

IMA or thoracodorsal arteries (TDA), such as from prior surgery or radiation, or underlying vasculitis, which may make them unsuitable for anastomosis.[37] Some have suggested a role for preoperative imaging of the recipient site itself to calculate a breast–abdominal flap volume ratio that could provide better matching of flap harvest sizing with needed tissue volume for the recipient site reconstruction.[35] Although adding thoracic CTA comes with inherent increased patient radiation dose, in selected patients, the benefit may outweigh the risk, particularly for those in whom thoracic vascular pathology is suspected or flap sizing mismatches are anticipated.

In our practice, thoracic imaging is included in selected protocols at the discretion of the treating plastic surgeon. The technical addition is straightforward, and simply requires extending the volume of acquisition cephalad above the clavicles so as to include the both the IMA and TDA circulations. The direction of scanning still occurs in a caudal-to-cranial direction for maximal vascular filling of the inferior epigastric circulation. This delay may result in mild venous contamination of the thoracic vasculature, but larger relative vessel size of IMA and TDA versus abdominal wall perforator vessels generally renders this of little consequence. Additional curved multiplanar reformatted images and volume rendered may be obtained of the IMA and TDA circulation. Cases of iatrogenic and intrinsic vascular pathology have been seen in our practice, and have resulted in alterations to the surgical/management plan (**Figs. 13** and **14**).

SUMMARY

Breast reconstruction is a critical part of a comprehensive treatment plan for patients with breast cancer. There have been significant advancements in microvascular operative techniques, which have facilitated greater degrees of muscle-sparing flaps for breast reconstruction surgery, such as the modern DIEP flap, which minimizes abdominal donor site morbidity while preserving a cosmetic outcome. CTA now plays an important role in the preoperative planning for patients considering DIEP flap harvesting – the accurate localization and depiction of relevant abdominal wall perforators by CTA for treating plastic surgeons has resulted in improved operative performance and clinical outcomes. There is growing interest in using CTA to evaluate thoracic recipient vascular territories as well, particularly if there is clinical suspicion of prior occult vascular injury or intrinsic thoracic vascular disease.

REFERENCES

1. Mahmood U, Hanlon AL, Koshy M, et al. Increasing national mastectomy rates for the treatment of early stage breast cancer. Ann Surg Oncol 2013;20(5):1436–43.
2. Pesce CE, Liederbach E, Czechura T, et al. Changing surgical trends in young patients with early stage breast cancer, 2003 to 2010: a report from the National Cancer Data Base. J Am Coll Surg 2014;219(1):19–28.
3. Balch CM, Jacobs LK. Mastectomies on the rise for breast cancer: "the tide is changing". Ann Surg Oncol 2009;16(10):2669–72.
4. Koshima I, Soeda S. Inferior epigastric artery skin flaps without rectus abdominis muscle. Br J Plast Surg 1989;42(6):645–8.
5. Tseng CY, Lipa JE. Perforator flaps in breast reconstruction. Clin Plast Surg 2010;37(4):641–54, vi–ii.
6. Allen RJ, Treece P. Deep inferior epigastric perforator flap for breast reconstruction. Ann Plast Surg 1994;32(1):32–8.
7. Atisha D, Alderman AK. A systematic review of abdominal wall function following abdominal flaps for postmastectomy breast reconstruction. Ann Plast Surg 2009;63(2):222–30.
8. Shridharani SM, Magarakis M, Stapleton SM, et al. Breast sensation after breast reconstruction: a systematic review. J Reconstr Microsurg 2010;26(5):303–10.
9. Nahabedian MY, Tsangaris T, Momen B. Breast reconstruction with the DIEP flap or the muscle-sparing (MS-2) free TRAM flap: is there a difference? Plast Reconstr Surg 2005;115(2):436–44 [discussion: 445–6].
10. Nahabedian MY, Momen B, Galdino G, et al. Breast reconstruction with the free TRAM or DIEP flap: patient selection, choice of flap, and outcome. Plast Reconstr Surg 2002;110(2):466–75 [discussion: 476–7].
11. Man LX, Selber JC, Serletti JM. Abdominal wall following free TRAM or DIEP flap reconstruction: a meta-analysis and critical review. Plast Reconstr Surg 2009;124(3):752–64.
12. Garvey PB, Buchel EW, Pockaj BA, et al. DIEP and pedicled TRAM flaps: a comparison of outcomes. Plast Reconstr Surg 2006;117(6):1711–9 [discussion: 1720–1].
13. Egeberg A, Rasmussen MK, Sorensen JA. Comparing the donor-site morbidity using DIEP, SIEA or MS-TRAM flaps for breast reconstructive surgery: a meta-analysis. J Plast Reconstr Aesthet Surg 2012;65(11):1474–80.
14. Khansa I, Momoh AO, Patel PP, et al. Fat necrosis in autologous abdomen-based breast reconstruction: a systematic review. Plast Reconstr Surg 2013;131(3):443–52.
15. Chun YS, Sinha I, Turko A, et al. Comparison of morbidity, functional outcome, and satisfaction following bilateral TRAM versus bilateral DIEP flap breast reconstruction. Plast Reconstr Surg 2010;126(4):1133–41.
16. Karunanithy N, Rose V, Lim AK, et al. CT angiography of inferior epigastric and gluteal perforating arteries before free flap breast reconstruction. Radiographics 2011;31(5):1307–19.
17. Malhotra A, Chhaya N, Nsiah-Sarbeng P, et al. CT-guided deep inferior epigastric perforator (DIEP) flap localization – better for the patient, the surgeon, and the hospital. Clin Radiol 2013;68(2):131–8.
18. Phillips TJ, Stella DL, Rozen WM, et al. Abdominal wall CT angiography: a detailed account of a newly established preoperative imaging technique. Radiology 2008;249(1):32–44.
19. Mathes DW, Neligan PC. Current techniques in preoperative imaging for abdomen-based perforator flap microsurgical breast reconstruction. J Reconstr Microsurg 2010;26(1):3–10.
20. Rozen WM, Ashton MW. Improving outcomes in autologous breast reconstruction. Aesthetic Plast Surg 2009;33(3):327–35.
21. Teunis T, Heerma van Voss MR, Kon M, et al. CT-angiography prior to DIEP flap breast reconstruction: a systematic review and meta-analysis. Microsurgery 2013;33(6):496–502.
22. Schaverien MV, Ludman CN, Neil-Dwyer J, et al. Contrast-enhanced magnetic resonance angiography for preoperative imaging of deep inferior epigastric artery perforator flaps: advantages and disadvantages compared with computed tomography angiography: a United Kingdom perspective. Ann Plast Surg 2011;67(6):671–4.

23. Cina A, Barone-Adesi L, Rinaldi P, et al. Planning deep inferior epigastric perforator flaps for breast reconstruction: a comparison between multidetector computed tomography and magnetic resonance angiography. Eur Radiol 2013;23(8):2333–43.

24. Casey WJ 3rd, Chew RT, Rebecca AM, et al. Advantages of preoperative computed tomography in deep inferior epigastric artery perforator flap breast reconstruction. Plast Reconstr Surg 2009;123(4): 1148–55.

25. Ghattaura A, Henton J, Jallali N, et al. One hundred cases of abdominal-based free flaps in breast reconstruction. The impact of preoperative computed tomographic angiography. J Plast Reconstr Aesthet Surg 2010;63(10):1597–601.

26. Masia J, Larranaga J, Clavero JA, et al. The value of the multidetector row computed tomography for the preoperative planning of deep inferior epigastric artery perforator flap: our experience in 162 cases. Ann Plast Surg 2008;60(1):29–36.

27. Rozen WM, Anavekar NS, Ashton MW, et al. Does the preoperative imaging of perforators with CT angiography improve operative outcomes in breast reconstruction? Microsurgery 2008;28(7):516–23.

28. Smit JM, Dimopoulou A, Liss AG, et al. Preoperative CT angiography reduces surgery time in perforator flap reconstruction. J Plast Reconstr Aesthet Surg 2009;62(9):1112–7.

29. Rozen WM, Ashton MW, Whitaker IS, et al. The financial implications of computed tomographic angiography in DIEP flap surgery: a cost analysis. Microsurgery 2009;29(2):168–9.

30. Rozen WM, Whitaker IS, Stella DL, et al. The radiation exposure of computed tomographic angiography (CTA) in DIEP flap planning: low dose but high impact. J Plast Reconstr Aesthet Surg 2009;62(12):e654–5.

31. See MS, Pacifico MD, Harley OJ, et al. Incidence of 'incidentalomas' in over 100 consecutive CT angiograms for preoperative DIEP flap planning. J Plast Reconstr Aesthet Surg 2010;63(1):106–10.

32. Liu PS, Platt JF. CT angiography in the abdomen: a pictorial review and update. Abdom Imaging 2014; 39(1):196–214.

33. Rozen WM, Ashton MW, Stella DL, et al. The accuracy of computed tomographic angiography for mapping the perforators of the deep inferior epigastric artery: a blinded, prospective cohort study. Plast Reconstr Surg 2008;122(4):1003–9.

34. Casares Santiago M, Garcia-Tutor E, Rodriguez Caravaca G, et al. Optimising the preoperative planning of deep inferior epigastric perforator flaps for breast reconstruction. Eur Radiol 2014;24(9): 2097–108.

35. Kim H, Lim SY, Pyon JK, et al. Preoperative computed tomographic angiography of both donor and recipient sites for microsurgical breast reconstruction. Plast Reconstr Surg 2012;130(1):11e–20e.

36. Fansa H, Schirmer S, Cervelli A, et al. Computed tomographic angiography imaging and clinical implications of internal mammary artery perforator vessels as recipient vessels in autologous breast reconstruction. Ann Plast Surg 2013;71(5):533–7.

37. Rozen WM, Alonso-Burgos A, Murray AC, et al. Is there a need for preoperative imaging of the internal mammary recipient site for autologous breast reconstruction? Ann Plast Surg 2013;70(1):111–5.

Computed Tomography Angiography of the Neurovascular Circulation

 CrossMark

Suyash Mohan, MD, PDCC[a], Mohit Agarwal, MD[b],
Bryan Pukenas, MD[a],*

KEYWORDS

- CT angiography • Aneurysm • Pseudoaneurysm • Arteriovenous malformation • Stroke

KEY POINTS

- Computed tomography angiography (CTA) is a proven modality for the evaluation of head and neck vascular pathologies.
- CTA interpretation should be done in a methodical way, without rushing.
- Despite its utility, some vascular lesions, particularly shunting lesions, may remain occult.

INTRODUCTION

Multidetector computed tomography angiography (CTA) is an extensively used technique for the noninvasive evaluation of the neurovascular circulation. It has replaced conventional catheter angiography as the initial examination for most neurovascular indications and is now the first-line imaging study for a variety of neurovascular applications, including the evaluation of carotid steno-occlusive disease, acute ischemic and hemorrhagic stroke, subarachnoid hemorrhage (SAH), and craniocervical trauma.[1,2] The expanding clinical applications of CTA in the past decade can be attributed to the development of advanced helical multidetector CT (MDCT) scanners, which enable the CTA acquisition with increased speed and quality.[1] However, because of the increase in the number of image slices per study and the difficulty of depicting the complex neurovascular tree with CTA, 3-dimensional (3D) postprocessing has become increasingly important for the accurate interpretation of CTA examinations. This article provides a comprehensive description of current neurovascular applications of CTA with an overview of postprocessing techniques. It also provides a brief outline of a suggested reporting format and an imaging checklist to empower the CTA readout sessions.

TECHNIQUE
Patient Selection and Preparation

Patients without absolute contraindication to the administration of iodinated contrast media are candidates for neurovascular CTA. If a relative contraindication to the administration of iodinated contrast medium is present, measures to reduce the possibility of contrast medium reactions or nephrotoxicity should be followed, as defined in the American College of Radiology (ACR)/Society for Pediatric Radiology's Practice Parameter for the Use of Intravascular Contrast Media, or an alternative vascular imaging modality, such as an magnetic resonance angiography (MRA), should be considered.[3]

Disclosures: The authors report no relevant disclosures.
[a] Division of Neuroradiology, Department of Radiology, Perleman School of Medicine, University of Pennsylvania, 3400 Spruce Street, Philadelphia, PA 19104, USA; [b] Division of Neuroradiology, Department of Radiology, Medical College of Wisconsin, 9200 W Wisconsin Avenue, Milwaukee, WI 53226, USA
* Corresponding author.
E-mail address: bryan.pukenas@uphs.upenn.edu

Radiol Clin N Am 54 (2016) 147–162
http://dx.doi.org/10.1016/j.rcl.2015.09.001
0033-8389/16/$ – see front matter © 2016 Elsevier Inc. All rights reserved.

radiologic.theclinics.com

Patients are asked to wear comfortable, loose-fitting clothing, preferably hospital gowns, before undergoing a CTA. Metal objects, including jewelry, eyeglasses, removable dental work, hairpins, hearing aids, bras containing metal underwire, and body piercings, may affect the CT images and should be removed before the examination. The CT technologist and the approving radiologist should carefully review the request and the clinical history to demonstrate the medical necessity of the examination. All current medications and a list of allergies must also be reviewed. Steroid premedication is considered if there is a known allergy according to the ACR's current guidelines.[3] Female patients of childbearing age should always be questioned if there is any possibility that they may be pregnant. The ACR's current guidelines suggest that only a very small percentage of contrast material is excreted in the breast milk, and available data suggest that it is safe for the mother and infant to continue breastfeeding after receiving iodinated contrast. However, if there is any concern whatsoever, breastfeeding women may want to pump breast milk ahead of time and keep it on hand for use after contrast material has cleared from your body, about 24 hours after the test. There is no value in stopping breastfeeding after 24 hours.[3]

When possible, patients should be well hydrated, and intravenous (IV) access should be established. A 20-gauge or larger antecubital IV catheter should be placed, ideally on the right side, to accommodate an optimal rate of 4 or 5 mL per second of iodinated contrast media. Medical personnel trained in the rapid recognition of IV extravasations should monitor the injection site. Department procedures for care of IV extravasations should be documented.

Equipment Specifications and Technique

For diagnostic-quality CTA, the CT scanner should meet or exceed the following specifications:

1. Neurovascular CTA: MDCT scanner, preferably with greater than or equal to 4 active detector rows
2. Gantry rotation: 1 second or less
3. Tube heat capacity that allows for a single 10-second or greater acquisition
4. Minimum section thickness: no greater than 3 mm, preferably no greater than 1.5 mm

To maximize the information available from the CT scan and, thus, derive the full diagnostic benefit for patients following x-ray irradiation, any CT scanner used for CTA must allow display and interpretation of the full 12 bits (from −1000–3095 HU) of attenuation information. Additionally, the display field of view must be sufficient to allow an assessment of the vasculature of interest, the end organ, and adjacent tissues. Appropriate emergency equipment and medications must be immediately available to treat adverse reactions associated with administered medications. The equipment and medications should be monitored for inventory and drug expiration dates on a regular basis. The equipment, medications, and other emergency support must also be appropriate for the range of ages and sizes in the patient population.

A good-quality CTA requires rapid acquisition of thin section images while optimizing opacification of the head and neck vasculature. CTA of the neck is obtained from the aortic arch to just above the skull base, whereas a CTA of the circle of Willis extends from the C2 level to the top of the vertex. If a complete evaluation of the head and neck vasculature is indicated, the scan is obtained from the aortic arch to the vertex. The scan is acquired from caudal to cephalad to minimize the total contrast dose and venous opacification. The patients' chin is placed in a neutral position to allow for adequate visualization of the anterior circulation because the gantry is not tilted.[1]

Usually a slice thickness of 0.5 to 1.25 mm is used for advanced MDCT scanners to optimize spatial resolution. In addition, maximizing the gantry rotation rate is preferred, although some artifacts may be induced when using the fastest settings. Generally, a 4- or 8-slice scanner uses a rate of 0.7 seconds per rotation; a 16-slice scanner uses 0.5 to 0.6 seconds per rotation; and a 64-slice scanner uses 0.4 seconds per rotation. This rate can vary with specific vendors. Some manufacturers dynamically alter the gantry speed, allowing for faster acquisitions in the neck where the vessels are generally larger and slower acquisitions in the circle of Willis where the vessels are smaller. Most current scanners use a maximally overlapping pitch of less than 1. A tube voltage of 120 kVP is usually used for CTA. The tube load is adjusted based on the gantry rate, patient weight and size, and region scanned. For example, an average-sized patient requires a milliampere second (mAs) range of 200 to 240 mAs. The milliampere is increased through the shoulders to decrease the streak artifact from the great vessels. The newer 16- or 64-slice scanners, however, have automatic milliampere adjustments that are based on in-plane and Z-axis attenuation correction.[4]

Optimizing vascular visualization involves adequate contrast delivery. This delivery is affected by certain injection parameters and physiologic factors. The preferred site of injection is the right antecubital vein that minimizes artifacts from dense contrast in the left brachiocephalic vein. Artifacts related to left-sided venous injection include artifact from dense contrast in the brachiocephalic vein obscuring adjacent arteries, reflux of contrast into the jugular veins simulating filling defects, and simple reflux into the internal jugular vein and/or vertebral veins or vertebral venous plexus reaching the dural venous sinuses and possible retrograde brain parenchymal enhancement.[5] There are multiple suggested causes for the left-sided predominance of venous reflux.[6] Anatomic differences in the course of the brachiocephalic veins may be a factor. The right brachiocephalic vein is more parallel to the ascending aorta, whereas the course of the left crosses the aorta and is, therefore, more susceptible to anatomic compression. An aberrant right subclavian artery may compress the left brachiocephalic vein.[7] Hypertension or age-related ectasia and tortuosity of the aorta may also compress the left brachiocephalic vein. In addition, retrosternal narrowing can also predispose to jugular venous reflux with left-sided injections.[8]

IV contrast is administered using at least a 20-gauge catheter at a rate of 4 mL/s to minimize the risk of vascular injury at the IV site.[9] Seventy to 110 mL of high-concentration contrast medium (370 mg I/mL or greater) provides an earlier and higher peak enhancement, improves opacification of smaller vessels, and can minimize venous contamination.

Contrast optimization is also affected by physiologic factors that affect the transit time of the contrast from the injection site to the targeted vessel. Some of these factors include patient weight, cardiac output, and recirculation of the blood pool.[10,11] For instance, poor cardiac output and arterial or venous stenosis result in delayed arterial enhancement but a greater peak of enhancement because of delayed washout. Synchronizing scan acquisition with peak opacification of the targeted vasculature is one of the main challenges to CTA.

Three techniques are used for timing:

1. Fixed time to injection: one size fits all: 20 seconds for CTA, 45 seconds for computed tomographic venography (CTV)
2. Imaging trigger: place region of interest (ROI) at a specific anatomic location, for example, aortic arch or internal carotid artery (ICA), and watch for increase in Hounsfield unit (HU) (also used for MRA)
3. Test bolus: IV injection of 10 to 20 mL with saline flush and calculate maximum attenuation in vessel

Generally, low kilovolt for timing bolus, low milli-ampere, and fixed delay (10 seconds) before starting a monitoring slice or imaging trigger slice is used to reduce the radiation dose in the neck. Currently bolus tracking and test bolus techniques are used to calculate the optimal scan delay. The bolus tracking and automatic triggering method involves monitoring an ROI placed in the aortic arch and triggering the scan when the contrast density reaches a preset value. For neck CTA, scanning is begun when a predetermined HU is reached. This threshold may be automatically set by the manufacturer or determined by the operator. For brain CTA, the same trigger is used with the delay in table movement to scanning area providing a short delay.[12] A test bolus method can also be used by injecting a small amount of contrast as a bolus (10–15 mL) to determine the length of time it takes for peak enhancement of the aortic arch. This time is then used for the prep delay for the injection while scanning.

Which attenuation in CTA allows the best evaluation of the presence and severity of vessel disease is not well studied. It is generally recommended that the mean and minimum attenuations of more than 250 and 200 HU, respectively, may be high enough for an excellent interrogation of the vessel, owing to a better contrast with calcifications in the vessel wall or atherosclerotic plaque. This may have an effect on both visual analysis and semi-quantitative analysis of the vessel dimensions.[13]

Intravenous Contrast

The use of nonionic iodinated contrast material has been shown to be safe in the setting of cerebral ischemia in animal models[14] and clinical studies.[15] However, patients who have diabetes, preexisting renal dysfunction, or both at baseline are at an increased risk for contrast-induced nephropathy (CIN). Nevertheless, several recent studies with large numbers of patients with acute ischemic and hemorrhagic stroke evaluated with CTA have found that the incidence of acute CIN in this patient population is low (ranging from 2% to 7%) and that this risk is not higher in patients whose baseline creatinine value is unknown at the time of scanning.[16–18]

In addition, the risk of CIN can be reduced by adopting several strategies. First, adequate pre-procedure and postprocedure hydration is considered by most experts to be the most important factor in preventing CIN. Second, because nephrotoxicity from contrast material is dose dependent, CTA protocols are designed to use the smallest amount of contrast possible. At the authors' institution, a routine CTA for neurovascular evaluation is performed by administering a total volume of 100 mL of nonionic low-osmolar iodinated contrast material with a concentration of 370 mg I/mL and is similar to or slightly lower than the typical contrast load of a conventional 4-vessel catheter angiogram. However, the authors have performed high-quality neurovascular CTAs with 60 to 70 mL of nonionic low-osmolar iodinated contrast (370 mg I/mL).

In patients with neurologic emergencies requiring rapid evaluation of the neurovascular circulation, emergent CTA evaluation with adequate preexamination and postexamination hydration and administration of the lowest possible dose of a low-osmolar iodinated contrast agent has been found safe with respect to the nephrotoxicity related to the iodinated contrast material, even in the setting of preexisting renal dysfunction.

In patients with a prior history of allergic reactions to iodinated contrast material, premedication with antihistamines and steroids can blunt the anaphylactoid response.[3] However, in the setting of an acute stroke, there is not enough time to complete a course of steroid administration. In this difficult situation, an MRA using gadolinium contrast agent may be used as an alternative to iodinated contrast for CTA evaluation.[19] The use of gadolinium may result in lesser peak vessel opacification compared with iodinated contrast agents, though the imaging remains diagnostic. A documented glomerular filtration rate of 30 mL/min is still a prerequisite in these patients with poor renal function, in light of the potential risk of nephrogenic systemic fibrosis.[20]

Postprocessing (Interpretation/Independent Thin Client/Workstation)

Image quality and accuracy of image interpretation improves when postprocessing techniques are combined with careful evaluation of the thin-section source images. Postprocessing techniques for CTA include maximal intensity projection (MIP) (**Fig. 1**), multiplanar reconstruction (MPR) (**Fig. 2**), and volume rendering (VR) (**Fig. 3**) that are generated on a 3D workstation. Surface-shaded displays have largely been replaced with VR imaging. The workstation should also allow the direct measurement of vascular diameters and stenosis estimations as applicable to the study (**Fig. 4**).

These postprocessed images are especially useful in outlining the length of the carotid artery, trimming out overlapping venous vasculature and bones. This outlining helps improve visualization of the carotid bifurcation where atherosclerotic disease predominates. MIP images are obtained from selecting the highest-density pixels, whereas

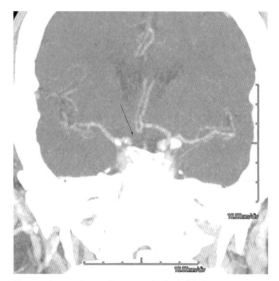

Fig. 1. Coronal MIP (20-mm thick slab) demonstrating a normal variant aplastic right A1 anterior cerebral artery (*arrow*).

MPR images are obtained from selecting the mean density of all the pixels. VR projects all the pixels and uses all data in a 3D display. Usually, the 3D image is significantly surface shaded so that the vessel interface is well demonstrated. VR surface-shaded 3D images have difficulty delineating calcium from vessel lumen and work best when vessels have little calcification, such as the intracranial vessels or when there is minimal atherosclerotic disease. MIP and MPR methods are more accurate than 3D images in evaluating stenoses with calcified plaques and occlusions. MPR images are the most accurate in demonstrating the lumen and wall of a vessel and revealing any intimal flaps, plaques, and intraluminal defects.[21]

Radiation Dose and Safety Issues

CTA exposes patients to ionizing radiation and should only be performed under strict medical supervision to optimize patient safety. It should be performed only for a valid medical reason and with the minimum exposure that provides the image quality necessary for adequate diagnostic information.

The radiation-related stochastic risk of a diagnostic cerebral angiography examination is primarily focused on the brain and the salivary glands.[22] The increased risk of benign and malignant tumors of the brain is small in comparison with the likelihood of developing malignancy in elderly patients who usually undergo such examinations.[23] Nevertheless, increased cancer risk exists for children and younger patients.

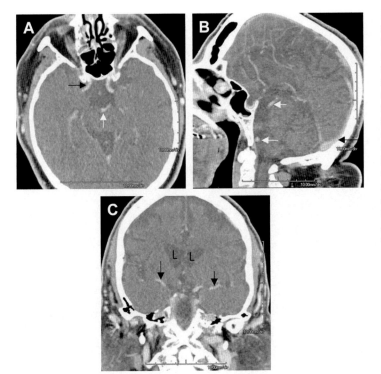

Fig. 2. Axial source images (*A*) with sagittal (*B*) and coronal (*C*) multiplanar reconstructed images of the intracranial vasculature. (*A*) Black arrow delineates the right internal cerebral artery. White arrow delineates the basilar artery. (*B*). Black arrow delineates the superior sagittal sinus as it forms a confluence with the torcular. White arrow delineates the basilar artery. (The basilar artery is mildly ectatic in this patient, which accounts for the apparent separation of the proximal and distal portions.) (*C*) Black arrows delineate the middle cerebral arteries. *L* delineates the lateral ventricles.

At the authors' institution, the dose length product (DLP) for a CTA of the head is about 900 mGy-cm and the DLP for a CTA of the neck is about 1100 mGy-cm, but this is scanner dependent. A recent study showed that radiation exposure with CTA examinations for the cerebral vessels yields a 5 times lower effective dose for patients than the same examination performed with digital subtraction angiography (DSA). The craniocervical CTA protocol causes a one-third higher effective dose compared with the same examination with DSA.[24] This study reveals that the absorbed doses to the skin, brain, salivary glands, and eyes during diagnostic CTA examinations are lower than those for DSA. Improvements in automatically controlling the tube current will potentially reduce radiation exposure to patients, a significant patient safety issue particularly in pediatric patients.

INDICATIONS

The common indications for neurovascular CTA include, but are not limited to, the diagnosis, characterization, and/or surveillance of the following:

1. Arterial and venous aneurysms or pseudoaneurysms

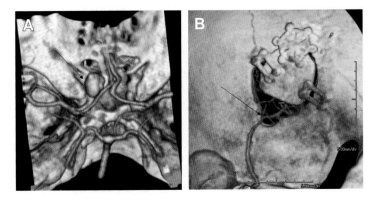

Fig. 3. (*A*) VR image of a left periophthalmic aneurysm (*arrow*). This view is a top-down view, and one must be cognizant of anatomic left versus right when viewing VR images. (*B*) VR image of a pial synangiosis demonstrating patency of the superficial temporal artery as it enters the craniotomy defect (*arrow*).

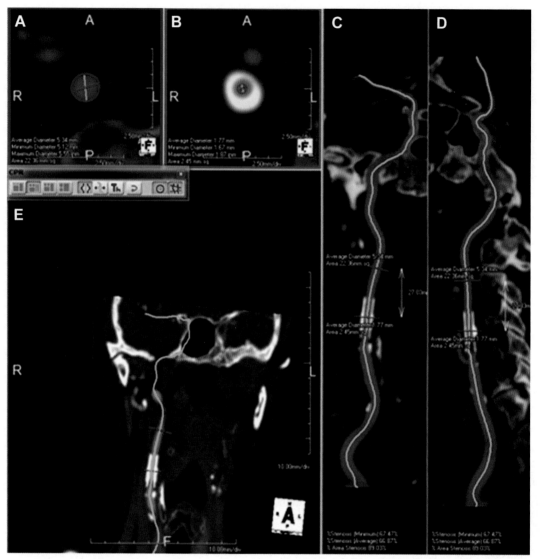

Fig. 4. Calculating stenosis. Axial images corresponding to the blue (*A*) and red (*B*) levels depicted on the curved planar reconstructed (CPR images). CPR images (*C–E*) of a right common and internal carotid artery. The presence of a stent in the carotid artery makes exact measuring difficult.

2. Stroke and vasospasm
3. Atherosclerotic occlusive disease
4. Nonatherosclerotic, noninflammatory vasculopathy
5. Traumatic injuries to arteries and veins
6. Arterial dissection and intramural hematoma
7. Venous and dural sinus thrombosis
8. Congenital vascular anomalies
9. Vascular anatomic variants
10. Vascular interventions (percutaneous and surgical)
11. Vasculitis and collagen vascular diseases
12. Vascular infection
13. Head and neck tumors of vascular origin, with rich vascular supply or invading vascular structures

COMPUTED TOMOGRAPHY ANGIOGRAPHY IN THE EVALUATION OF CAROTID ARTERY STENOOCCLUSIVE DISEASE

Atherosclerosis is the major cause for carotid steno-occlusive disease. This disease can occur by progressive buildup of atherosclerotic plaque in the arterial wall or in some cases by a spontaneous tear in the arterial wall causing the blood to leak in between the arterial layers, producing a false lumen and narrowing the parent vessel, a phenomenon known as spontaneous dissection.

The selection criteria for patients who should be evaluated for carotid occlusive disease include clinical presence of carotid bruit, an episode of transient ischemic attack, or an episode of ischemic stroke.[25] Evaluation of carotid stenosis is important to stratify patients who would benefit from medical versus surgical treatment. An assessment of carotid steno-occlusive disease includes consideration of 2 factors, the degree of stenosis and plaque morphology.

The most common method used to quantify the degree of stenosis is percent stenosis, also used by the North American Symptomatic Carotid Endarterectomy Trial (NASCET) (Fig. 5). Other methods are measurement of residual lumen area or residual lumen diameter. The significance of measuring the degree of stenosis lies in the fact that NASCET reported a significant benefit from carotid endarterectomy in symptomatic patients with more than 70% carotid stenosis. The results are less beneficial for asymptomatic patients or for symptomatic patients with 50% to 69% stenosis. There was no clear surgical benefit for symptomatic patients with less than 50% stenosis or for asymptomatic patients with 50% to

69% stenosis.[25,26] The measurement in the NASCET method is done by taking the smallest vessel diameter at the stenosis divided by the diameter of the normal-sized vessel. There are 3 potential pitfalls in measuring percent stenosis. If the window and level settings are not optimized at the time of measurement, a calcific plaque may bloom and lead to an erroneous overestimation of stenosis.[1,25] To increase diagnostic confidence, measurement of percent stenosis can be done in different planes if the presence of calcium is thought to hinder accuracy.[1,25] The second potential pitfall in the NASCET method of measurement is the reference diameter of the distal ICA. ICA diameters vary widely among individuals, and similar residual lumen diameters will result in a significantly different percent stenosis if the reference diameter of the distal ICA is different. This difference can cause underestimation of disease in persons with smaller reference diameters.[27] Studies have shown that a residual lumen diameter of less than 1 mm narrows the distal ICA by decreasing the perfusion pressure. This decrease can be appreciated on a CTA by a decreased caliber of the affected vessel compared with its contralateral counterpart.[25] For this reason, some centers routinely report a residual lumen diameter alongside percent stenosis while evaluating

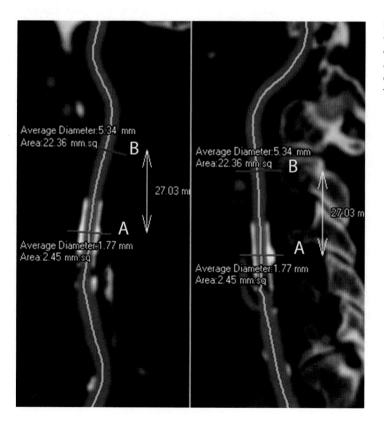

Average Diameter:5.34 mm
Area:22.36 mm.sq
B

27.03 mm

A

Average Diameter:1.77 mm
Area:2.45 mm.sq

Average Diameter:5.34 mm
Area:22.36 mm.sq
B

27.03 m

A

Average Diameter:1.77 mm
Area:2.45 mm.sq

Fig. 5. Measuring stenosis by NASCET criteria. 1- A/B × 100. In this case there is 67% stenosis. However, artifacts within the stent make exact vessel measurement within the stented segment difficult.

carotid stenosis. The third potential pitfall pertains not to measurement of residual lumen but simply recognizing the correct artery. The ascending pharyngeal artery runs along the internal carotid artery; in some cases with complete carotid occlusion, it may mimic the ICA (**Fig. 6**). This potential pitfall can be avoided by bearing in mind that the ascending pharyngeal artery does not quite reach the skull base.[27]

Plaque morphology is an important consideration in the evaluation of carotid steno-occlusive disease. Ulceration, fibrous cap, lipid core, and hemorrhage within the plaque are all associated with increased stroke risk.[27,28] In some studies, arterial wall enhancement around the plaque also correlates well with stroke symptoms.[29] Increased soft plaque thickness has also been correlated with increased stroke risk[30,31] with each 1-mm increase in soft plaque thickness associated with approximately 3.7 times more likelihood of a prior stroke in a retrospective study.[32] Plaque density can be quantified by CTA with soft plaque measuring at 20 to 60 HU, fibrous plaque at 60 to 130 HU, and calcified plaque more than 150 HU.[1]

COMPUTED TOMOGRAPHY ANGIOGRAPHY IN THE EVALUATION OF ACUTE ISCHEMIC STROKE

Ischemic stroke is a major cause of morbidity and mortality in the United States and accounts for 87% of all strokes. According to the Centers for Disease Control and Prevention, 130,000 Americans die every year of stroke and one American dies every 4 minutes of this disease.[33]

If given within the therapeutic time window, thrombolytic therapy and endovascular procedures remain the mainstay for the treatment of acute ischemic stroke. These treatments can reperfuse potentially salvageable brain parenchyma and reduce long-term disability.[27] After hemorrhage has been excluded from a noncontrast head CT, the following information guides management and helps predict the response:

1. Presence, length, and location of intra-arterial thrombus
2. Presence of irreversibly infarcted tissue and, more importantly, the presence/absence of potentially salvageable brain tissue
3. Presence/absence of antegrade flow past the site of occlusion
4. Presence/absence of collateral circulation

These questions can be answered by CTA. It is important to know if there is a thrombus that can be targeted for thrombolysis. This goal is adequately achieved by looking at the thin-slice CTA data and the multiplanar orthogonal reformats that are an integral part of a CTA study.[27] Thick-slab MIP images in 3 planes make it possible to identify a thrombus or occlusion as far as the A3, M3, and P3 division branches of the anterior cerebral artery, middle cerebral artery (MCA), and posterior cerebral artery (PCA), respectively. In some cases, a thrombus beyond these vessels can also be demonstrated. The length and location of a thrombus helps to predict the therapy response. Studies show that larger clots are more resistant to thrombolytic therapy, likely because of their lower surface-to-volume ratio.[34] Also, clots in distal arteries are more amenable to thrombolytic therapy than those in proximal arteries (**Fig. 7**).[35]

Although it is important to determine the area of irreversibly infarcted brain tissue, it is more important to determine if there is any reversible ischemia or potentially salvageable brain parenchyma that can be reperfused with thrombolytic therapy. Initiation of thrombolytic therapy in cases with all the area being infarcted, without an ischemic penumbra, could worsen the outcome by precipitating intracranial hemorrhage.[27] The attenuation and enhancement of brain tissue on CT depends on the water content and perfusion. Brain parenchyma with low perfusion appears hypodense with delayed contrast enhancement on CTA source images and is correlated with irreversible tissue damage.[36,37] This appearance can be

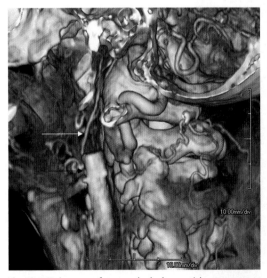

Fig. 6. VR image of an occluded carotid artery stent (*black arrow*). The ascending pharyngeal artery (*white arrow*) can mimic a partially collapsed carotid artery.

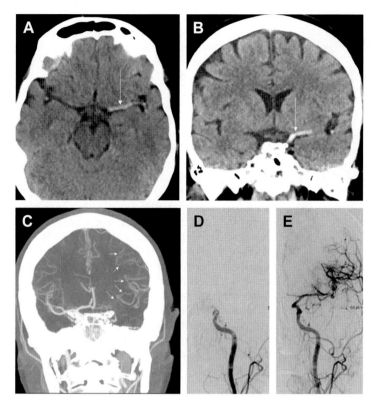

Fig. 7. Unenhanced axial (*A*) and coronal MPR (*B*) CT of the head showing a dense left MCA and ICA, confirmed on CTA (*C*). Notice the left hemispheric collaterals, which extend almost to the site of occlusion in the MCA (*arrows*). The patient failed IV tissue plasminogen activator therapy but was successfully treated with intra-arterial therapy (*D, E*).

used to determine the area of infarcted tissue. CT perfusion can help to find out if there is an area of salvageable brain tissue. A mismatch between the area with delayed mean transit time on CT perfusion versus the hypodense area on CT source images or the area with normal or increased blood volume on cerebral blood volume (CBV) images can help delineate the area of ischemic penumbra.

The angiographic appearance of delayed antegrade contrast opacification distal to the occlusion site has been associated with improved recanalization after endovascular procedures and intra-arterial thrombolytic therapy.[34,38] Four-dimensional (4D) CTA, which enables the noninvasive evaluation of flow dynamics of the intracranial vasculature by multiple subsequent CT acquisitions or a continuous-volume CT acquisition for a period of time, has been comparable with DSA in discriminating antegrade and retrograde flow across a cerebral artery occlusion.[34,39] The presence of antegrade flow on 4D CTA is associated with an increased chance of early vessel recanalization.[34]

The extent of collateral circulation is another factor that predicts the response to thrombolytic therapy (see **Fig. 7**). Patients with poor collateral flow and paucity of leptomeningeal collaterals on CTA have poor clinical outcomes.[34,40]

Revascularization of patients with poor collateral circulation may result in significant harm with higher infarct volume, increased malignant brain edema, and higher rates of intracerebral hemorrhage. Recognition of these patients, thus, becomes important on CTA to predict the overall outcomes.[41]

COMPUTED TOMOGRAPHY ANGIOGRAPHY IN THE EVALUATION OF ACUTE HEMORRHAGIC STROKE

Hemorrhagic stroke is the lesser common form of stroke but carries a worse prognosis than ischemic stroke. Hemorrhagic stroke may or may not be caused by underlying vascular lesions. The fact that underlying lesions may be potentially treatable makes their detection important. The traditional approach of patient selection for cerebral angiography for intracerebral hemorrhage stems from the risks of DSA outweighing the diagnostic yield.[42] The advent of noninvasive angiographic techniques has markedly lessened that risk. Prediction of hematoma expansion is possible with the identification of a spot sign on CTA,[43,44] which is a sign of active ongoing hemorrhage. Newer hemostatic treatments and vigorous control of blood pressure to reduce hematoma

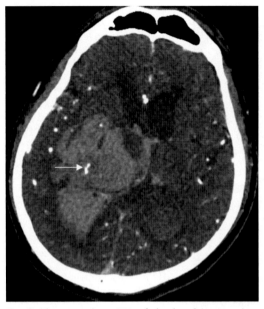

Fig. 8. The spot sign. CTA of the head in a patient with a large parenchymal hematoma demonstrating a spot sign within the hematoma (*arrow*).

expansion may be guided by the physician's awareness of ongoing hemorrhage.[45] Also, total volume of extravasated blood and expansion of hematoma are indicators of poor outcome and mortality.[27,46–48] CTA can, therefore, be useful even in patients without underlying vascular lesions and argues in favor of early CTA for the management of acute hemorrhagic stroke.[45]

From the earlier discussion, the authors can infer the following 2 major uses of CTA in hemorrhagic stroke:

1. Detection of underlying vascular lesions
2. Detection of spot sign

Detection of a vascular lesion, such as an AVM or aneurysm, is usually straightforward and

prompts focused definitive therapy. Younger age, lobar or infratentorial hemorrhage, absence of known hypertension, and impaired coagulation are independent predictors for a higher yield of vascular lesions on CTA.[49]

The evaluation of a spot sign deserves some discussion here. A spot sign (**Fig. 8**) is the visualization of a region of active contrast extravasation within the hematoma on CTA. These areas are not visible on nonenhanced scans, and on CTA they at least have an attenuation of 120 HU. These areas are separately visualized from adjacent vasculature. The first 2 criteria allow the reader to make the important differentiation between spot signs and spot sign mimics, such as choroidal calcifications (**Fig. 9**), aneurysms (**Fig. 10**), and arteriovenous malformations (AVMs) (**Fig. 11**), whereas the third criterion minimizes the likelihood that hematoma heterogeneity and inherent CTA noise may be misdiagnosed as a spot sign.[27] Various characteristics of the spot sign have been used to calculate a spot sign score. Studies have shown a correlation between a higher spot sign score and a poor clinical outcome.[50] Number, size, and density of the spot sign are the 3 criteria used for scoring. One to 2 spot signs get 1 point, whereas more than 2 spot signs get 2 points. A spot sign of 4 mm or less gets no extra point, whereas a spot sign more than 4 mm gets an additional point. Another additional point is given if the density of the spot is greater than 180 HU. Spots between 120 and 179 HU get no additional points.[50] Of the 3 characteristics, spot sign number is the most important predictor of hematoma expansion and overall clinical outcome.[51]

Some studies have described the appearance of a spot sign on delayed CTAs, which carry the same prognostic value as those seen in the first-pass CTAs.[50,52] Delayed CTAs may also be useful to differentiate a spot sign from a small aneurysm or AVM, if such distinction was doubtful on the

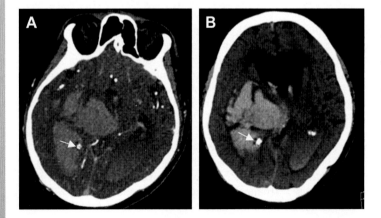

Fig. 9. CTA (*A*) demonstrating a parenchymal hematoma (same patient as in **Fig. 8** but more inferior level) and a hyperdense focus in the medial aspect of the hematoma (*arrow*). (*B*) Unenhanced CT at the same level as *A* shows this hyperdense focus is calcified choroid plexus (*arrow*), a potential pitfall/mimic of the spot sign.

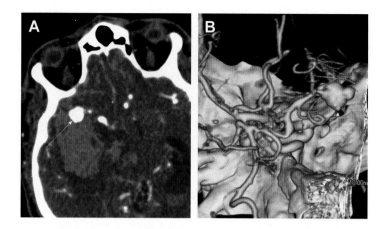

Fig. 10. (A) Axial CTA of the head showing a right parenchymal hematoma and an apparent spot sign (*arrow*). (*B*) VR image of the same patient showing the spot sign is a large MCA bifurcation aneurysm (*arrow*).

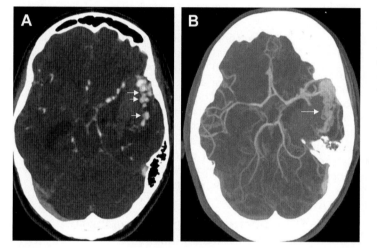

Fig. 11. (*A*) Axial CTA of the head showing a large left parenchymal hematoma with hyperdense lateral foci (*arrows*). (*B*) Axial MIP shows these foci to be the nidus and draining veins of an arteriovenous malformation (*arrow*).

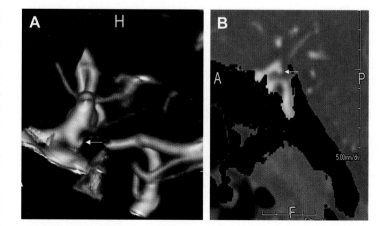

Fig. 12. (*A*) VR images of the internal carotid artery demonstrate a PCA infundibulum versus small aneurysm. (*B*) Sagittal MPR shows the PCA originates from the dome of the less-than-2-mm rounded outpouching, indicating that this is an infundibulum (*arrows*).

first-pass CTA. A vascular lesion will continue to show the same morphology on the delayed CTA, which might change with a spot sign.[27]

COMPUTED TOMOGRAPHY ANGIOGRAPHY IN THE EVALUATION OF SUBARACHNOID HEMORRHAGE AND CEREBRAL VASOSPASM

Trauma and aneurysm rupture are the 2 most common causes of subarachnoid hemorrhage. On occasions, SAH can be caused by a vascular malformation. The presence of blood in the subarachnoid space acts as an irritant to the intracranial arteries and can cause vasospasm with resultant cerebral ischemia or infarct. CTA may serve the following purposes in cases of subarachnoid hemorrhage:

1. Detect cerebral aneurysm and its characteristics such as size, shape, neck, and so forth
2. Detect residual aneurysm/neck in clipped aneurysms
3. Diagnose cerebral vasospasm

The detection of cerebral aneurysms by CTA is fraught by 2 potential pitfalls. Tiny arteries originating from infundibula may not be resolved (**Fig. 12**), and they may be confused with aneurysms. Small aneurysms may not be resolved by CTA, decreasing the overall CTA sensitivity versus DSA for cerebral aneurysm detection. Debate continues over the use of CTA in aneurysm detection, especially if a DSA is not performed after a negative CTA.[27,53] With that being stated, CTA with 3D rendering is a very useful tool in detecting aneurysms and outlining their characteristics for management decisions.[54,55] Artifacts from aneurysm coils may hinder detection of residual necks. However, in cases with surgical clipping, CTA may be of use in visualization of residual aneurysm neck.[56–58]

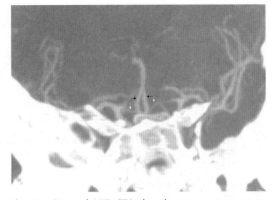

Fig. 13. Coronal MIP CTA showing severe vasospasm of the proximal anterior cerebral arteries. Notice the diameter of the A1 segments (*white arrows*) is smaller than the diameter of the A2 segments (*black arrows*).

Cerebral vasospasm and secondary ischemia or infarct are ominous complications of SAH (**Fig. 13**). The superb anatomic detail of CTA for outlining intracranial vasculature can detect vasospasm early on and help prevent cerebral infarction by tailoring further therapy. Detection of severe vasospasm is easier than mild or moderate spasm. However, comparison with prior examinations/baseline studies may prove useful.[27] Combining CTA with CT perfusion may be of further benefit and may increase diagnostic yield by showing areas of ischemia.[27]

DOCUMENTATION/STANDARDIZED REPORTING FORMAT
Imaging Checklist

Reporting should be in accordance with the ACR Practice Parameter for Communication of Diagnostic Imaging Findings (**Boxes 1–3**).[59]

Box 1
CTA interpretation and reporting

- Provided history/reason for examination
  - Any relevant and known risk factors or allergies
  - Review of electronic medical records for any additional pertinent clinical information
- Technique
- Contrast: amount, route of administration, and type
- Comparison studies (relevant)
  - Date and type of previous examinations available and reviewed, as applicable
- Findings
  - Image quality: artifacts/motion, and so forth

- ○ Scout films review
- ○ Vascular anatomy
  - ▪ Visualized segment of aortic arch
  - ▪ Origin of great vessels (classic vs variant anatomy)
  - ▪ Common carotid, carotid bifurcation, internal and external carotid arteries
  - ▪ Subclavian arteries and origin of vertebral arteries
  - ▪ Distal cervical internal carotid and vertebral arteries
  - ▪ Intracranial internal carotid arteries (petrous carotid artery, cavernous carotid artery, supraclinoid internal carotid artery, communicating segment internal carotid artery, and carotid terminus)
  - ▪ Anterior cerebral arteries and region of anterior communicating artery
  - ▪ Middle cerebral arteries
  - ▪ Intracranial vertebral arteries
  - ▪ PICAs (origin as well as distal PICA)
  - ▪ Basilar artery and tip
  - ▪ Anterior inferior cerebellar artery
  - ▪ Superior cerebellar artery
  - ▪ PCA
- ○ Possible pathologies: normal, absent, degree of narrowing (mild, moderate or severe), dissection (flow limiting vs nonflow limiting), irregularity (focal or diffuse), aneurysms (size, morphology, number), occlusion (extent, location, consequence), obvious vascular malformations, normal variants, and so forth
- ○ Postprocessing: multiplanar reformats and 3D VR
- • Blind spots
  - ○ Brain: hemorrhage, herniation, hydrocephalus, ischemia, mass effect, and midline shift
  - ○ Neck: aerodigestive tract, lymph nodes, glands, skull base
  - ○ Spine: bone windows as well as soft tissue windows for intraspinal contents and spinal cord status
  - ○ Lungs: lung windows
- • Impression: (itemized with most important actionable items)
- • Suggested recommendations, if any
- • Documented communication (as warranted)

Abbreviation: PICA, posterior inferior cerebellar artery.

Box 2
CTA interpretation pearls

- • Do not read a CTA in a rush. It requires a diligent and competent reader.
- • Think of it as a combination of head CT, CT neck, CT chest, CT spine, and of course an angiogram, so take your time and review it all.
- • Use all available tools: thin client, MIPs, MPRs, bone and soft windows, and surface-rendered images.
- • Keep in mind that even with an experienced reader, CTA has limitations.

Box 3
CTA interpretation pitfalls

- • There can be left arm injection and contrast reflux.
- • There can be poor bolus timing and inadequate vascular opacification.
- • There can be thrombosed aneurysms.
- • Remember that small vascular malformations may remain occult.
- • Do not forget the source images.
- • CTA is not equivalent to a contrast-enhanced CT of the brain or neck soft tissues.
- • Do not forget the nonvascular pathologies.

SUMMARY

CTA is a powerful and reliable tool to demonstrate the vasculature of the head and neck with proven utility for the detection and characterization of vascular diseases particularly in the acute setting.[1] It may be used as the primary modality for detecting disease or as an adjunct tool for better characterizing known disease or assessing changes in the disease state over time. With the proliferation of CT scanners in the emergency departments, CTA examinations will continue to grow in numbers, helping to guide intervention in the emergency setting of neurovascular diseases.

ACKNOWLEDGMENTS

The authors would like to thank Alexander C. Mamourian, MD and Dasha Pechersky, MD (University of Pennsylvania, Philadelphia, PA, USA) for providing their insights and experience in the preparation of this article.

REFERENCES

1. Enterline DS, Kapoor G. A practical approach to CT angiography of the neck and brain. Tech Vasc Interv Radiol 2006;9(4):192–204.
2. Mohan S, Lee W, Tan JT, et al. Multi-detector computer tomography angiography in the initial assessment of patients acutely suspected of having intracranial aneurysm rupture. Ann Acad Med Singapore 2009;38(9):769–73.
3. American College of Radiology. Manual on contrast media. Version 10.1. Available at: http://www.acr.org/Quality-Safety/Resources/Contrast Manual; http://www.acr.org/~/media/ACR/Documents/PDF/Quality Safety/Resources/Contrast%20Manual/2013_Contrast_Media.pdf/#page=103. Accessed October 19, 2015.
4. Enterline D, Lowry CR, Tanenbaum LN. Multidetector computed tomography (MDCT): brain, and head and neck applications in multidetector CT protocols developed for GE scanners. Princeton (NJ): BDI; 2005. p. E1–57.
5. Chen JY, Mamourian AC, Messe SR, et al. Pseudopathologic brain parenchymal enhancement due to venous reflux from left-sided injection and brachiocephalic vein narrowing. Am J Neuroradiol 2010; 31(1):86–7.
6. McCarthy J, Solomon NA. The effects of injection site, age, and body position on cervical venous reflux. Radiology 1979;130:536–67.
7. Tanaka T, Uemura K, Takahashi M, et al. Compression of the left brachiocephalic vein: cause of high signal intensity of the left sigmoid sinus and internal jugular vein on MR images. Radiology 1993;188: 355–61.
8. Tseng TC, Hsu HL, Lee TH, et al. Venous reflux on carotid computed tomography angiography: relationship with left-arm injection. J Comput Assist Tomogr 2007;31:360–4.
9. Herts BR, O'Malley CM, Wirth SL, et al. Power injection of contrast media using central venous catheters: feasibility, safety, and efficacy. AJR Am J Roentgenol 2001;176:447–53.
10. Cademartiri F, van der Lugt A, Luccichenti G, et al. Parameters affecting bolus geometry in CTA: a review. J Comput Assist Tomogr 2002;26:598–607.
11. Brink JA. Use of high concentration contrast media (HCCM): principles and rationale—body CT. Eur J Radiol 2003;45:53–8.
12. Enterline DS. CT angiography of the neck and brain. In: Saini S, Rubin GD, Kalra MK, editors. MDCT: a practical approach. Milan (Italy): Springer; 2006. p. 151–66.
13. de Monyé C, Cademartiri F, de Weert TT, et al. Sixteen-detector row CT angiography of carotid arteries: comparison of different volumes of contrast material with and without a bolus chaser. Radiology 2005;237(2):555–62.
14. Doerfler A, Engelhorn T, von Kummer R, et al. Are iodinated contrast agents detrimental in acute cerebral ischemia? An experimental study in rats. Radiology 1998;206:211–7.
15. Palomäki H, Muuronen A, Raininko R, et al. Administration of nonionic iodinated contrast medium does not influence the outcome of patients with ischemic brain infarction. Cerebrovasc Dis 2003;15:45–50.
16. Krol AL, Dzialowski I, Roy J, et al. Incidence of radiocontrast nephropathy in patients undergoing acute stroke computed tomography angiography. Stroke 2007;38:2364–6 [Erratum appears in Stroke 2007; 38:e97].
17. Dittrich R, Akdeniz S, Kloska SP, et al. Low rate of contrast-induced nephropathy after CT perfusion and CT angiography in acute stroke patients. J Neurol 2007;254:1491–7.
18. Hopyan JJ, Gladstone DJ, Mallia G, et al. Renal safety of CT angiography and perfusion imaging in the emergency evaluation of acute stroke. Am J Neuroradiol 2008;29:1826–30.
19. Henson JW, Nogueira RG, Covarrubias DJ, et al. Gadolinium-enhanced CT angiography of the circle of Willis and neck. Am J Neuroradiol 2004; 25:969–72.
20. Morcos SK, Thomsen HS. Nephrogenic systemic fibrosis: more questions and some answers. Nephron Clin Pract 2008;110:c24–31.
21. Takhtani D. CT neuroangiography: a glance at the common pitfalls and their prevention. AJR Am J Roentgenol 2005;185:772–83.
22. Norbash AM, Busick D, Marks MP. Techniques for reducing interventional neuroradiologic skin dose: tube position rotation and supplemental beam filtration. Am J Neuroradiol 1996;17:41–9.

23. Miller DL. Overview of contemporary interventional fluoroscopy procedures. Health Phys 2008;95:638–44.

24. Manninen AL, Isokangas JM, Karttunen A, et al. A comparison of radiation exposure between diagnostic CTA and DSA examinations of cerebral and cervicocerebral vessels. AJNR Am J Neuroradiol 2012;33(11):2038–42.

25. Romero JM, Ackerman RH, Dault NA, et al. Noninvasive evaluation of carotid artery stenosis: indications, strategies, and accuracy. Neuroimaging Clin N Am 2005;15:351–65.

26. Barnett HJM, the North American Symptomatic Carotid Endarterectomy Trial Collaborators. Beneficial effect of carotid endarterectomy in symptomatic patients with high-grade carotid stenosis. N Engl J Med 1991;325:445–53.

27. Delgado Almandoz JE, Romero JM, Pomerantz SR, et al. Computed tomography angiography of the carotid and cerebral circulation. Radiol Clin North Am 2010;48:265–81.

28. Pacheco FT, Littig IA, Gagliardi RJ, et al. Multidetector computed tomography angiography in clinically suspected hyperacute ischemic stroke in the anterior circulation: an etiological workup in a cohort of Brazilian patients. Arq Neuropsiquiatr 2015;73(5):408–14.

29. Romero JM, Babiarz LS, Forero NP, et al. Arterial wall enhancement overlying carotid plaque on CT angiography correlates with symptoms in patients with high grade stenosis. Stroke 2009;40:1894–6.

30. Trellers M, Eberhardt KM, Buchholz M, et al. CTA for screening of complicated atherosclerotic carotid plaque—American Heart Association type VI lesions as defined by MRI. Am J Neuroradiol 2013;34:2331–7.

31. Gupta A, Baradaran H, Kamel H, et al. Evaluation of computed tomography angiography plaque thickness measurements in high-grade carotid artery stenosis. Stroke 2014;45:740–5.

32. Gupta A, Mtui EE, Baradaran H, et al. CT angiographic features of symptom-producing plaque in moderate-grade carotid artery stenosis. Am J Neuroradiol 2015;36:349–54.

33. Available at: http://www.cdc.gov/Stroke/index.htm.

34. Kortman HGJ, Smit EJ, Oei MTH, et al. 4D-CTA in neurovascular disease: a review. Am J Neuroradiol 2015;36:1026–33.

35. Porelli S, Leonardi M, Stafa A, et al. CT angiography in an acute stroke protocol: correlation between occlusion site and outcome of intravenous thrombolysis. Interv Neuroradiol 2013;19:87–96.

36. Schramm P, Schellinger PD, Fiebach JB, et al. Comparison of CT and CT angiography source images with diffusion-weighted imaging in patients with acute stroke within 6 hours after onset. Stroke 2002;33:2426–32.

37. Puetz V, Sylaja PN, Hill MD, et al. CT angiography source images predict final infarct extent in patients with basilar artery occlusion. AJNR Am J Neuroradiol 2009;30:1877–83.

38. Christoforidis GA, Mohammad Y, Avutu B, et al. Arteriographic demonstration of slow antegrade opacification distal to a cerebrovascular thromboembolic occlusion site as a favorable indicator for intra-arterial thrombolysis. AJNR Am J Neuroradiol 2006;27:1528–31.

39. Frolich AM, Psychogios MN, Klotz E, et al. Antegrade flow across incomplete vessel occlusions can be distinguished from retrograde collateral flow using 4-dimensional computed tomographic angiography. Stroke 2012;43:2974–9.

40. McVerry F, Liebeskind DS, Muir KW. Systematic review of methods for assessing leptomeningeal collateral flow. AJNR Am J Neuroradiol 2012;33:576–82.

41. Elijovich L, Goyal N, Mainali S, et al. CTA collateral score predicts infarct volume and clinical outcome after endovascular therapy for acute ischemic stroke: a retrospective chart review. J Neurointerv Surg 2015;1–4.

42. Aviv RI, Kelly AG, Jahromi BS, et al. The cost-utility of CT angiography and conventional angiography for people presenting with intracerebral hemorrhage. PLoS One 2014;9(5):e96496.

43. Wada R, Aviv RI, Fox AJ, et al. CT angiography "spot sign" predicts hematoma expansion in acute intracerebral hemorrhage. Stroke 2007;38:1257–62.

44. Goldstein JN, Fazen LE, Snider R, et al. Contrast extravasation on CT angiography predicts hematoma expansion in intracerebral hemorrhage. Neurology 2007;68:889–94.

45. Khosravani H, Mayer SA, Demchuk A, et al. Emergency noninvasive angiography for acute intracerebral hemorrhage. Am J Neuroradiol 2013;34:1481–7.

46. Davis SM, Broderick J, Hennerici M, et al. Hematoma growth is a determinant of mortality and poor outcome after intracerebral hemorrhage. Neurology 2006;66:1175–81.

47. Becker KJ, Baxter AB, Bybee HM, et al. Extravasation of radiographic contrast is an independent predictor of death in primary intracerebral hemorrhage. Stroke 1999;30:2025–32.

48. Kim J, Smith A, Hemphill JC III, et al. Contrast extravasation on CT predicts mortality in primary intracerebral hemorrhage. AJNR Am J Neuroradiol 2008;29:520–5.

49. Delgado Almandoz JE, Schaefer PW, Forero NP, et al. Diagnostic accuracy and yield of multidetector CT angiography in the evaluation of spontaneous intraparenchymal cerebral hemorrhage. AJNR Am J Neuroradiol 2009;30:1213–21.

50. Delgado Almandoz JE, Yoo AJ, Stone MJ, et al. The spot sign score in primary intracerebral hemorrhage

identifies patients at highest risk of in-hospital mortality and poor outcome among survivors. Stroke 2010;41:54–60.

51. Huynh TJ, Demchuk AM, Dowlatshahi D, et al. Spot sign number is the most important spot sign characteristic for predicting hematoma expansion using first-pass computed tomography angiography. Stroke 2013;44:972–7.

52. Delgado Almandoz JE, Yoo AJ, Stone MJ, et al. Systematic characterization of the computed tomography angiography spot sign in primary intracerebral hemorrhage identifies patients at highest risk for hematoma expansion. The spot sign score. Stroke 2009;40:2994–3000.

53. Kallmes DF, Layton K, Marx WF, et al. Death by nondiagnosis: why emergent CT angiography should not be done for patients with subarachnoid hemorrhage. AJNR Am J Neuroradiol 2007;28: 1837–8.

54. Hoh BL, Cheung AC, Rabinov JD, et al. Results of a prospective protocol of computed tomographic angiography in place of catheter angiography as the only diagnostic and pretreatment planning study for cerebral aneurysms by a combined neurovascular team. Neurosurgery 2004;54:1329–40.

55. Wang H, Li W, He H, et al. 320-Detector row CT angiography for detection and evaluation of intracranial aneurysms: comparison with conventional digital subtraction angiography. Clin Radiol 2013; 68:e15–20.

56. Dehdashti AR, Binaghi S, Uske A, et al. Comparison of multislice computerized tomography angiography and digital subtraction angiography in the postoperative evaluation of patients with clipped aneurysms. J Neurosurg 2006;104:395–403.

57. Uysal E, Ozel A, Erturk SM, et al. Comparison of multislice computed tomography angiography and digital subtraction angiography in the detection of residual or recurrent aneurysm after surgical clipping with titanium clips. Acta Neurochir (Wien) 2009;151:131–5.

58. Gerardin E, Tollard E, Derrey S, et al. Usefulness of multislice computerized tomographic angiography in the postoperative evaluation of patients with clipped aneurysms. Acta Neurochir (Wien) 2010;152(5): 793–802.

59. ACR Practice Parameter for Communication of Diagnostic Imaging Findings. Available at: http://www.acr.org/~/media/ACR/Documents/PGTS/guidelines/Comm_Diag_Imaging.pdf. Accessed October 19, 2015.

Pediatric Considerations in Computed Tomographic Angiography

 CrossMark

David Saul, MD[a], Andrew Mong, MD[a,b],
David M. Biko, MD[a,b],*

KEYWORDS

• Pediatrics • Cardiovascular disease • CT angiography

KEY POINTS

• Although noninvasive vascular imaging modalities such as magnetic resonance angiography and ultrasound lack ionizing radiation, with improving technology and an increased focus on radiation dose reduction, computed tomographic angiography (CTA) continues to have a role in evaluating cardiovascular disease in pediatric patients.
• Two considerations that are more important in the pediatric population when considering what imaging modality to use are (1) radiation dose and (2) need for sedation.
• An important step to obtaining high-quality CTA in the pediatric population is to establish a warm, comforting, and engaging atmosphere for the child.
• Assessing whether a child will require sedation depends on developmental stage and age of the child.

Cardiovascular disease in children comprises a diverse collection of diseases involving multiple organ systems. Abnormality in children is predominately congenital but also may be acquired. Although noninvasive vascular imaging modalities such as magnetic resonance angiography (MRA) and ultrasound (US) lack ionizing radiation, with improving technology and an increased focus in radiation dose reduction, CT angiography (CTA) continues to have a role in evaluating cardiovascular disease in pediatric patients.

IMAGING CHOICES: HOW DOES COMPUTED TOMOGRAPHIC ANGIOGRAPHY COMPARE TO OTHER MODALITIES?

Indications for computed tomographic angiography (CTA) in pediatric patients may differ based on age (**Table 1**). Depending on the organ system, age of the patient, and clinical question, CTA may be the correct imaging modality to properly evaluate abnormality in the safest and most effective manner. Two considerations that are more important in the pediatric population when considering what imaging modality to use are (1) radiation dose and (2) need for sedation.

In general, imaging modalities that do not use ionizing radiation, such as US or MR imaging, are preferred in the pediatric population. Unlike adults, children are uniquely sensitive to ionizing radiation. The Law of Bergonié and Tribondeau states that ionizing radiation has a greater effect in rapidly dividing cells (as in children) than in slowly dividing ones.[1,2] In addition, children have a longer lifespan within which to manifest these adverse effects. The cancer-related risk of death from a single

Disclosure Statement: The authors have nothing to disclose.
[a] Department of Radiology, The Children's Hospital of Philadelphia, 34th and Civic Center Boulevard, Philadelphia, PA 19104, USA; [b] Department of Radiology, Perelman School of Medicine, University of Pennsylvania, Philadelphia, PA, USA
* Corresponding author. Department of Radiology, The Children's Hospital of Philadelphia, 34th and Civic Center Boulevard, Philadelphia, PA 19104.
E-mail address: bikod@email.chop.edu

Radiol Clin N Am 54 (2016) 163–176
http://dx.doi.org/10.1016/j.rcl.2015.08.006
0033-8389/16/$ – see front matter © 2016 Elsevier Inc. All rights reserved.

Table 1
Examples of indications for computed tomographic angiography in children

Organ System	Indication
Head/neck	Vascular trauma, arterial occlusive disease, vascular dissection, arteriovenous malformation, vasculitis, veno-occlusive disease
Chest	Congenital heart disease, coronary anomalies, Kawasaki disease, coarctation of the aorta, vascular rings, pulmonary veno-occlusive disease, pulmonary embolism, congenital pulmonary airway malformation (CPAM), sequestration, pulmonary arteriovenous malformation
Abdomen	Vascular trauma, renal artery stenosis, vasculitis, gastrointestinal bleeding, mesenteric ischemia, liver/renal transplant evaluation, ureteropelvic junction obstruction
Extremity	Vascular trauma, vasculitis, veno-occlusive disease

abdominal CT performed on a neonate is estimated at 0.14%.[3] Although CT scans in children only accounted for 7% of the total CT volume in 2007 in the United States, their radiation burden is expected to account for up to 15% of iatrogenically induced cancers.[4] Another study estimates that there are 4 million pediatric CT scans performed per year in the United States, with 0.4% to 2.0% of all cancers attributable to radiation from CT studies.

A second consideration when deciding on if CTA is the best imaging modality is the need for sedation. Imaging modalities such as US rarely need sedation to obtain a diagnostic study. CTA may or may not require sedation, but comparatively, MR imaging requires a pediatric patient to remain still for longer periods of time, and sedation is more often necessary.

Modalities other than CTA that are routinely used to image pediatric cardiovascular disease include US (including echocardiography), MR angiography (MRA), and catheter angiography.

Computed Tomographic Angiography or Echocardiography?

Echocardiography is often the first-line imaging study for children with heart disease, and it has many advantages. Importantly, it does not require ionizing radiation or iodinated contrast material. Other advantages of echocardiography over CTA are that it is portable, provides more complete functional information, and has better temporal resolution. However, echocardiography is more time-consuming and operator-dependent and requires sedation for transesophageal imaging.[5]

CTA has greater utility for global assessment of the cardiovascular system in comparison to echocardiography; this is especially true when evaluating branch pulmonary arteries, pulmonary veins, and great vessels (**Fig. 1**). Anterior structures such as the free wall of the right ventricle are also seen better with CTA.[5] Echocardiography

has traditionally been used as the primary diagnostic modality for neonates with complex congenital heart disease, as CTA has only been thought feasible in older children due to neonatal rapid heart rates and the need for sedation. However, with advances in scanner technology allowing for subsecond scans, nonsedated cardiac CTA has been performed in neonates with high diagnostic accuracy.[6]

For the evaluation of the noncardiac vascular structures, US is typically the first imaging modality, particularly in the extremities and solid organs of the abdomen due to its availability and portability. There is no ionizing radiation as in CT, no need for sedation, and no nephrotoxic effects of intravenous (IV) contrast media. US provides real-time evaluation of flow dynamics in the vascular structures, but as in the evaluation of the heart with echocardiography, CT provides a more global assessment and can evaluate vessels that cannot be visualized due to lack of a proper acoustic window (**Fig. 2**).

Computed Tomographic Angiography or MR Angiography?

MRA is an ideal test to provide a complete evaluation of cardiovascular morphology and cardiac function without the use of ionizing radiation. Disadvantages of MRA compared with CTA include greater need for sedation, longer scan time, greater vulnerability to motion, greater expense, and greater image degradation from the inability to scan with certain metallic implants (**Fig. 3**).[5]

When increased spatial resolution is desired, CTA is preferred because of its submillimeter isotropic voxel/spatial resolution. However, the spatial resolution of MRA has improved and can be comparable in some applications (**Fig. 4**).[7] In addition, gadofosveset (Ablavar) has become a valuable option for blood pool imaging.[8] CTA remains the modality of choice for combined evaluation of the pulmonary vasculature and lung parenchyma/bronchial structures.

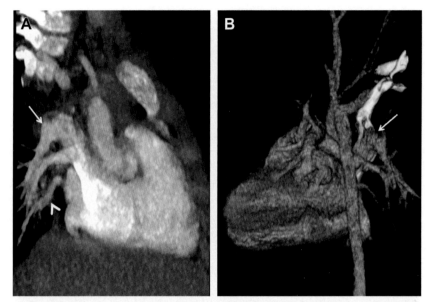

Fig. 1. A 4-year-old boy with a history of repaired congenital diaphragmatic hernia who presented with pulmonary hypertension. Oblique sagittal 10-mm maximum intensity projection image (*A*) demonstrates the upper lobe pulmonary vein (*arrow*) draining into the superior vena cava, consistent with partial anomalous pulmonary anomalous pulmonary venous return. The right lower lobe pulmonary vein is noted emptying normally into the left atrium (*arrowhead*). Volume rendering (VR, *B*) again demonstrates the anomalous return of the right upper lobe pulmonary vein (*arrow*).

Thin-section virtual tracheobronchoscopic images allow 3-dimensional evaluation of the airway that is not yet possible using MRA (**Fig. 5**).[9–11]

Computed Tomographic Angiography or Catheter Angiography?

Catheter angiography has long been regarded as the gold standard for cardiac evaluation. It has extremely high temporal resolution, allows for real-time indirect visualization of cardiac chamber and vessel lumens, and can provide physiologic pressure measurements. Most importantly, therapeutic interventions are possible (**Fig. 6**).

Disadvantages include the need for sedation in all age groups, invasive technique, greater expense and health care personnel utilization, and higher radiation doses. In one study of 70 children with coronary disease, doses ranged from 3.5 to 5.6 mSv. The comparative dose for CTA performed in that cohort ranged from 0.97 to 1.20 mSv, with no discrepancies between techniques.[12]

PATIENT PREPARATION FOR COMPUTED TOMOGRAPHIC ANGIOGRAPHY

Before engaging in CTA in any child, the radiology practitioner should first determine whether the study is indicated and if the clinical question could be answered via another imaging modality without ionizing radiation. Understanding of the clinical indication can also guide the decision of how much anatomy to include. For example, a situs evaluation in a new patient will require scanning the chest and upper abdomen, whereas a patient referred for evaluation of pulmonary arterial anatomy may only need to have that segment of the chest included in the scan. If CTA is the best test to answer the clinical question, the patient should then be assessed for contraindications as follows.

Screening for Renal Disease and Contrast-induced Nephropathy

Contrast-induced nephropathy (CIN) is defined as an increase in creatinine level of 0.5 mg/dL or 25% above baseline within 3 days after administration of iodinated contrast material. It is thought to occur due to vasoconstriction in the outer portion of the renal medulla, leading to acute tubular necrosis.[13] Renal failure is less common in the pediatric population than in adults.[13] As such, CIN is also less common. Rates of CIN after cardiac catheterization in children can be as high as 12%,[14] but CIN in CTA is less common due to smaller injected contrast volumes.[15] However, the same precautions exercised in the adult population apply in the pediatric setting. Pediatric patients should be screened for renal disease and, if present, should be evaluated with renal function tests. NGAL (neutrophil gelatinase-associated

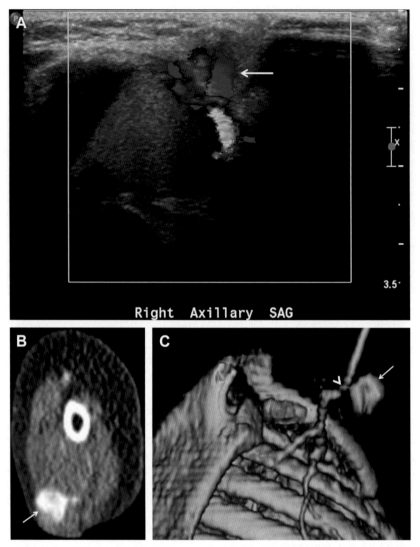

Right Axillary SAG

Fig. 2. A 2-year-old with a history of right axillary cut down who presented with enlarging right axillary mass. Color Doppler US image (*A*) of the right axilla demonstrates a pseudoaneurysm (*arrow*) with "to-and-fro" flow. Axial image (*B*) and VR (*C*) from a CT angiogram demonstrates an extravascular blush of contrast consistent with a pseudoaneurysm (*arrow*) arising from the proximal brachial artery. Adjacent brachial artery narrowing was due to vasospasm (*arrowhead*).

lipocalin) has shown promise as a biomarker for children at greater risk of CIN, but its occurrence is still unpredictable.[14] Creatinine levels can be used as a screening test, but its absolute value has limited utility in children. Creatinine values are lower in children owing to lower levels of muscle mass, and upper levels of normal vary drastically from the newborn to the teenage period. Glomerular filtration rate (GFR) is a more accurate indicator of renal function and can be calculated by the Schwarz equation.[16]

If the child has reduced GFR, the clinical team should readdress the risk-benefit ratio for administration of iodinated contrast material to answer the clinical question. If CTA is still the best test, proper hydration should be the first step. Nephrotoxic medications such as nonsteroidal anti-inflammatory drugs and metformin should be discontinued if possible 48 hours before the study. In the setting of grade 4 or 5 chronic renal failure (GFR 15–29 or 0–14 mL/min), pediatric patients will usually undergo dialysis after the study.

Intravenous Contrast Reactions in Pediatric Patients

Contrast reactions in children are rare.[17] In a report from 2007 in 11,000 patients less than the age of

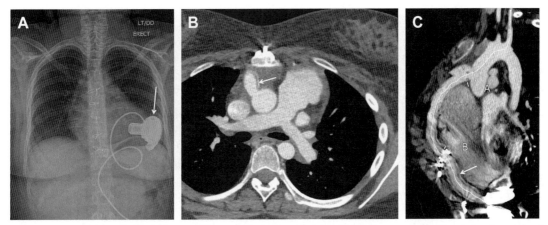

Fig. 3. A 14-year-old girl with a history of heart failure secondary to giant cell myocarditis. Frontal radiograph of the chest (*A*) demonstrates the left ventricular assist device in place (*arrow*). Axial image from a CT angiogram (*B*) of the chest demonstrates no evidence of outflow stenosis with eccentric thrombus (*arrow*) lining the cannula at the insertion into the aorta. Curved planar reconstructed image (*C*) demonstrates thrombus throughout the cannula (*arrow*).

19, the total frequency of contrast reactions was 0.18%. Severe reactions occurred in 0.03%, moderate reactions in 0.009%, and mild reactions in 0.14%.[18] For comparison, the rate of adult contrast reactions at the same institution was 0.6%.[17] The general management for children with contrast reactions is the same as in adults, but medication dosages differ by patient weight. A complete listing of medication doses for various contrast reactions in children can be found in the American College of Radiology Manual on Contrast Media.[17]

Atmosphere

The next step to consider in obtaining high-quality CTA in the pediatric population is to establish a warm, comforting, and engaging atmosphere for the child.[19] This atmosphere will mitigate stress for the child who is in a strange and potentially frightening new setting and can help reduce motion by decreasing anxiety. Loud beeping, dark lighting, and other strange sensations are more frightening to a child than to an adult. They should be given an age-appropriate explanation of what they may feel, see, hear, or taste. Rehearsing breathing instructions and practicing remaining motionless can help improve scan quality and should be reinforced by liberal praise from radiology personnel. Depending on the age, pacifiers, toys, movies, or music can be used as distractions to help the patient relax. Having an appropriately shielded parent in the room can also be very comforting, and the

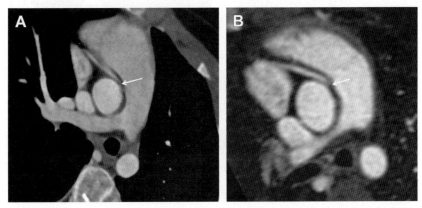

Fig. 4. A 10-year-old with intermittent chest pain. CT angiogram of the coronary arteries (*A*) demonstrates an anomalous right coronary artery arising from the left sinus of Valsalva above the level of the sinotubular junction. The right coronary artery courses between the right ventricular outflow tract and the aorta and narrows proximally (*arrow*). MR angiogram following the injection of IV gadofosveset (Ablavar) of the same patient (*B*) demonstrates similar findings (*arrow*).

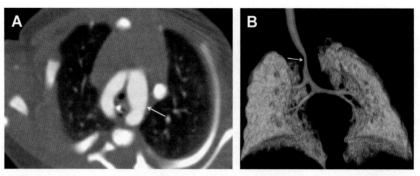

Fig. 5. A 1-day-old girl with known double aortic arch. Axial image (*A*) from a CT angiogram demonstrates a double aortic arch with a more dominant left component (*arrow*). VR of the same CT angiogram (*B*) demonstrates associated smooth narrowing of the distal trachea (*arrow*).

parent can participate in reinforcing breathing technique and motionlessness.[19]

The personal atmosphere created by the staff is not the only component that children experience in the CT suite. The physical (visual, auditory, tactile) atmosphere is equally important (**Fig. 7**). One investigator created a comprehensive protocol to alter the physical atmosphere to provide greater comfort for pediatric patients. This protocol allowed the child patient to have control over the lighting and sound in the room. The child could also choose which cartoon to watch, which would explain what they would experience during the study. Use of a toy patient and a miniature toy

CT scanner ("kitten scanner") provided familiarity before encountering the real scanner, and the cartoon praised the child at the end of the examination. These measures yielded a 16% decrease in need for sedation under 18 months and a 28% decrease under 4 years.[20]

Sedation

The next step in patient preparation is to assess if the child will be able to participate in the study without sedation, or if the child will need added measures to remain motionless; this depends on the developmental stage and age of the child.

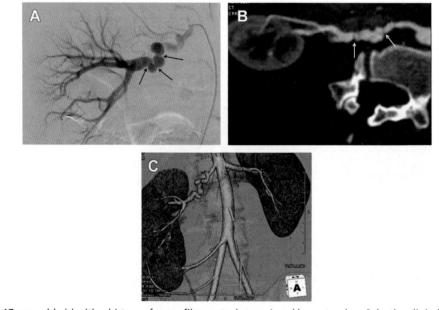

Fig. 6. A 17-year-old girl with a history of neurofibromatosis type 1 and hypertension. Selective digital subtractive angiography of the right renal artery (*A*) demonstrates multifocal stenoses of the right renal artery (*arrows*). There are small aneurysms within the right renal artery but absence of intrarenal aneurysms. Curved planar reconstruction (*B*) and VR (*C*) of a CT angiogram demonstrate similar findings with multiple areas of stenosis within the right renal artery and small aneurysms.

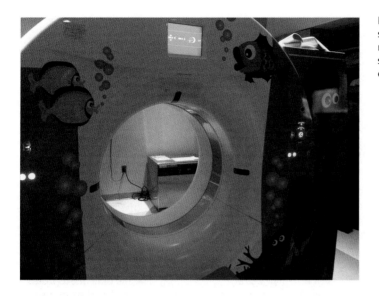

Fig. 7. Pediatric CT scanner demonstrates child-friendly decorations that may be create a welcoming atmosphere for a child receiving a CT examination.

Depending on the institution and pediatric population demographics, about 1% to 10% of CT studies will require sedation.[21]

Sedation should be avoided when possible. Respiratory compromise and aspiration, especially if oral contrast administration is considered, are both concerns.[22] Cardiac arrest is a rare but significant risk, occurring in 1.4/10,000 anesthetics. More than half of arrests occur in children less than 1 year old.[23] These rates are even higher with pre-existing heart disease, with an incidence of cardiac arrest greater than 50% in children with cardiomyopathy or aortic stenosis.[24] Exposure to anesthesia at a young age (less than 4 years) could be associated with learning disability.[25]

Neonates and young infants can often successfully complete a CTA in the absence of pharmacologic sedation by utilization of a technique called "feed-and-sleep." This technique has also been called "feed-and-wrap" or "feed-and-swaddle." It involves fasting and sleep-depriving the baby for a period of time (2–4 hours), followed by feeding just before scan acquisition. The patient is then wrapped in one or a few sheets, placed in an immobilizer, and scanned.[21] Many patients in this age group will sleep and remain motionless and can be scanned during quiet respiration without sedation.

Older children and adolescents can often be verbally coached to remain motionless in order to obtain a good-quality examination, but young children (1–3 years old) are more apt to require sedation.[26,27] They are too old for successful use of the "feed-and-swaddle" technique, but are not yet old enough to understand and cooperate in the unfamiliar setting of the CT scanner.

A full discussion of the technique of pediatric sedation for CTA is beyond the scope of this review, especially because sedation in the current era is rarely performed by the radiologist.[21] However, several points warrant specific comment.

The first is the question of who will perform the sedation; this can include pediatricians, emergency medicine physicians, hospitalists, critical care physicians, nurses, nurse practitioners, or anesthesiologists. The level of supervision depends on the complexity of the patient and the type of anesthetic required as well as the need for endotracheal intubation. Some medications such as ketamine and dexmedetomidine may be administered by nonanesthesiologist practitioners. Others, such as propofol, require supervision by an anesthesiologist due to the potential for respiratory and myocardial depression.[21]

Another important consideration is which practitioner should ultimately be responsible for quality assurance of a particular institution's sedation program. As recommended by the Joint Commission on the Accreditation of Healthcare Organizations, it is usually the anesthesiologist who will make the final decision regarding level of supervision for the various types of sedation and who will be in charge of continuing practice review for quality control.[21,28]

A common anesthesia-related problem that arises during CTA for combined evaluation of thoracic vascular and pulmonary abnormality (such as evaluation of pulmonary hypertension or congenital lung lesions) is that of anesthesia-induced atelectasis. Anesthesia-induced atelectasis can occasionally be addressed by prone positioning or by ventilating at higher lung volumes, but these techniques are not uniformly successful. Another option is to perform lung recruitment maneuvers in conjunction with controlled ventilation, which can yield a significant increase in quality of inspiration (in one study, the proportion of very good to excellent-quality chest CTA studies increased from 24% to 70%).[29]

βBlockade in Pediatric Cardiac Computed Tomographic Angiography

Rapid heart rates and arrhythmias can pose a problem for obtaining high-quality cardiac CTA, especially in young children. Cardiac motion can cause blurring; rapid circulation can make timing difficult, and prospective gating is difficult to perform at high heart rates. The decision to administer β-blockers for cardiac CTA in children is at the discretion of the institution performing the study. The authors do not routinely use β-blockade at their institution, but use of this technique in children has been described by others. According a survey of the members of the Society for Pediatric Radiology in 2006, 15 of 41 practices used β-blockers for cardiac CTA. A protocol described by Han and colleagues[12] is noted in **Table 2**.

COMPUTED TOMOGRAPHIC ANGIOGRAPHY TECHNIQUE

For reasons stated above, radiation dose is a major concern in pediatric imaging. The Alliance for Radiation Safety in Pediatric Imaging, through the Image Gently campaign, has published universal pediatric CT protocols with recommendations on technical parameters and radiation dose.[30,31] For cardiac CTA, average effective dose should be in the range of 1 to 3 mSv[32] and can be lower, with some authors citing effective doses as low as 0.15 mSv.[6]

Tube Current

The tube current (mA) and potential (kVp) will affect both dose and noise levels. Acceptable contrast-to-noise ratio (CNR) and signal-to-noise ratio will vary between readers, but the institution performing pediatric CTA should strive for technical factors that yield as low a dose as possible. Many radiologists will often accept a higher noise level for pediatric CTA than for adult CTA.[33]

Tube current used should be as low as possible to yield a diagnostic study and can be achieved by several techniques. First, positioning of the patient's arms such that they are out of the field

Table 2 Protocol for pediatric β-blockade	
Outpatient	
One hour before scan	HR 50–60 bpm; metoprolol 2 mg/kg, maximum of 50 mg by mouth HR >60 bpm; metoprolol 2 mg/kg, maximum of 100 mg by mouth
Immediately before scan	HR >60 bpm; metoprolol 0.25 mg/kg, maximum of 1 mg/kg IV (<30 kg) or metoprolol mg, maximum 30 mg IV (>30 kg)
General anesthesia	
Oral premedication	HR >60 bpm; metoprolol 1 mg/kg, maximum 50 mg by mouth
Immediately before scan	HR >60 bpm; metoprolol 0.25 mg/kg, maximum of 1 mg/kg IV (<30 kg)

Abbreviations: bpm, beats per minute; HR, heart rate.

Adapted from Han BK, Lindberg J, Overman D, et al. Safety and accuracy of dual-source coronary computed tomography angiography in the pediatric population. J Cardiovasc Comput Tomogr 2012;6(4):259.

of view will allow scanning at lower mAs. For chest and abdomen CTA, the arms will be up, and for head and neck imaging, the arms should be down.

Second, automated tube current modulation can achieve significant reduction in dose. By adjusting the mA in real time based on the patient's size from the scout image, the scanner will automatically decrease the tube output when imaging less attenuating portions of anatomy, such as the chest and extremities, and increase output when imaging more attenuating regions, such as the shoulders and pelvis. This technique can yield dose savings of 40% to 50% or greater.[33,34] In addition, consultation with a medical physicist and testing image quality on phantoms can help determine the lowest acceptable settings for tube output in patients of various sizes. Similarly, mA can be automatically modulated during cardiac scanning according the phase of the cardiac cycle, a process known as electrocardiogram-dependent mA modulation.[35] The scanner will increase the tube output during middiastole when the heart is most still and decrease output during the remainder, allowing for acquisition of high signal images during the most motionless portion of the R-R interval, but with a decrease in overall dose.[32,35,36]

Tube Potential

Another major factor that impacts radiation dose is the tube potential, or kVp. Typical kVp settings available for CTA are 80, 100, 120, and 140 kVp.[18] However, the higher energy spectra (and higher radiation doses) produced at the higher kVp values are often not necessary to penetrate small pediatric patients. In addition, scanning at lower kVp values brings the mean photon energy production closer to the k-edge of iodine (33.2 keV). For comparison, the mean photon energy produced at 140 kVp is about 76 keV, whereas that produced at 80 kVp is about 56 keV. This amount translates to a higher proportion of photon attenuation by iodinated contrast media via the photoelectric effect in the lower energy spectrum.[37]

In other words, scanning at a lower kVp will yield both a higher CNR and a lower radiation dose to the pediatric patient (**Fig. 8**). Some practices have described scanning neonates and smaller infants at 70 kVp, with up to 100% technically diagnostic studies and age- and size-adjusted effective dose of less than 1 mSv.[6,38] Phantom studies have suggested that optimal voltage in children should be closer to 60 kVp.[39] It should be noted that scanning at lower kVp for CTA does necessitate an increase in mA by about 30% to 60% on average compared with conventional CT, although overall radiation dose will still be lower.[5,38]

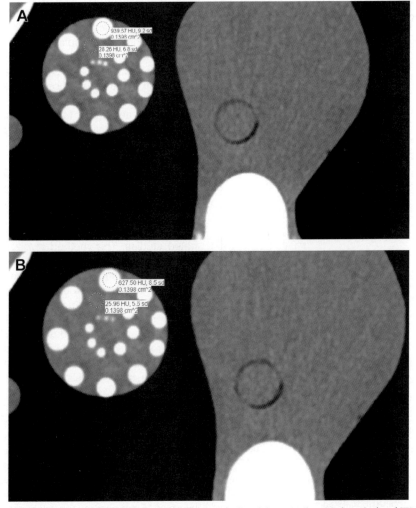

Fig. 8. A 5-year-old phantom at 2 different tube potentials (kVp) but similar CT dose index (CTDI) measuring 1.36 mGy. Axial image at 80 kVp and 93 mAs (*A*) demonstrates a calculated CNR of 134. Axial image at 120 kVp and 25 mAs (*B*) demonstrates a calculated CNR of 107. In this example, lowering the kVp with similar radiation exposure (CTDI) produces better CNR.

Table 3 shows rough guidelines for radiation parameters for CTA in pediatric patients. These guidelines are meant to serve as a starting point for dose calibration and standardization, as individual doses will differ depending on the type of scanner, individual patient size, clinical question, and radiologist preference.

Pitch and Temporal Resolution

Pitch is defined as the distance of table translation in the z-axis per rotation of the scanner

Weight (kg)	kVp	mA
Table 3		
Guideline for pediatric radiation exposure parameters		
A. Guideline for tube parameters in pediatric head CTA. Compared with other body regions, higher kVp is needed to penetrate the calvarium		
<10	120	129
10–12	120	160
13–20	120	211
21–74	120	269
75	120	340
B. Guideline for tube parameters in pediatric chest CTA		
<10	80	70
10–20	80–100	80
20–30	100	90
30–40	100	120
40–50	120	140
50–75	120	160–180
>75	120	>200
C. Recommended tube parameters for pediatric abdomen CTA		
<7.5	80	100
7.5–9.4	80	110
9.5–11.4	80	120
11.5–14.4	100	130
14.5–18.4	100	140
18.5–23.4	100	150
23.5–29.4	120	160
29.5–36.4	120	180
>36.4	120	>200

Adapted from [A] The Alliance for Radiation Safety in Pediatric Imaging. Image gently development of pediatric CT protocols 2014. Available at http://www.imagegently.org/Procedures/Interventional-Radiology/Protocols; [B] Frush DP, Herlong JR. Pediatric thoracic CT angiography. Pediatr Radiol 2005;35(1):9; and [C] Frush DP. Pediatric abdominal CT angiography. Pediatr Radiol 2008;38(Suppl 2):S262.

gantry. Gantry rotation in older scanners is usually 0.5 second, but can be less than 0.3 second in newer-generation scanners. Given that this value is relatively fixed on any particular scanner, pitch will be mostly determined by table translation speed.[32]

In pediatric CTA, the highest possible pitch should be used that still results in diagnostic image quality. Typical values for single source scanners range from about 1.4 to 1.5, whereas dual-source scanners perform well at pitch up to 3.0 to 3.4.[32] This range has 3 distinct advantages. First, using a higher pitch will decrease the total scan time, which will decrease mAs, resulting in a lower effective dose. The second advantage is that the shorter scan time can help to mitigate respiratory and cardiac motion, especially in non-sedated patients and young children with higher heart and respiratory rates. The third advantage to higher pitch value is a more uniform contrast bolus during the scan.[33]

The potential disadvantage to utilization of high pitch values is that, beyond a certain point, sections of anatomy will not be included in at least 180° of the gantry rotation and detail will be lost.[40] A reference table of typical pitch values and gantry and table translation speed values can be found in Hellinger and colleagues.[32]

Scanning Mode

Image acquisition in CT can be performed in several ways. Older scanners used to exclusively scan with axial ("step-and-shoot") technique, although this can still be used for prospectively gated studies. This method involves scanning a volume of tissue corresponding to the detector thickness and then powering off the beam, translating the table to a new tissue volume, and scanning another section of anatomy.[41]

Newer scanners use a helical scan technique, which features continuous and simultaneous gantry rotation during table translation. This technique enables faster scanning and reconstruction of variable thickness slices, without step-ladder artifact.

A third technique is known as volumetric scanning. This technique is similar to axial scanning in that the table remains still during scan acquisition, but the difference is that the entire scan is completed in a single table position during one gantry rotation. This technique is well suited to pediatric imaging, because a typical detector width of 16 cm can cover a relatively large proportion of the anatomy of a small infant or child. For example, cardiac CTA or CTA of the entire neonatal thorax can be performed in one gantry rotation, allowing scan times as low as 0.5 second (or 0.25 second in a dual-source scanner).[32,36,42] In one pediatric study, volumetric scanning yielded a dose reduction of 68% for prospectively gated and 46% for retrospectively gated cardiac CTAs compared with helical technique. Volumetric scan acquisition is so rapid that diagnostic studies can be obtained without gating, yielding an average effective dose of 0.9 mSv in the same study (69% dose reduction compared with helical).[43]

Intravenous Access and Contrast Administration

As in adult CTA, selection of IV access is critical to performing a high-quality study. Selection of IV access may be even more important in children given the relatively small size of their veins, smaller volumes of contrast material administered, higher heart rates, and more rapid circulation. Both the size and the location of the access line are important to consider.[32] Most commonly, 20- or 22-gauge access will be achievable. However, very small children (<10 kg) can be successfully imaged with a 24-gauge line and larger children and adolescents (>60 kg) can often be accessed with an 18-gauge catheter[32] (Table 4).

When considering location of IV access, the antecubital fossa is preferred given the presence of relatively larger veins in this location and its proximity to the heart. However, published studies and the authors' own personal experience have shown that successful angiography can be performed with peripheral lines in the hand or foot.[32,44] CTA has been successfully performed with a 24-gauge hand IV via both manual injection[44] and power injection.[45] Rates of approximately 1 mL/s can be achieved by manual injection.[44]

The side of IV access should also be considered. If the clinical question pertains to the aortic arch, imaging through the right arm is recommended to avoid streak artifact obscuring the aorta. If the question involves the right upper extremity, injecting through the left arm will likely be more effective. For unique indications such as assessing the inferior cavopulmonary shunt in a child with a Fontan repair for congenital heart disease, injection through a lower extremity catheter may yield better contrast opacification of the area of concern.[5]

Another option for cases in which more than one phase of opacification is desired (ie, pulmonary arteries and liver portal venous phase) is to administer a split bolus. A CTA technique has been described in children in which two-thirds of the bolus volume is administered initially, and the remaining one-third is administered after a prescribed delay. The time between boluses is typically 45 to 65 seconds, depending on the child's weight. Scanning was initiated 15 to 25 seconds after the initial bolus, allowing for enhancement of the pulmonary arterial system. This technique yielded greater than 95% success rate for good or optimal vascular and parenchymal enhancement.[46]

A contrast volume of 1.5 to 2.0 mL/kg is sufficient to obtain good vascular opacification for most CTA indications, but doses up to 3.0 mL/kg can be administered without increased concern for renal injury.[5,18] In patients with renal failure, a lower volume of contrast can be administered. Low osmolality iodinated contrast media are available in concentrations of 300, 350, and 370 mg/mL. Higher concentrations of iodine will yield higher levels of contrast and can also be useful if fluid restriction is an issue, but 300 mg/mL is often sufficient for clinical use.[18]

CTA scan timing can be complicated in the pediatric population. Unlike in adult imaging, empiric timing delays are difficult to use in pediatric CTA due to the large variability in patient size and contrast doses. Bolus tracking should be used when possible in older children, with a threshold of 150 to 300 HU depending on institutional preference.[18,32] In neonates and younger children with small-volume contrast boluses, manual triggering may be preferred to avoid the possibility of triggering too early, too late, or not at all (if the contrast density does not reach the threshold HU value).

Table 4
Guideline for intravenous line size and recommended flow rate for pediatric computed tomographic angiography

Weight (kg)	IV Gauge	Flow Rate (mL/s)
<10	24	1.5–2.0
11–30	22	2.0–4.0
31–60	20	3.0–5.5
>60	18	3.0–7.0

Adapted from Frush DP. Pediatric abdominal CT angiography. Pediatr Radiol 2008;38(Suppl 2):S263; and Hellinger JC, Pena A, Poon M, et al. Pediatric computed tomographic angiography: imaging the cardiovascular system gently. Radiol Clin North Am 2010;48(2):447.

PITFALLS OF PEDIATRIC COMPUTED TOMOGRAPHIC ANGIOGRAPHY

There are many factors that may cause diagnostic pitfalls in the evaluation of cardiovascular disease in pediatric patients. Most children are smaller than adults and may have a smaller-gauge IV

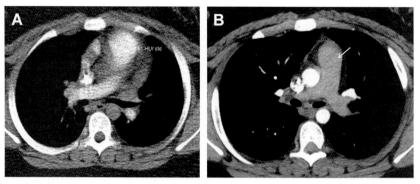

Fig. 9. Example of transient interruption of contrast phenomenon in a 13-year-old girl with a history of Ewing sarcoma who presented with tachypnea, tachycardia, and suspected pulmonary embolism. Premonitoring axial CT image (*A*) of the chest demonstrates opacification of the main pulmonary artery to 161 HU. Axial image (*B*) from a subsequent CT angiogram performed immediately following the premonitoring scan demonstrates poor opacification of the main pulmonary artery (*arrow*), measuring only 80 HU and producing a nondiagnostic scan in this patient with transient interruption of contrast. This is due to rapid inflow of unenhanced blood from the inferior vena cava during deep inspiration.

line; this in turn may necessitate a slower contrast rate injection and even a manual contrast injection in some cases. Given their smaller size, the volume of IV contrast boluses may be very small. Due to the short injection, the contrast bolus can be missed if not triggered at the right time, which may yield a nondiagnostic scan. In healthy older children and adolescent patients, forceful inspiration may cause transient interruption of contrast, resulting in a nondiagnostic imaging study (**Fig. 10**).

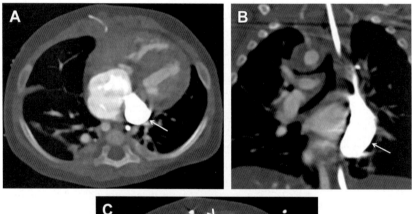

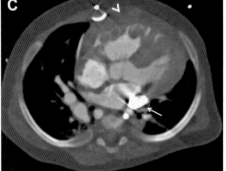

Fig. 10. A 6-month-old with a history of tetralogy of Fallot. Axial (*A*) and coronal (*B*) CT angiogram images demonstrate dense contrast within a left superior vena cava entering the right atrium through a dilated coronary sinus (*arrow*). Given the poor right heart function, the dense contrast obscured the left pulmonary veins, which were not visualized on this examination. The left superior vena cava was not known before imaging. Axial CTA image (*C*) demonstrates marked right ventricular hypertrophy (*arrowhead*) and dilated coronary sinus (*arrow*).

In this phenomenon, large negative intrathoracic pressure results in increased unopacified blood inflow from the inferior vena cava, which can severely dilute the contrast column.[47] Pediatric patients may also have difficulty with breath-holding instructions or be unable to breath hold at all, making the examination more challenging.

Variations in anatomy may also cause difficulty in the evaluation of certain structures due to streak artifact from dense contrast bolus (**Fig. 10**). The artifact may also be exacerbated given a lower kVp, which can accentuate streak artifact and beam hardening.[33] Children also have less abdominal fat to provide internal contrast. Although radiologists will often tolerate lower CNRs in children, some CTA applications may demand very high spatial resolution, which mandates lower noise levels to successfully interpret. For example, a noise level of 12 HU in the liver of an adult may be adequate, but it is unacceptably high for diagnosis in a 6-year-old child.[33]

SUMMARY

Many aspects of pediatric CTA are unique to children in comparison to adults. Given that pediatric patients are more sensitive to radiation effects, alternative imaging modalities that do not use ionizing radiation should always be considered first when imaging children. When a CTA is performed, the radiologist should have a thorough understanding of CT dose parameters in order to perform the highest quality study with the least amount of ionizing radiation. The need for sedation is also a challenge that is much more prevalent than in the adult population. The small size of the patient can place some restrictions on IV contrast administration, including the volume of contrast, the route of administration, and the rate of injection. Overall, the benefits of performing CTA versus the risks of radiation exposure and sedation should be considered to provide the best possible care for the pediatric patient.

ACKNOWLEDGMENTS

The authors thank to Winnie Zhu for her assistance with **Fig. 8**.

REFERENCES

1. Haber AH, Rothstein BE. Radiosensitivity and rate of cell division: "Law of Bergonié and Tribondeau". Science 1969;163(3873):1338–9.
2. Dougeni E, Faulkner K, Panayiotakis G. A review of patient dose and optimisation methods in adult and paediatric CT scanning. Eur J Radiol 2012; 81(4):e665–83.
3. Brenner DJ, Hall EJ. Computed tomography–an increasing source of radiation exposure. N Engl J Med 2007;357(22):2277–84.
4. Berrington de González A, Mahesh M, Kim K-P, et al. Projected cancer risks from computed tomographic scans performed in the United States in 2007. Arch Intern Med 2009;169(22):2071–7.
5. Frush DP, Herlong JR. Pediatric thoracic CT angiography. Pediatr Radiol 2005;35(1):11–25.
6. Han BK, Overman DM, Grant K, et al. Non-sedated, free breathing cardiac CT for evaluation of complex congenital heart disease in neonates. J Cardiovasc Comput Tomogr 2013;7(6):354–60.
7. Biko DM, Chung C, Hitt DM, et al. High-resolution coronary MR angiography for evaluation of patients with anomalous coronary arteries: visualization of the intramural segment. Pediatr Radiol 2015;45(8):1146–52.
8. Chan FP, Hanneman K. Computed tomography and magnetic resonance imaging in neonates with congenital cardiovascular disease. Semin Ultrasound CT MR 2015;36(2):146–60.
9. Heyer CM, Nuesslein TG, Jung D, et al. Tracheobronchial anomalies and stenoses: detection with low-dose multidetector CT with virtual tracheobronchoscopy—comparison with flexible tracheobronchoscopy. Radiology 2007;242(2):542–9.
10. Katz M, Konen E, Rozenman J, et al. Spiral CT and 3D image reconstruction of vascular rings and associated tracheobronchial anomalies. J Comput Assist Tomogr 1995;19(4):564–8.
11. Watanabe N, Hayabuchi Y, Inoue M, et al. Tracheal compression due to an elongated aortic arch in patients with congenital heart disease: Evaluation using multidetector-row CT. Pediatr Radiol 2009; 39(10):1048–53.
12. Han BK, Lindberg J, Overman D, et al. Safety and accuracy of dual-source coronary computed tomography angiography in the pediatric population. J Cardiovasc Comput Tomogr 2012;6(4):252–9.
13. Karcaaltincaba M, Oguz B, Haliloglu M. Current status of contrast-induced nephropathy and nephrogenic systemic fibrosis in children. Pediatr Radiol 2009;39(Suppl 3):382–4.
14. Hirsch R, Dent C, Pfriem H, et al. NGAL is an early predictive biomarker of contrast-induced nephropathy in children. Pediatr Nephrol 2007; 22(12):2089–95.
15. Nash K, Hafeez A, Hou S. Hospital-acquired renal insufficiency. Am J Kidney Dis 2002;39(5):930–6.
16. Cohen M. What is the normal serum creatinine concentration in children? Pediatr Radiol 2008;38(11):1265.
17. Cohan RH, Dillman JR, Hartman RP, et al. American College of Radiology manual on contrast media version 9 ACR manual on contrast media. Reston, VA: American College of Radiology; 2013.
18. Frush DP. Pediatric abdominal CT angiography. Pediatr Radiol 2008;38(Suppl 2):259–66.

19. Linder JMB, Schiska AD. Imaging children: tips and tricks. J Radiol Nurs 2007;26(1):23–5.

20. Anastos JP. The ambient experience in pediatric radiology. J Radiol Nurs 2007;26(2):50–5.

21. Slovis TL. Sedation and anesthesia issues in pediatric imaging. Pediatr Radiol 2011;41(Suppl 2):514–6.

22. Sanborn PA, Michna E, Zurakowski D, et al. Adverse cardiovascular and respiratory events during sedation of pediatric patients for imaging examinations. Radiology 2005;237(1):288–94.

23. Morray JP, Geiduschek JM, Ramamoorthy C, et al. Anesthesia-related cardiac arrest in children. Anesthesiology 2000;93:6–14.

24. Ramamoorthy C, Haberkern CM, Bhananker SM, et al. Anesthesia-related cardiac arrest in children with heart disease: data from the pediatric perioperative cardiac arrest (POCA) registry. Anesth Analg 2010;110(5):1376–82.

25. Kalkman CJ, Peelen L, Moons KG, et al. Behavior and development in children and age at the time of first anesthetic exposure. Anesthesiology 2009; 110(4):805–12.

26. Sacchetti A, Carraccio C, Giardino A, et al. Sedation for pediatric CT scanning: is radiology becoming a drug-free zone? Pediatr Emerg Care 2005;21(5):295–7.

27. Keeter S, Benator R, Weinberg S, et al. Sedation in pediatric CT: national survey of current practice. Pediatr Radiol 1990;175:745–52.

28. Mason KP. The pediatric sedation service: who is appropriate to sedate, which medications should I use, who should prescribe the drugs, how do I bill? Pediatr Radiol 2008;38(Suppl 2):218–24.

29. Newman B, Krane EJ, Gawande R, et al. Chest CT in children: anesthesia and atelectasis. Pediatr Radiol 2014;44(2):164–72.

30. Goske MJ, Applegate KE, Boylan J, et al. The image gently campaign: working together to change practice. AJR Am J Roentgenol 2008;190(2):273–4.

31. Goske MJ, Applegate KE, Boylan J, et al. The "Image Gently" campaign: increasing CT radiation dose awareness through a national education and awareness program. Pediatr Radiol 2008;38(3):265–9.

32. Hellinger JC, Pena A, Poon M, et al. Pediatric computed tomographic angiography: imaging the cardiovascular system gently. Radiol Clin North Am 2010;48(2):439–67, x.

33. Yu L, Bruesewitz MR, Thomas KB, et al. Optimal tube potential for radiation dose reduction in pediatric CT: principles, clinical implementations, and pitfalls. Radiographics 2011;31(3):835–48.

34. Herzog C, Mulvihill DM, Nguyen SA, et al. Pediatric cardiovascular CT angiography: radiation dose reduction using automatic anatomic tube current modulation. AJR Am J Roentgenol 2008;190(5):1232–40.

35. Meinel FG, Henzler T, Schoepf UJ, et al. ECG-synchronized CT angiography in 324 consecutive pediatric patients: spectrum of indications and trends in radiation dose. Pediatr Cardiol 2014; 36(3):569–78.

36. Jadhav SP, Golriz F, Atweh LA, et al. CT angiography of neonates and infants: comparison of radiation dose and image quality of target mode prospectively ECG-gated 320-MDCT and ungated helical 64-MDCT. AJR Am J Roentgenol 2015;204(2): W184–91.

37. Cho E-S, Chung T-S, Kun Oh D, et al. Cerebral computed tomography angiography using a low tube voltage (80 kVp) and a moderate concentration of iodine contrast material. Invest Radiol 2012;47(2): 142–7.

38. Niemann T, Henry S, Duhamel A, et al. Pediatric chest CT at 70 kVp: a feasibility study in 129 children. Pediatr Radiol 2014;44(11):1347–57.

39. Nievelstein RA, van Dam IM, van der Molen AJ. Multidetector CT in children: current concepts and dose reduction strategies. Pediatr Radiol 2010;40(8): 1324–44.

40. Strauss KJ, Goske MJ, Kaste SC, et al. Image gently: ten steps you can take to optimize image quality and lower CT dose for pediatric patients. AJR Am J Roentgenol 2010;194(4):868–73.

41. Hausleiter J, Meyer TS, Martuscelli E, et al. Image quality and radiation exposure with prospectively ECG-triggered axial scanning for coronary CT angiography: the multicenter, multivendor, randomized PROTECTION-III study. JACC Cardiovasc Imaging 2012;5(5):484–93.

42. Sorantin E, Riccabona M, Stücklschweiger G, et al. Experience with volumetric (320 rows) pediatric CT. Eur J Radiol 2013;82(7):1091–7.

43. Greenberg SB, Bhutta S, Braswell L, et al. Computed tomography angiography in children with cardiovascular disease: low dose techniques and image quality. Int J Cardiovasc Imaging 2012; 28(1):163–70.

44. Schooler GR, Zurakowski D, Lee EY. Evaluation of contrast injection site effectiveness: thoracic CT angiography in children with hand injection of IV contrast material. AJR Am J Roentgenol 2015; 204(2):423–7.

45. Yang M, Mo XM, Jin JY, et al. Image quality and radiation exposure in pediatric cardiovascular CT angiography from different injection sites. AJR Am J Roentgenol 2011;196(2):117–22.

46. Thomas KE, Mann EH, Padfield N, et al. Dual bolus intravenous contrast injection technique for multiregion paediatric body CT. Eur Radiol 2014;25(4): 1014–22.

47. Gosselin MV, Rassner UA, Thieszen SL, et al. Contrast dynamics during CT pulmonary angiogram: analysis of an inspiration associated artifact. J Thorac Imaging 2004;19(1):1–7.

Index

Note: Page numbers of article titles are in **boldface** type.

Radiol Clin N Am 54 (2016) 177–183
http://dx.doi.org/10.1016/S0033-8389(15)00217-1
0033-8389/16/$ – see front matter © 2016 Elsevier Inc. All rights reserved.

Moving?

Make sure your subscription moves with you!

To notify us of your new address, find your **Clinics Account Number** (located on your mailing label above your name), and contact customer service at:

Email: journalscustomerservice-usa@elsevier.com

800-654-2452 (subscribers in the U.S. & Canada)
314-447-8871 (subscribers outside of the U.S. & Canada)

Fax number: 314-447-8029

Elsevier Health Sciences Division
Subscription Customer Service
3251 Riverport Lane
Maryland Heights, MO 63043

*To ensure uninterrupted delivery of your subscription, please notify us at least 4 weeks in advance of move.

ELSEVIER